# The Parent's Guide
# to Childhood Eating Disorders

# · THE ·
# PARENT'S GUIDE TO CHILDHOOD EATING DISORDERS

MARCIA HERRIN, Ed.D., M.P.H., R.D.,

AND

NANCY MATSUMOTO

AN OWL BOOK

HENRY HOLT AND COMPANY · NEW YORK

Henry Holt and Company, LLC
*Publishers since 1866*
115 West 18th Street
New York, New York 10011

Henry Holt® is a registered trademark of
Henry Holt and Company, LLC.

Library of Congress Cataloging-in-Publication Data
Herrin, Marcia.
 The parent's guide to childhood eating disorders / Marcia Herrin
and Nancy Matsumoto.—1st ed.
  p.  cm.
 Includes index.
 ISBN 0-8050-6649-7
 1. Eating disorders in children.  2. Eating disorders in adolescence.
3. Children—Nutrition—Psychological aspects.  I. Matsumoto, Nancy.  II. Title.

RJ506.E18 H475    2002
618.92'8526—dc21                                              2001039837

Henry Holt books are available for special promotions
and premiums. For details contact: Director, Special Markets.

First Edition 2002

Designed by Victoria Hartman

Printed in the United States of America
1  3  5  7  9  10  8  6  4  2

*To Alan, Branch, and Gretta*

—MH

*To Grant and Sandy*

—NM

# Contents

## Part Two: Taking Action

## Part Three: Healthy Eating Guide

# *Foreword*

Eating disorders pose a tremendous challenge to society, health care professionals, parents, and individuals either suffering from these disorders or at risk for developing them. It is estimated that more than six million women and perhaps over half a million men have a clinical eating disorder at some point in their lives. Increasingly it is the preteen, or even younger child, who first begins to struggle with food, exercise, and weight issues. Those who are most at risk are often exceptionally talented, intelligent, and capable in every other area of their lives. Why should some of our most gifted have such low self-esteem, and engage in disordered-eating behaviors that rob them of many pleasures and put them in medical danger? What role can parents play to reduce the liklihood of their children becoming anorexic or bulimic, and what can they do when they notice unhealthy eating behaviors in their child? *The Parent's Guide to Childhood Eating Disorders* answers these questions.

Over the past thirty years we have learned a great deal about the causes, complications, and treatment of eating disorders. There are now several scientific journals dedicated solely to disseminating the latest research and important clinically relevant information on these disorders to researchers and clinicians. Popular magazines, newspapers, TV news magazines, and TV movies make meaningful attempts to inform the public about unhealthy role models in the media, the neurobiological and genetic underpinnings to eating disorders, and their all-too-often tragic outcomes. However, as this book does so well, literature for a nonclinical readership is needed to supplement these contributions so that these readers are adequately informed by relevant scientific research findings.

I became interested in the study and clinical care of the anorexic patient in the late 1970s. At that time few medical schools had lectures on eating disorders, anorexia nervosa was largely an unfamiliar term (known only as a teenage problem), and bulimia was unheard of. As a pediatrician and child psychiatrist, I created a multidisciplinary eating disorders unit at Massachusetts General Hospital. Over the years parents uniformly asked what I would recommend they read on the subject. Though there has been a proliferation of good books on eating-disorders care, *The Parent's Guide to Childhood Eating Disorders* is exceptional in several ways. Replete with sound information, it is also well organized and easy to read. Most important, with its focus primarily on nutritional interventions that can be used at home within the family, it is uniquely directed to parents of children struggling with eating and body-related conflicts.

Marcia Herrin is the consummate clinician who has built one of the best college eating-disorders programs in the country. Her many years of clinical practice treating children and their families, her dedication to her patients, her passion for acquiring and disseminating knowledge, and her practical, no-nonsense approach all make this book an important resource. Nancy Matsumoto interviewed me for several articles for *People* magazine, and I was struck by her dedication to get the information right and present it in the most accurate fashion possible.

*The Parent's Guide to Childhood Eating Disorders* is a welcome addition to the library of the clinician working in the field of eating disorders and is an invaluable guide for the parent eager to learn how to battle often frightening eating-disordered attitudes and behaviors.

David Herzog, M.D.
Professor of Psychiatry and Pediatrics, Harvard Medical School
President and Founder, Harvard Eating Disorders Center

# Acknowledgments

We are greatly indebted to the many patients and their parents whose stories and struggles have both taught and inspired us; we hope this book succeeds in passing on some of their accumulated wisdom.

We thank Carole Stashwick, M.D., and Hilary Coons, Ph.D., for their invaluable clinical collaboration, and for their helpful editorial advice. Thanks go to Marcia's Dartmouth College Health Service colleagues, who worked with her to develop Dartmouth's Eating Disorder Prevention, Education and Treatment Program, Heidi Fishman, Ph.D., and Jack Turco, M.D. A special acknowledgment to the sustaining support of Gabrielle Lucke, M.S., head of Dartmouth's Health Resource Department, and to Leslie Clancy and Molly St. Sauveur.

We also wish to thank Joan Gussow, Ed.D., Marcia's mentor and doctoral dissertation advisor at Columbia Teachers College, who made her realize she might have something important to offer the world.

Our collaboration on this book would not have happened without the April 1999 *People* magazine cover story ("Wasting Away: Eating Disorders on Campus") that introduced us to each other. At *People*, we thank Jack Kelley and Maria Eftimiades for supporting and guiding Nancy during her years as a correspondent for the magazine, and Carol Wallace and Bonnie Johnson for caring about eating disorders and launching the story that led to this book.

Thanks to our agent, Elaine Koster, and our editor at Henry Holt, Deborah Brody, for seeing the potential in our book, encouraging us, and guiding us through the editorial process with a sure hand. We thank Michaela

Hamilton for her welcome editorial advice, Michael Lockshin, M.D., for his valuable medical insights and support, and Lisa Lazzarini for her generous administrative assistance.

Finally, we thank those who sacrificed the most to make this book possible, our families. We are especially grateful to our husbands, Alan and Grant, who believed in us and helped us believe in ourselves. To our children, Branch, Gretta, and Sandy, who let their moms sit in front of the computer screen far longer than any of them would have wished, we offer our thanks, and (temporarily) turn over our keyboards to them.

# Preface: Marcia's Story

When I was coming of age in the sixties and early seventies, eating disorders were not the commonly diagnosed disease they are today. There was only one diet soda on the market, Tab. Packaged foods listing calories and fat grams on their wrappings did not exist yet. But there was the impossibly thin model, Twiggy. She was the first supermodel, the original waif, five-foot-six and only 91 pounds. Twiggy was the face of the mod sixties, ushering in an era of fake eyelashes, miniskirts, and androgynous, childlike bodies. To young girls like me who were both eager to grow up but anxious about leaving behind the safety of childhood, Twiggy represented our ideal of feminine beauty. The physical attribute that I coveted most was her amazing "no thigh" legs.

It is hard to imagine now what an impact Twiggy had on a generation of teens like me. The only person remotely comparable today might be the actress Calista Flockhart, who is also known for her short skirts and waiflike dimensions. But the difference between the two is that much of the talk that Flockhart generates is about whether or not she has an eating disorder. In the sixties there was none of that, just wonder and envy over how Twiggy managed to stay so thin.

At fifteen, I was the oldest of five teenage girls, just beginning to develop hips. I began starving myself in an attempt to feel special and stand out in a family of competitive Montana horseback riders. I developed ritualistic methods of eating, carefully counting out portions of lettuce leaves and raisins, two of my favorite no-fat foods. When I look back at family pictures today, I see that I looked a lot like Twiggy. And yet my success at losing weight was never enough. Still, I thrived on the compliments and the obvious envy of my sisters, and took more pride in my weight loss than anything else. I know now that I became a classic anorexic, dropping down to 100 pounds on a five-foot-six-inch frame. On paper, I possessed the same measurements as my role model. But now, when I look at pictures of me from that period of my life, they look awful to me. I have dark circles under my eyes, and my hair is stringy. I look pretty spaced out. Yet I vividly remember how thrilled I was with the way I looked, absolutely thrilled. My boyfriend at the time, who himself was very thin, also liked my thinness, even though my anorexia made me so withdrawn socially that at its peak, I really had no friends other than him.

At the same time that my dramatic weight loss was taking place, a classmate of mine was exhibiting the same signs of rapid weight loss. Later, I found out that she had been pregnant and was starving herself to end the pregnancy. Eventually, depleted of sustenance, she miscarried. I remember being shocked that her dieting could kill. Still, I never linked her experience to mine. After all, her self-starvation killed her baby; she herself survived.

As often happens in families of anorexics, no one voiced their concerns directly to me, which might have helped turn my disorder around earlier. At the urging of my grandmother, my mother took me to our aging family physician, who happened to be close to retirement. Though my family had noticed my changed eating habits, we really did not know that my restrictive eating and the resulting weight loss were dangerous. Assuming that if there were a problem, the doctor would diagnose it, neither Mom nor I mentioned the fact that I had virtually stopped eating meals, only that I was losing my hair, had stopped getting my period, and looked tired and unhealthy. Even these symptoms, disturbing as they might seem, did not trouble me. I was just too pleased with how thin I had become. I never once thought about future health problems that could result from my starvation.

I was reassured when our doctor found no cause for alarm and recommended that I put olive oil in my hair. When I tell this story now, I always say, "He should have told me to add the olive oil to my food." He really didn't understand what was going on. But we weren't giving him all the information. In fact, very few health professionals in the mid-sixties would have recognized my symptoms as an eating disorder.

Times have changed since then, certainly. But it still surprises me how often eating disorders are overlooked, or misdiagnosed. How my large, supportive family could have spawned an eating disorder is another source of wonder for me. Looking back now as an eating disorders expert, I realize that my family, ideal as it was in many ways, had despite itself primed me for an eating disorder.

When the youngest of my five siblings, Keith, was born, the whole family was delighted to finally have a boy in the family. We doted on him, and we were devastated when we discovered that he had developed a disease known as retinal blastoma when he was only nine months old. Although it is now quite treatable, at the time, it was quite often fatal. By the time Keith was six years old, he had lost both eyes to the disease. My mother and grandmother learned Braille and translated all of his schoolbooks so he could continue at our country school. My mother also learned and then taught him mobility training so he could negotiate the barnyard and school grounds. He was a great kid. I don't remember him ever complaining. Instead, as he got sicker, he drew us all closer together. He loved to listen to my sisters' and my girl talk about boyfriends and other topics that normally would bore a young boy silly. During the last six months of his illness, Keith moved into the bedroom off the living room. I would spend hours just lying with him, and I think my sisters did the same.

Since my family's main activity was raising and riding horses, it never occurred to us that Keith would not continue to be involved and compete, even as he lost first one eye, and then the other. He adored his horse, Cutie, the half-Shetland, half-quarter horse that we all learned to ride on. Cutie was a pretty, round little bay with the most amazing arched neck. Keith inherited Cutie from my sister Laura when she moved up to a faster horse. Like all of us, Keith started riding early, first sitting behind an older sibling, then alone. By the time he lost his second eye at age six, he was an accomplished rider, so it did not seem like a big stretch to continue riding. In barrel racing and pole-bending competitions, I would sit behind him on his horse, coaching him through the patterned races and making sure he was safe. I would hold my arms outstretched to show the judges that I was not guiding the horse.

Keith died when he was only twelve. Six months before that, my parents had divorced. Against this backdrop of loss and sorrow, my anorexia was a project for me. It gave me focus when my world was coming apart.

Away at college, my anorexia gave way to periods of bingeing followed by even more stringent fasting. For a while I maintained my stick figure, but eventually the bingeing won out, and I gained 60 pounds. I hated myself and everything about the eating disorder: the eating in secret, the crumbs in my bathrobe pocket, the lack of control. I began taking food from my roommate, stealing food from the dining halls, even shoplifting food from local stores. All of this is common behavior for a bulimic. Stolen food does not "count" for the eating-disordered person. I would stay up late bingeing on my stash of pilfered food, which made me groggy in classes the next day. As I gained weight, I felt less and less attractive, assuming that people wouldn't like me because of my size. My thoughts were so centered on food- and size-related issues that I had little time to develop any other thoughts. My self-confidence slowly eroded as I became more and more one-dimensional.

I eventually, gradually, shook free of my eating disorder without any professional help, but I regret the seven years I lost doing so. I realize now how damn lucky I was. It might not have gone that way. Most people do not gradually recover on their own. I would love to do those early years in high school and college over, years I squandered amid the chaos of an eating disorder. I missed out on relationships, on learning how to make good friends. I was just a skinny body, a hollow shell; I didn't have much of a personality, I didn't have the energy to develop one.

Partially to pull my life back together while recovering from my eating disorder, I dropped out of college and helped start a natural foods cooperative. After five years of talking to customers about food, I became interested in what science had to say about food and nutrition issues, and decided to return to school and work toward an undergraduate degree in nutrition.

Ironically, I did not connect the interest in studying nutrition to my own past and my eating disorder; to me, those bygone problems with food were ancient history, a dim memory. But when in my first nutrition course, I was assigned a term paper on anorexia nervosa, something clicked. This was an unfamiliar topic to all of us in the mid-seventies, and neither I nor my fellow students knew that anorexia was about to become a major public concern. As I combed the medical literature, researching my assigned topic, it hit me: *I had been an anorexic.* Still, although I found this revelation an interesting insight into my own past, I did not know that eating disorders would become my professional focus.

I completed my undergraduate degree at the University of Montana and was accepted into the graduate program of my dreams, at the University of California at Berkeley. In the intellectually charged atmosphere of Berkeley in the seventies, I began to learn more about the political, cultural, and social issues that contribute to the development of eating disorders. In a society where body size is overvalued, dieting and fear of food, we were beginning to realize, were in fact "women's issues." All of this was critical in the development of my thinking about eating disorders.

After earning my master's degree in public health and completing a dietetic internship at Berkeley, I returned to the University of Montana and taught nutrition part-time. Eating disorders were still considered a curious offshoot of the field, hardly a subject worthy of adopting as a specialty. Yet I found myself teaching a whole unit on them in my introductory nutrition class, often bringing in as guest speakers students who had sought me out to discuss their personal struggles with an eating disorder. The response of my students was overwhelming. Many shared openly, in large classes, their own experiences with eating disorders. Each semester, several students would seek my advice on whether it was possible to recover from their disorder, and what steps they needed to take to do so.

Just as my own teaching experiences were showing me how serious a problem eating disorders were among college students, research and interest in the field accelerated in the 1980s. I took all of this in, avidly staying on top of the latest scientific findings. The top nutrition textbooks by this time included chapters on eating disorders and weight control. Students, and even faculty members, came to me for individual help with these issues. The topic of eating disorders seemed almost to choose me.

Several years later, my university department generously gave me leave to enter Columbia University's doctoral program in nutrition education. I jumped at the chance to earn a degree that I knew would open doors for me professionally. At Columbia, I was exposed to the latest thinking about food, society, women's issues, food production and the environment, and yes, eating disorders. It was an amazing education that taught me how to think critically and to develop my own ideas about eating disorders and how to treat them. A number of the doctoral students were from other countries, including Africa, China, and South America. I learned a lot from them about how parenting and culture affects how we feel about food and our bodies. Columbia's graduate program specialized in nutrition education for children and was also one of the few programs at the time that focused on the connection between nutrition and exercise physiology. I was lucky enough to work with the best thinkers and researchers in those fields. Looking back, I see now how all of these factors steered me toward, and prepared me for, working with eating-disordered children.

Within a year of completing my degree at Columbia, my entire academic department at the University of Montana was eliminated, a victim of severe budget cuts. As I searched the country for a position that appealed to me, one job stood out. It involved developing a new program in nutrition education focusing on eating disorders, sports nutrition, and wellness at Dartmouth College in New Hampshire. It seemed the ideal place for me. At Dartmouth, I found myself spending most of my working hours with students who had serious struggles with anorexia, bulimia, and binge eating. I knew I had found my life's work.

Several years later, a professor came to me and asked me to treat her anorexic daughter, who was not responding to traditional treatment and was fast becoming seriously ill. After helping her recover, word of my work spread, and soon in addition to my job at Dartmouth I had a private practice treating patients with eating disorders.

I learned an immense amount from both the Dartmouth students I treated, and the children and adults in my private practice. I read every scientific article I could find on eating disorders, and was pleased to find that the strategies I developed were extraordinarily successful, even on patients other professionals had written off as hopeless cases. While I was encountering a wide range of eating-disordered youths in my work, at home, my husband and I were attempting to raise our own two children free of eating disorders. Thankfully, our efforts have been successful, but that success was by no means a foregone conclusion. Raising my daughter, Gretta, especially has taught me a great deal about the challenges of parenting a child with healthy attitudes toward food. I know that the traits that made me susceptible to an eating disorder are part of her genetic inheritance, and I see her confronting the same issues that I stumbled over in my adolescence. Unlike me and my Twiggy-worship of twenty-five years ago, though, Gretta knows that Calista Flockhart is too thin, and that her own natural body size and shape are nothing to be ashamed of.

Raising my own children has taught me that parents play a crucial role in shaping the attitudes of their children toward food and eating. In a society where eating disorders are rampant, it often takes special awareness, vigilance, and effort to raise children who will come to the dinner table free of the modern food-related phobias: fear of fat, fear of excess calories, obsession with physical appearance. If you do not know what I mean, take a look at the following statistics from recent surveys:

- More than 70 percent of adolescents are dissatisfied with their bodies and want to lose weight.
- On any given day approximately two-thirds of all teenaged girls and one-fifth of all teenaged boys are dieting.
- Among *preadolescents,* 60 percent of all girls and 25 percent of all boys report having dieted recently.
- One study found that 13 percent of the girls surveyed and 7 percent of the boys surveyed binged and purged a few times a week or more.
- Recent findings indicate that girls who smoke to suppress their appetite are the highest group of new nicotine addicts.

Because the first line of defense in combating an eating disorder is at home, with the child's family, I involve the parents of my patients in their treatment far more than most other professionals. I give families assignments to work on at home with their child, I suggest new ways of managing food at home, and I take careful note of parents' insight into and feelings about what is happening in the home. Often simply providing families with information about how eating disorders begin, how they take root, and the practical steps they can take to help put their child on the path to recovery is what turns a desperate situation around. It is not unusual for you as parents to have a hard time mustering the empathy that is crucial to bringing your eating-disordered child back to health. You feel angry, scared, frustrated, hopeless. But once you begin to understand the insidious nature of the disease, you are better able to direct these emotions toward the disorder, not toward the child. You become more sympathetic to your child's plight, which puts you in a better position to help.

My success in treating the patients in my clinical practice, as well as my husband's and my success at home with our children has been gratifying. In recent years, as my work with eating-disordered children has become more widely known, I have been inundated with calls from worried parents from across the country asking for advice and help. Many of them ask for a good book, a practical guide to help them cope with their child's eating disorder. Although there are many books on the topic, none are completely satisfactory to me. So I have decided to write my own, along with Nancy Matsumoto, a journalist and mother of a six-year-old boy. Nancy's voice is that of the parent who shares the concerns of parents everywhere that their children grow up with healthy attitudes toward food and eating.

## What You Will Find in This Book

*The Parent's Guide to Childhood Eating Disorders* is the first book to address the eating problems of children and adolescents from the practical point of view of a nutritionist. Because eating disorders are no longer strictly the province of teenagers and adults, but afflict ten-, eight-, even five-year-olds who come home from school one day and announce they need to go on a diet, this book is designed primarily for parents or caregivers who are concerned about the eating patterns of their child. It is you who are the first to become aware of an emerging problem, and it is you who spend the most time with your child, preparing meals, trying to get her to eat, worrying about your child's health. As the people closest to your child, you can also have the strongest impact on her life. It is our belief, and one that is supported by the latest research in the field, that the family can play a critical role in turning around an emerging or full-blown eating disorder.

*The Parent's Guide to Childhood Eating Disorders* focuses on what you as a family can do to help your child. Not every family can afford (and fewer and fewer insurance companies are willing to pay) thousands upon thousands of dollars in expensive inpatient treatment. It is also not always necessary to spend huge sums of money to turn around an eating disorder. This book is proof that effective solutions can begin in the home, at virtually no cost to you other than a healthy investment in time, effort, and love.

Because being well-informed is an important first step in successfully helping your child, our book begins with a thorough briefing on the different types of eating disorders and disordered eating. We offer concrete strategies for parents and siblings who want to help, discuss the ramifications of gender and culture, and include a comprehensive overview of the medical symptoms and findings associated with the various eating disorders. We then guide you through the difficult process of intervention, and describe in detail the food and exercise plans that form the therapeutic heart of our book. Our approach is predicated on normalizing both eating and exercise, and is designed to, over time, return control of these areas of your child's life back to her or him.

This book will help you become an integral part of your child's recovery process, whether you are taking it on single-handedly or need to involve a professional or a team of professionals. There are many books that delve into the psychology of eating disorders, the many and complex reasons *why* young people develop eating disorders. This book is the nutritional and practical counterpart to those books, offering advice and guidelines on how to respond to one of the most life-threatening hazards of adolescence.

Even with a strictly nutritional approach, as ours is, however, it benefits you as parents to understand the psychological foundations upon which our method is built. In chapter 14, "When You've Done All You Can," we will discuss the different types of psychotherapy that have been found to be the most useful in treating eating disorders, and explain how we have drawn upon those theories to create our practical nutritional guidelines. If you are seeking a psychotherapist as part of your child's treatment, this chapter will help you select the best psychotherapist for your child. For the child who is currently in therapy, it will help you better understand the psychotherapist's approach.

Eating disorder survivors and health care professionals often say that like alcoholism, an eating disorder is never cured. At best, they say, sufferers are perpetually "in recovery." This book, based on my years of study, fifteen years of clinical practice treating eating disorders, as well as my own personal experience as a recovered sufferer and seasoned parent, aims to turn that myth on its head and demonstrate that with sustained, effective effort from all involved, including you, your child, and the professionals you engage, you can be successful in banishing the eating disorder from your child's life.

*The Parent's Guide to Childhood Eating Disorders* is dedicated to helping you as parents prevent the immeasurable losses—of time, of opportunities to love and be loved, of health—that accrue to children with eating disorders.

### A Note about the Text

To protect the confidentiality of my patients and their parents, whose many and diverse stories we tell in this book, we have changed their names and other telltale, superficial details. We hope, however, that the anecdotes we relate are an accurate reflection of their struggles with an eating disorder, and their hopes, fears, and triumphs.

This book is addressed to "you," meaning you parents, either married or single, adoptive, straight, or gay, who are concerned about an eating-disordered child. "You" can also be a relative, a friend, a guardian, a teacher. In short, our book is addressed to anyone who cares for a child who is struggling with food problems and wants to know how to help.

Our use of the pronouns "he," "she," and "they" is more problematic. As we note in the book, more girls than boys suffer from eating disorders. Yet eating disorders among boys and men is a growing problem. To use either the feminine pronoun or the masculine pronoun, "she" or "he," exclusively seems to us an unfair slighting of the opposite sex, especially when many boys and men struggling with an eating disorder feel the added burden of shame about having a "girl's problem." Yet the use of "they" or "them" to refer to indefinite singular antecedents is undeniably clumsy, and to some perhaps even offensive. Our solution, for which we ask your forbearance, is to use both "he" and "she" in an effort to make the point that contrary to popular perception, eating disorders know no gender boundaries.

Finally, we have written this book using both the first-person singular "I," and the first-person plural "we." Here again, we ask your forbearance. While perhaps confusing, this combination of voices nevertheless reflects the collaborative nature of our effort. "I" is the voice of Marcia, whose clinical experience, case histories, and copious research have supplied the rich material for this book. "We" refers to Marcia and Nancy, who together labored to bring this book forth.

# The Parent's Guide
# to Childhood Eating Disorders

# PART ONE

# IDENTIFYING AN
# EATING DISORDER

# At Risk: Recognizing an Eating Disorder and Spotting Early Warning Signs

Ruth, age thirteen, is well adjusted, at the top of her class academically, and loves to play soccer. Her mother, Susan, has been somewhat worried about Ruth's recent weight loss, but reassures herself that Ruth looks nothing like the images of girls suffering from eating disorders that she has seen on television talk shows and in magazines. Instead of ghoulishly skeletal, Ruth really looks cute, athletic, slim, and energetic. One day, however, while straightening up Ruth's room, Susan comes across a diary in an open drawer. She can't resist taking a peek, thinking that it might shed light on Ruth's recent weight loss. Susan learns that Ruth has thrown up for the first time the night before. Although she has been trying to self-induce vomiting for a number of weeks up until now, this is her first success. Ruth writes that she is relieved that vomiting is not very hard to do once you figure it out, and that she is confident she can continue doing it. Susan replays recent changes in Ruth's behavior—occasional dizziness, the significant reduction in her food intake, the way she was eager to bake a birthday cake for her brother but refused to eat any of it herself. She realizes that she has been oblivious to the early signs of an eating disorder in her daughter, a disorder which, left untreated, could become life threatening.

Most people know what the extreme emaciation of full-blown anorexia looks like, and some of us might even be able to recognize some of the telltale signs of chronic bulimia, the swollen cheeks, or trips to the bathroom after every meal. But recognizing an eating disorder before it reaches these stages is trickier. In this chapter, we will describe the different types of eating disorders and provide checklists of early warning signals.

As we note throughout this book, although we separate anorexia, bulimia, and binge-eating disorder into neat categories, often people will go from being an anorexic to a bulimic, or the reverse, or even exhibit all the hallmarks of both disorders at the same time. I advise parents not to get distracted trying to figure out which diagnosis is correct, but simply to take action as early as possible if they suspect their child has an eating disorder.

## Anorexia Nervosa

The anorexic child refuses to maintain even a minimally normal body weight. (See the growth chart, Appendix B, for guidance on how to assess your child's body build and weight history.) She is intensely afraid of gaining weight, a fear that is fueled by a distorted perception of her body's shape and size. No matter how thin she gets, she sees herself as fat and unattractive, and this distortion in perception usually becomes more severe the more weight she loses. Some anorexics who have not yet reached adulthood will not necessarily lose weight. Instead, they may fall short of expected weight gains while still increasing in height. Others will not grow at all and may be permanently stunted in height unless they begin to eat better.

Anorexic girls who have already begun menstruating stop getting their periods due to their starving bodies' abnormally low levels of estrogen. Among girls who have not yet reached puberty, menstruation may be delayed or completely inhibited by anorexia. In all of these cases, lack of estrogen poses serious risks to bone health of girls. Boys' bones can also be affected by starvation-induced hormonal changes. In anorexic boys, lowered levels of testosterone can lead to reduced bone density.

### The History of Anorexia and Anorexia-like Behaviors

Self-imposed starvation is an ancient disorder that dates back to medieval times. In the Europe of the thirteenth century, historical records tell of women saints who fasted and refused food as part of their religious practice. In 1689, one of the earliest cases of what is now known as anorexia involved a sixteen-year-old English boy.

By the 1870s the term *anorexia nervosa,* meaning loss of appetite due to emotional reasons, had been coined to describe the self-starvation found primarily among upper-middle-class western European and American girls. The historian Joan Jacobs Brumberg, author of the book *Fasting Girls,* argues that modern anorexia is distinct from early cases because of its body-image concerns triggered by "mass cultural preoccupation with dieting and a slim female body."

## Anorexia Subtypes

There are two subtypes of anorexics. The first is the restricting type. The anorexic of this subtype loses weight simply by reducing her food intake, fasting, or engaging in excessive and lengthy periods of exercise as a means of working off calories. The second subtype is the binge-eating/purging type. She restricts her intake as well, but alternates this behavior with bouts of binge eating and often purging. The purging can take the form of self-induced vomiting or the abuse of laxatives, diuretics, or enemas. Some anorexics of this type don't binge, but still purge after consuming even small amounts of food.

## Common Triggers

Often anorexia nervosa is triggered by a stressful life event—leaving home for the first time to enter boarding school, summer camp, or college, being teased about one's weight, breaking up with a boyfriend, not getting chosen for a sports team, or problems within the family, such as divorce. Other risk factors include affluent and well-educated parents, early feeding problems, low self-esteem, high neuroticism (overly moody, sensitive, or fearful), an overprotective mother, having a relative with anorexia or bulimia, especially a parent or sibling (identical twins are particularly at risk in that if one develops an eating disorder, the other is at high risk), and childhood sexual abuse. (For more information on eating disorders and sexual abuse, see p. 248.)

## Anorexia among Children

Although it was at one time thought that anorexia rarely develops before puberty, this appears to be changing, despite the lack of firm data to support what therapists, nutritionists, and other professionals have observed in their own practices. While researchers have not yet documented a rise in childhood anorexia, they *have* shown that girls as young as six years old equate thinness with "goodness," worry about being too fat, and initiate dieting for self-improvement.

Because my clinical practice focuses on children ages five through college age, I have seen many children with anorexia. While experts agree that eating disorders are usually caused by a combination of genetic (see "Genetics and Eating Disorders," p. 126) and environmental causes, among those children I have treated precipitating events range from attempting to get attention in a family where communication has broken down to home schooling the child against his or her wishes, the difficulty of adjusting to being an only child after an older sibling goes off to college, divorce in the family, a sick sibling, mother's dieting, father's bulimia, an insensitive comment by a coach, friend, or sibling about the child's weight, or to the simple fact that other girls at school are restricting their eating. I recently had a thirteen-year-old patient tell me that her introduction to bulimia was at summer camp where one girl showed their group how to purge, after which they all purged together.

Despite the suspected increase in childhood anorexia, parents can take heart from the fact that research has shown that those who become anorexic during childhood and early adolescence may have a better prognosis than those whose disorder starts later.

## Common Traits and Beliefs of the Anorexic

The child who is becoming anorexic often becomes obsessive about counting calories and fat grams and begins to exclude foods she perceives as fattening. Sometimes she will turn to vegetarianism, ostensibly to "eat more healthily," but in fact as a way of controlling her intake of high-fat foods. Often the anorexic exhibits an increased interest in food labels and extreme concern, even fear, of eating fat. Other anorexics, however, especially younger anorexics, simply restrict food intake, seemingly with little interest or awareness about how many calories or fat grams those foods contain. It is not uncommon for the anorexic to eventually eat only a limited number of foods and approach those foods in a ritualistic, programmed way. She may cut up her food into small pieces, or chew each bite of food a certain number of times, or she may constantly sip diet sodas or other no-calorie drinks to fill her stomach.

The anorexic does not always believe that she is overweight. She may acknowledge that she is thin, but wants to be even thinner, and is still bothered by certain aspects of her body that she insists are too big. Prime areas of dissatisfaction are the abdomen, buttocks, and thighs. (For more on body image and anorexia, see pp. 131–32.). The anorexic often weighs herself obsessively, constantly assesses her figure in the mirror, or makes up other ingenious ways of measuring fat. A patient of mine was convinced she was too fat unless she could see prominent veins on her arms. Another of my patients was only satisfied when a coin fit in the hollow of her collarbone. The regular taking of thigh or waist measurements with a tape measure is another commonly used method, along with lying down to assess how sunken the anorexic's stomach is compared to her hipbones. Patients have told me that they do this by putting a ruler across their abdomen and making sure that the stomach and the ruler do not touch.

As the above examples illustrate, anorexics often have obsessive personalities, are perfectionistic and driven to achieve. Although they may be highly intelligent and accomplished, their self-esteem gradually comes to be largely based on the shape and weight of their body. Weight loss becomes a sign of self-discipline, a huge achievement. Conversely, they view weight gain as a sign of failure, the result of a pitiable lack of self-control. Although anorexics often perceive themselves to be very well educated in matters of nutrition and exercise, they may in fact harbor many misconceptions about these topics. Those that are aware of the serious medical consequences of anorexia often find it hard to believe that their own case is dire enough to result in such problems. When they finally do realize it is, the patterns of self-starvation are often too entrenched, and the anorexic tries to hide his or her disorder and deny any medical problems.

Because anorexics are unlikely to cry out for help, but more apt to deny a problem, parents and siblings need to be especially observant when they suspect an eating disorder, and willing to step in and intervene in a sensitive, constructive manner.

### Mood and Behavioral Problems Associated with Anorexia
The secondary problems that result from self-starvation include depression, social withdrawal, irritability, and insomnia.

Obsessive-compulsive behavior is common, leading the anorexic to think constantly of food, even to develop an interest in cooking, collect recipes, and hoard food but not eat it. Teenagers with eating disorders who have jobs often find themselves working in food-related establishments. One reason, of course, is that these are the positions most readily available to teenagers. Yet it also seems that eating disorders often propel affected teenagers toward these jobs.

Bethany told me that while working in the local ice-cream shop she would slip into the walk-in ice-cream freezer to surreptitiously eat ice cream, even though her extreme thinness made the cold almost unbearable, and even though she would never allow herself to do such a thing in the presence of others. As Bethany's story illustrates, the mind of the starving adolescent naturally focuses on food, almost to the exclusion of everything else.

While anorexics often have obsessive or perfectionistic personalities *before* the onset of their disorder, and indeed are at higher risk to become anorexic because of those traits, this is not always the case. Researchers believe that obsessive-compulsive behaviors like Bethany's can also be caused or magnified by the effects of starvation on the body and are not necessarily characteristics of the anorexic herself.

For this reason, standard practice calls for a psychological assessment if these behaviors persist once the anorexic has returned to normal weight.

The anorexic may dislike eating in public, suffer from feelings of ineffectiveness, and be inflexible and controlling of her environment. She also often has difficulty expressing herself emotionally. The anorexic of the binge-eating/purging subtype is more apt to have difficulty controlling her impulses, therefore is more likely to abuse alcohol or other drugs, engage in activities such as shoplifting, and exhibit more mood swings.

There is some evidence that the secondary mental disturbances among those whose anorexia does develop before puberty are more serious. In younger anorexics, who are less likely to have been affected by peer or cultural pressure to diet, it is more likely that the eating disorder is an indication of underlying emotional problems (overly perfectionistic nature, low self-esteem, or obsessive-compulsive traits, for example), rather than the emotional problems being a by-product of the eating disorder.

Yet in most cases, after the eating disorder is resolved, these children regain their emotional equilibrium. They have learned to better manage these emotional issues and are more resilient for having endured the disorder. As painful, dangerous, and difficult as these disorders can be, many of my patients have described overcoming an eating disorder as a character-building experience.

### How Prevalent Is Anorexia?

There has been a remarkable increase in anorexia among teenagers in recent years, making it the third most common chronic condition among adolescent girls after obesity and asthma. Among adults, the prevalence of anorexia has remained constant in recent years, with possibly as high as 4 percent of American girls and women suffering from anorexia at some time during their lives.

Anorexia among children, although less well documented, appears to be increasing as well. Parents should also be aware that contrary to popular belief, boys are not immune to anorexia. Although only one-tenth of the adult population of anorexics are men, among adolescents, boys account for up to one-third of all anorexics. This means that parents of boys should not be complacent about early signs of an eating disorder. (See chapter 5 for more information.)

### The Course of Anorexia

The course of anorexia among different patients is extremely variable, especially if no treatment is provided. Some anorexics recover after a brief episode, some will experience alternating bouts of weight gain and then relapse, and others' condition will steadily decline over many years. Others may move quickly into life-threatening anorexia with little forewarning. Some will go on to develop bulimia or binge-eating disorder. Having anorexia increases a person's risk of dying by more than twelve times the expected rate, with deaths most often resulting from starvation, suicide, or severely low potassium levels. Because anorexia is such a dangerous and potentially life-threatening disorder, early detection and prevention is critical. Research, in fact, has shown that early, aggressive treatment protects against mortality. Effective treatments for eating disorders are now available, yet because anorexics will often deny their illness or attempt to conceal it, it is not uncommon for there to be significant and costly delays between the onset of the disorder and the beginning of treatment.

## Bulimia Nervosa

Instead of the self-starvation that is characteristic of anorexics, bulimics engage in periodic bouts of binge eating. These are always followed by a period of contrition during which the bulimic tries to undo the effects of the binge, either by purging, abusing diuretics or laxatives, or fasting and/or exercising to the extreme.

### The History of Bulimia

Although there are scattered references to bulimia-like behavior from the ancient Greeks onward (the Roman vomitorium was the designated site for forced vomiting between banquet courses), bulimia is a modern and quite recent phenomenon. The word *bulimia* is derived from a Greek word that can be literally translated as "ox hunger." The word has been used medically for hundreds of years to describe excessive, ravenous hunger. Descriptions resembling what we know as bulimia today—bingeing followed by purging—began to emerge in the 1930s. The incidence of this behavior increased after World War II, and by the 1960s bulimia was described as a feature of some anorexic patients. An epidemic-sized increase in the 1970s among college-aged women led to the recognition of bulimia as a distinct eating disorder. In 1979 the term *bulimia nervosa* was officially coined to describe an eating disorder that is related to anorexia, with the added clinical features of bingeing and purging.

### Bulimia Subtypes

There are two subtypes of bulimia, the purging type and the non-purging type. In the first, the bulimic regularly engages in self-induced vomiting or the abuse of laxatives or diuretics after a binge. The non-purging subtype refers to someone who binges, but compensates by fasting or excessive exercise instead of vomiting or taking laxatives or diuretics.

### Common Triggers

The triggers to a binge can vary from depressed mood to the extreme hunger that results from stringent dieting or feelings of self-loathing related to the bulimic's own weight or shape. Often the onset of bulimia is preceded by a stressful or traumatic event, such as leaving home for the first time, being criticized for being fat, a death or illness in the family, breaking up with a boyfriend, starting high school, starting to menstruate, suffering a disfiguring accident, a first sexual experience, or an abortion.

Having siblings or a parent who suffers from bulimia, depression, or alcoholism increases a child's risk of becoming bulimic, most likely because of a potent combination of both genetic and environmental triggers.

### Common Traits and Beliefs of the Bulimic

Like the anorexic, the bulimic's self-esteem is based to an excessive degree on her own body shape and weight. Like the anorexic, the bulimic tries to restrict food intake, but eventually fails, usually by engaging in a binge. (We should note that such a "failure" is perfectly normal behavior after a period of self-starvation, although the bulimic does not see this.) A period of often severe restriction follows, usually ending in another binge. Binges are defined as eating far more than most people would eat during a discrete period of time. Binges can begin in one place and continue in another; for example, at a party at a restaurant, and then in the privacy of the bulimic's bedroom or bathroom. Different people binge on different sorts of food, but the binge usually includes sugary, high-calorie foods.

Unlike the anorexic, who may be proud of her ability to restrict her intake of food, the bulimic is usually mortified by and ashamed of her own behavior. She tries to hide her problem, and is often highly effective at doing so. She may steal food to binge on in secret, use her allowance money to buy binge food, or make sure to run the shower when throwing up so no one hears her.

Once a binge begins, the bulimic eats rapidly, almost without thinking, until she feels discomfort or even outright pain from her excessive consumption.

While anorexics revel in the feeling of total control over their own eating, bulimics during a binge feel a total lack of control. Their binges, especially during the early stages of the disorder, may put them into a state of frenzy, or even beyond that, trigger a sense of dissociation, the feeling of not even inhabiting the body that is doing such damage to itself. The binge is usually followed by a crash in mood, and the return of depressive or self-loathing feelings.

Bulimia can sometimes be harder for parents to detect because the typical bulimic is within normal weight range and because of the secretive nature of the eating and purging behaviors. Some research has indicated that before the onset of the disorder, the child (this is especially true of boys) is more likely to be overweight than his or her peers.

**Purging Behaviors**

Purging, or vomiting to compensate for a binge, is used by 80 to 90 percent of the bulimics who are treated in eating-disorder clinics. Purging offers immediate relief from the often acute feelings of discomfort that follow a binge, and the sense of "undoing" the caloric damage the bulimic has done to his or her body. It is after purging that bulimics once again feel in control and a sense of well-being returns. They feel light, their stomach is flat once again, and they feel they have fixed, or erased, their problem. Purging is usually followed by a period of dieting: restricting calories and avoiding fattening foods or foods the bulimic fears may trigger another binge. Purging may also be followed almost immediately by another binge, then another purge and so on. Most younger patients do not have enough unsupervised time to develop such a destructive pattern of behavior, but for those who do, this cycle can go on for hours. My college-age patients tell me their binge-purge cycles can last for a whole day or evening.

Bulimics induce vomiting most often by using their fingers or other instruments such as a spoon or toothbrush to stimulate the gag reflex. They may use laxatives and diuretics as another way of purging, and in rare cases even resort to enemas or, to induce vomiting, syrup of ipecac.

**Fasting and Excessive Exercise**

Bulimics may also compensate for their binges by fasting for a day or even longer, or exercising to excess. Exercise is considered excessive when it significantly cuts into important activities, when the child engages in it at odd times or in odd settings (getting up in the middle of the night to run in place, or on car trips, running around the car at rest stops), or when the child pursues a taxing regimen despite an injury or other medical complication. My advice to parents is that concern is warranted if exercise sessions last more than an hour, if your child exercises more than once a day, or if your child's exercise routine exceeds that suggested by their coach. (For more on exercise, see chapter 12.)

**Problems Associated with Bulimia**

Bulimics are more apt to suffer from depressive symptoms or anxiety disorders than the average person, but it seems that often the onset of the mood and anxiety disturbance coincides with the development of the disorder. Once the bulimia is effectively treated, these disturbances disappear. Adolescent bulimics are also more prone to substance abuse problems, which occur in about a third of all sufferers. Bulimics will often begin stimulant use, caffeine, nicotine, NoDoz, as a means of controlling their appetite. They may abuse diet pills or prescription medications belonging to friends or parents.

The physical health of most bulimics, unless they are underweight, is not as compromised as that of anorexics. Yet they tend to be more aware of and concerned about their physical symptoms, and they report more physical complaints than anorexics. They will often report nonspecific symptoms such as "heartburn" or feeling "bloated," without giving all the information necessary to make the diagnosis of bulimia. In some cases they don't link their symptoms to their bulimia. In others, they are torn between wanting to hide the disorder and wanting to be confronted about it by a physician or parent. Embarrassed by or ashamed of their problem, they throw out clues that fall short of a confession.

Kellie, a chronic bulimic, would spontaneously vomit when leaning over. Unaware that this is a very common occurrence with chronic bulimia, she was sure she had a serious intestinal disease. Kellie convinced her mother, who had suspected Kellie was struggling with bulimia but wasn't sure, to make an appointment with a gastroenterologist. Kellie's mom hoped the doctor would get to the bottom of the problem. As is often the case in such situations, however, Kellie's mom did not inform the doctor of her suspicions. Kellie accurately described her symptoms, but because she failed to mention her history of bulimia, she ended up with medicines and advice for a symptom that was caused by her bulimia, while the bulimia itself remained untreated.

### How Prevalent Is Bulimia?

The prevalence of bulimia among adolescent and young adult women is estimated to be as high as 5 percent of the population. The prevalence of bulimia in males has yet to be established, but researchers report that of all bulimic patients, 10 to 15 percent are male.

Unlike anorexia, which we suspect is on the increase among children, bulimia appears to be quite rare in younger children. Practitioners are, however, seeing younger and younger teenagers with bulimia. Until now, it was thought that bulimia usually strikes slightly older adolescents than does anorexia, commonly making its appearance from mid-adolescence through the college years. That may be changing as bulimia becomes more prevalent among quite young adolescents.

In my own practice, a number of my college-age patients tell me that they have been bulimic since sixth or seventh grade. One reason researchers may be overlooking bulimic children is that most bulimics wait a number of years before seeking treatment or before their illness is discovered.

### The Course of Bulimia

The binge eating of bulimia often begins during or after an episode of dieting. This restricted eating may lead to some weight loss, after which bingeing and purging begin to predominate. The course of bulimia ranges from chronic to intermittent bouts interspersed with periods of remission.

## Binge-Eating Disorder

Children and adolescents suffering from binge-eating disorder engage in periodic episodes of binge eating, but do not regularly follow it up with any of the compensatory measures described in the previous section on bulimia.

Binge eaters suffer the same inability to control their food intake as bulimics. They eat rapidly during a binge, almost without thinking, even when they are not hungry. They usually binge secretly, ashamed of and repulsed by their own behavior. Yet hard as they try, they are unable to stop bingeing. When a binge is over, they feel a combination of disgust at their behavior, guilt, and often depression. Most often, bingeing occurs as a consequence of repeated and unsuccessful efforts to diet.

Binge eating may be detected when there is evidence of eating in secret, lying about eating, or food disappearing, although some children without an eating disorder will engage in such behaviors if parents are overly restrictive in allowing them access to food. Being overly restrictive in turn increases the child's risk of developing an eating disorder.

Like bulimics, binge eaters suffer a great deal of distress over their inability to stop eating once they have started a binge. But the binge eater does not induce vomiting, does not misuse laxatives or diuretics, does not regularly fast or exercise excessively the way the bulimic does. Binge eaters may occasionally engage in some of these behaviors, but not regularly, as bulimics do.

### The History of Binge Eating

Albert Stunkard, one of the premier researchers in binge eating, pointed out that binge eating is the oldest of all the eating disorders, one that has deep historical roots and may go back more than two millennia. Binge eating was described by early writers like Homer and Hippocrates and is discussed in early medical literature. It was not until the mid-eighteenth centry, however, that binge eating was described as a pathology. By the turn of the nineteenth century, it was firmly established as an aberrant behavior.

When binge eating was first described in the modern medical literature in 1959 it was almost immediately classed as an occasional practice of anorexics. Later, when bulimia was identified, binge eating came to be considered characteristic of bulimia. Only since the mid-1990s has binge-eating disorder been recognized as a separate and unique eating disorder. Even now, however, more research must be done before binge-eating disorder becomes an official eating disorder diagnosis.

## Common Triggers

Binge eating may be triggered by depression and anxiety, feelings that often are put at bay or relieved by a binge. The binge eater may turn to food as a comfort in the face of a family disturbance, or trouble at school.

Often a child or adolescent begins bingeing after losing a significant amount of weight from dieting. Much research, in fact, has been done showing that habitual dieting leads to binge eating. Dieters attempt to restrict their food intake, only to overcompensate by bingeing. One study done on former World War II prisoners of war found that the veterans, who suffered dramatic weight loss while in captivity, reported significantly higher frequency of binge eating than those veterans who had not been imprisoned and starved. Largely based on studies such as these, the current medical opinion on binge eating is that often it is the body's natural response to starvation—or the modern-day equivalent, the weight-loss diet.

Elyse had always been on the "chunky" side, but was determined to enter high school at a lower weight. To do so, she had to reduce her intake of calories to less than 300 calories per day. Even then, she was unable to lose as much weight as she wanted. Eventually she found herself binge eating between bouts of dieting. Over time this pattern of diet-binge-diet caused her weight to creep up to even higher than it was when she started dieting.

## Characteristics of the Binge Eater

The onset of the disorder typically occurs in late adolescence or the early twenties, although in my practice I have seen an increasing number of younger adolescents and even children who are binge eating. Binge eaters tend to be more overweight than other eating-disordered patients and experience more dramatic fluctuations in weight. Binge-eating disorder does not necessarily lead to weight gain, however, particularly among adolescents with active metabolisms, or among young athletes. Parents can miss a serious problem of binge eating because their child is normal weight. Although the binge eating of the normal-weight child may not seem to be anything to worry about, vigilance is advised because binge eating can lead to other eating disorders. A common scenario is the binge eater who over time gains weight, which in turn triggers bulimia or anorexia. Binge eating can also lead to low self-esteem since most people who binge eat feel very guilty and ashamed about this behavior.

David, a fourteen-year-old patient of mine, tells me he feels physically addicted to binge eating. He desperately wants to stop, but finds that he cannot.

Binge eaters like David report that their disorder interferes with their relationships with other people and their ability to feel good about themselves, as well as higher rates of self-loathing, disgust about body size, depression, and anxiety about weight gain. Like bulimics, those who suffer from binge-eating disorder are more prone to substance abuse than the general population.

Latryce, who began bingeing after unsuccessfully trying a severely restrictive diet, eventually resorted to taking an herbal supplement containing ephedrine. An amphetamine stimulant that has been associated with cardiac problems, ephedrine has led to a number of deaths. Despite her therapist's warnings about the dangers of the supplement, Latryce found that she was unable to make herself stop taking it.

### How Prevalent Is Binge Eating?

Binge eating differs from anorexia and bulimia in that the incidence among females and males is closer to parity. Approximately 40 percent of binge-eating disorder cases occur in boys and men.

Among children, although there are no published scientific studies to back this up, my clinical experience has led me to believe that there is a clear increase in the number of those suffering from binge-eating disorder in recent years.

I have also noticed that although I treat about an equal number of girls and boys for binge eating in my practice, parents tend to be more concerned when a daughter binge-eats than a son. Because it is more socially acceptable for boys to have a big appetite than for girls, a serious binge-eating problem in a boy may be overlooked. (For a comparison of the different way in which parents react to boys' bulimia and anorexia, see chapter 5, p. 76.)

Brad, a young patient of mine, had to gain 50 pounds before his binge eating was recognized as a problem by his parents and pediatrician. Gina's parents, on the other hand, were quick to consult me after hearing that one of Gina's close friends dieted and binged at the summer camp both girls attended. They worried that Gina, a lovely, shapely fourteen-year-old, might be at risk. They knew she struggled with the fact she wasn't as thin as she wanted to be and they wanted advice on how to be proactive.

The tremendous rise in obesity among young people in our country has been well documented, but has been largely ascribed to lack of exercise, increase in junk food consumption, and super-sized American servings. The severely overweight kids that I see in my practice are also binge eating, which I believe is another reason for the significant increase in obesity among American children. (See chapters 10 and 11 for a nutritional approach that will help binge eaters control their eating and their weight.)

## Eating Disorders Not Otherwise Specified

Because so many people who are treated by eating disorders programs do not fit neatly into the category of anorexics or bulimics, the American Psychiatric Association has established another category, eating disorders not otherwise specified (EDNOS). EDNOS is the designation that professionals use for eating disorders that do not meet all the criteria for anorexia or bulimia and is considered a distinct class of eating disorder in and of itself.

People who fall into this category may, for example, exhibit all of the characteristics of anorexia including severe weight loss, but still have menstrual periods, or they may still manage to maintain a weight in the normal range in spite of radically reduced food intake. The latter happens most often with larger or obese children; no one suspects they have anorexia because even severe weight loss does not leave them visibly malnourished. In other cases of EDNOS, patients may binge by chewing and then spitting out rather than swallowing most of their food.

EDNOS is particularly common among adolescents with eating disorders, whose disorders might not be as dire or entrenched as those of older patients. Bulimia is diagnosed as EDNOS when it has occurred for less than three months or when binge-purge episodes occur less than twice a week.

I tell parents not to assume that just because their child is diagnosed as having EDNOS that the child's problem is insignificant and does not need treatment. They can be in as much physical danger as the classic anorexic or bulimic, and suffer just as much emotional distress.

## Anorexia, Bulimia, and Binge-Eating Disorders Are Not Mutually Exclusive

Parents should realize that although we have described three types of eating disorders as separate phenomena, in real life they are not always that clear-cut. An anorexic, as we have described, may alternate self-starvation with periods of bingeing, and even purging. It is quite common for a restricting-type anorexic, after engaging in months or years of fasting and superhuman self-restraint, to finally give in to her incessant thoughts and cravings about food and become a binge eater or a bulimic. In fact, up to 50 percent of patients with anorexia develop bulimic symptoms, and some people who start out as bulimics develop the symptoms of anorexia.

## Does Your Child Have an Eating Disorder?

We have so far described what a full-blown eating disorder looks like. It should also be clear to you now that eating disorders are most effectively and easily treated when they are caught early. This is a bigger challenge than recognizing a child in the midst of a crisis. How do you know if your child is at risk for an eating disorder? Here we offer you a series of check-lists of early warning signs. (For a checklist of criteria that will tell you if your child has a diagnosable eating disorder, see Appendix A.)

Ideally these checklists should make it clear when you need to worry about your child's eating behaviors, but because we are talking about early-warning signs it is difficult to say with certainty what total number of checks should cause you to become alarmed. By offering this exhaustive list of early warning symptoms, our aim is to outline the range of tip-off behaviors, attitudes, and symptoms to watch for. By encouraging you to use your own intuition about your child and her symptoms we hope to transform the process of early detection from an art into more of a science. However, it will always remain in large part an art, which requires knowing your child well, being observant, and trusting your instincts.

Having said that, here are some general guidelines. We begin with a checklist of symptoms found with all three disorders—anorexia, bulimia, and binge-eating disorder. If you check more than eight items on this list, you likely have a serious problem on your hands that warrants your atten-tion and a visit to the doctor. If you check between five and eight items, some preventive strategies are in order, which we will outline in chapter 3. Keep an eye on your child and make sure these symptoms do not increase in number. If your child exhibits only a few of these symptoms and yet you feel uneasy, you should at the very least share your concerns with your child's doctor, who can help you sort through the situation.

### What Are the Early Warning Signs of an Eating Disorder?

❑  Obvious changes in weight, both up and down.
❑  Going through puberty early, or being bigger or taller than average size (this can lead a child to become overly body conscious).
❑   Going on a diet.
❑  Pickiness in food choices, fear of fat in food.
❑  Sudden interest in nutrition and healthy eating.
❑  Interest in food labels, especially fat grams and calories.
❑  Deciding to become vegetarian.
❑  Avoiding desserts.
❑  Skipping meals, especially breakfast.
❑  Drinking excessive amounts of water, diet soda, coffee, or other non-caloric drinks.

❑ Frequent complaints of feeling full or bloated, constipation, diarrhea, stomach pain, nausea, and vomiting.
❑ Lying about food intake.
❑ Seems distressed and guilty about eating.
❑ Spends a lot of time worrying about size and shape.
❑ A newfound interest in sports, or exercising in addition to sports practice.
❑ A drive to excel in sports.
❑ Involvement in "thinness demand sports" such as dance, ballet, gymnastics, figure skating.
❑ Involvement in sports with weight classes such as wrestling, some martial arts.
❑ Involvement in sports in which weight can affect performance, such as running, cross-country skiing.
❑ A tendency to be a perfectionist.
❑ Low self-esteem.
❑ Development of moodiness, seems less happy in general.

The next three checklists cover anorexia, bulimia, and binge-eating disorder individually. Where the preponderance of your checks fall in these last three checklists will help you determine which type of eating disorder your child may have. (For a full explanation of the symptoms and laboratory findings associated with these eating disorders, see chapter 6.)

## What Are the Early Warning Signs of Anorexia?

❑ When regular well-child assessments show failure to gain weight or weight loss.
❑ Denying obvious thinness or weight loss.
❑ Complaints of being cold all the time, or wearing lots of layers of clothing.
❑ Hands and feet are cold to the touch much of the time and may be bluish in color.
❑ Evidence of increased hair loss; more hair on the pillow or in brushes. Hair looks thinner and drier.
❑ Lanugo hair on face or body (similar to body hair found on newborns).
❑ Crying without producing tears (due to dehydration).
❑ Yellowish skin tone due to elevated levels of carotene (caused by eating excessive amounts of vegetables and/or poor liver function).
❑ Complaints of dizziness.
❑ Fainting.

❑ Restricting fluids.
❑ Preparing food for others, but not eating it.

### What Are the Early Warning Signs of Bulimia?

❑ Finding evidence that the child has obtained laxatives, diuretics, or diet pills.
❑ Complaints on a regular basis of "stomach flu" or that certain foods "don't sit right."
❑ Complaints of heartburn-type symptoms (very rare in children without an eating disorder), chronic sore throat, hoarseness, difficulty swallowing.
❑ Puffy face or swollen cheeks.
❑ Redness or calluses on the back of hands.
❑ Redness around the mouth from exposure to stomach acid.
❑ Small red blood spots around the eyes, or bloodshot eyes (resulting from the pressure of self-inducing vomiting).
❑ Dental exam reveals large number of cavities when previously your child has always had good dental reports.

### What Are the Early Warning Signs of Binge-Eating Disorder?

The following can also be signs of bingeing behaviors that are associated with bulimia.
❑ On and off weight-loss diets.
❑ Out-of-control eating, wants to control eating, promises to control eating, but can't.
❑ Eats when not hungry.
❑ Often complains of being too full.
❑ Eats rapidly.
❑ Eats a lot when sad, mad, depressed.
❑ Secretive eating.
❑ Food missing from kitchen or refrigerator.
❑ At well-child visits has gained significant weight beyond what would have been expected.

If, after reading this chapter and going through these checklists, you are still unsure whether you should be concerned about your child's eating, I suggest reaching out to local experts. Therapists, nutritionists, and of course your own pediatrician will very likely be willing to talk with you about your concerns. My experience has been if a parent is concerned enough to call me for advice about the signs and symptoms they are noticing in their child, there is a good reason for their concern.

## In Summary

As you can see from the checklists, the most obvious signals an eating-disordered child will send will be of rapid and or significant weight loss or weight gain, or extreme changes in eating or exercise patterns. We remind you, however, that detecting an eating disorder in a child or adolescent can be trickier, since instead of losing weight, she may be failing to grow in height, or experiencing delayed onset of puberty. Detection can also be made difficult by the typical efforts of the eating-disordered child to hide her problem.

You should pay attention if your child is fearful of weight gain or of fatness in general, if your child restricts food intake for fear of gaining weight, or avoids foods because of their calorie and fat content.

When attempting to arrive at a diagnosis for your child's problem, you should be aware that there are both physical and psychological conditions that produce symptoms similar to those of an eating disorder. Physical conditions that can mimic an eating disorder include inflammatory bowel disease, Crohn's disease, Addison's disease, diabetes, and thyroid disease.

Psychiatric disorders such as obsessive-compulsive disorder or depression may lead to food refusal and weight loss as well. These disorders are treated primarily by medications and psychotherapy. This can be a tricky area. We have stressed in this chapter that psychological disturbances are usually caused by an eating disorder, and that standard practice is to restore nutritional status and wait to see if mood and behavioral problems resolve before treating these problems. Yet we must also point out that occasionally psychiatric disorders do occur with an eating disorder. In such cases, both problems should be treated. (For more on medications and eating disorders, see pp. 263–65.)

Your rule of thumb should be that if your child is not exhibiting some of the key symptoms of an eating disorder (clearly pursuing weight loss, body-image problems, or evidence they are bingeing or purposefully vomiting) but is losing weight or periodically vomiting, then further medical evaluation and tests should be done to rule out some other explanation. Whether your child ends up with a formal eating disorder diagnosis or is suffering from a milder form of disorganized or disordered eating (see next chapter), we recommend that you act immediately and effectively, as we outline in Part III, to correct your child's disordered eating, and prevent the development of a full-blown eating disorder.

# 2

# Bad Habit or Dangerous Behavior?: When to Worry about Disordered Eating

After reading descriptions of the various eating disorders, you may have decided that your child does not have a full-blown eating disorder. Yet you may be worried that she is heading in that direction, adopting eating behaviors that make you uneasy, possibly because they are clearly unhealthy and rigidly or fanatically held. If this describes your situation, your child may be exhibiting signs of disordered eating.

Disordered eating is a subclinical eating disorder, which, if left unaddressed, may develop into a full-blown eating disorder. Or it may continue to simmer just below the surface, quietly eroding the quality of your child's life. Though disordered eating is a term frequently used by professional and layperson alike, it has not been formally defined. It has come to refer to those whose body dissatisfaction is strong enough to lead them to diet and to experiment with other eating-disordered behaviors.

In this chapter, we will describe the different forms of disordered eating that children can exhibit, the risk factors that predispose a child to disordered eating, and some strategies for turning around a disordered-eating situation before it progresses any further. We will focus in particular on the number-one form of disordered eating, dieting, and explain why even though it is a common practice among millions of Americans, it is a behavior that puts the dieter at risk for an eating disorder. Some of you may think we are exaggerating when we assert that dieting is risky behavior. "How can that be," you might wonder, "when the weight-loss diet is so much a part of contemporary life? Who *hasn't* dieted at one time or another?" Yet for reasons that we will outline in detail in this chapter, this is exactly what many experts are concluding: dieting *is* a form of disordered eating, and it *does* put the dieter, especially if that dieter is a child or an adolescent, at risk for an eating disorder.

## How Does Disordered Eating Differ from a Full-Blown Eating Disorder?

Distinguishing disordered eating from a full-blown eating disorder can be difficult, and in one sense is not worth attempting since children who suffer from either should be helped. Those whose business it is to make such distinctions have argued that the difference between the two groups is that disordered eaters still retain some control over their eating, and do not let abnormal food behaviors interfere with their life in an appreciable way, while eating-disorder sufferers' lives are profoundly influenced by their eating problems.

## Why Worry about Disordered Eating?

Although it is true that many adolescents who suffer from disordered eating manage to live normal lives and go on to develop healthy and normal eating patterns, this is not always the case. If you are reading this book, you are probably already concerned that your child is not one of those who will simply outgrow her eating problems. We are devoting this chapter to disordered eating because those who suffer from it in one important respect do not differ from those suffering from full-blown disorders: they too can experience chronic and substantial distress and impairment. Disordered eating, in fact, can be as chronic as full-syndrome eating disorders. When a child's symptoms fall below the radar of doctors and other caregivers, the danger is that her subclinical behaviors may go unnoticed for months or even years, in some cases severely compromising the disordered eater's quality of life. My patient Rosalind is a case in point.

Rosalind, now in her mid-twenties, has been seriously dieting since she was thirteen, and is finally just beginning to get her periods for the first time. Even though her weight has never been low enough to classify her as an anorexic, she, like many disordered eaters whose diet is poor, suffered from lack of periods, a classic symptom of full-blown anorexia.

When she first began to restrict her eating as a child, she recalls, "My mom accused me of dieting just to get attention. After that, I went 'underground.' Mom still doesn't know about my food problems." (Keeping those problems from her mother was hardly difficult. Rosalind's mother was inattentive and uninterested in monitoring her daughter's health, and to the extent that she thought about it, unrealistically ascribed Rosalind's lack of periods to being a "late bloomer.") Although they are invisible to her family and friends, Rosalind's problems are significant. For the past ten years, Rosalind's life has revolved around her disordered eating. Though she has managed to maintain a low weight, she views her body so negatively that she refuses to date. Excited about her new job in an up-and-coming young advertising agency, Rosalind nevertheless finds it hard to make friends among colleagues because she never takes anyone up on their invitations for lunch or dinner. She admits to having a "secret rule": she turns down any social invitation that involves food. Though she looks totally put-together, hair stylishly cut, dressed head-to-toe in fashionable clothes, Rosalind admits she feels anything but at ease. Her kitchen is a mess, and at any given moment she is either dieting or living on junk food. Though her "binges" are small she feels miserable when she eats four croissants for dinner. Occasionally she makes herself throw up or uses laxatives to purge.

I see Rosalind after a recent doctor's visit at which her doctor assures her that her weight is fine as long as she does not lose any more. As usual, her laboratory values are normal. "See," Rosalind tells me, "my *doctor* doesn't even think my problems are serious." Because Rosalind has changed doctors several times, only recently has the effect of her lack of periods on bone density become a concern, and even now, it is not high on her doctor's list of concerns. (See pp. 87–88 for more on eating disorders and bone health.) The unfortunate truth is that doctors often fail to explore this issue with adults suffering from a chronic eating disorder.

Rosalind's experience is typical of many suffering from disordered eating—no one takes them seriously. I tell her, "Your doctor's remarks are simply a factual summary of your health status. Just because she says your weight is okay does not mean she's implying that your life is okay." Because most doctors do not delve into patients' eating behaviors in any detail, their comments should not be interpreted as an overall assessment of function. As a nutritionist, I wish that doctors like Rosalind's would put their comments in context so patients would be less apt to misinterpret their remarks. If her doctor had said, "I'm glad to say that you are not in any medical danger at the moment. But I am quite concerned that your disordered-eating habits have not been resolved," Rosalind might have been less likely to use her doctor's assessment as a rationale for accepting her bleak status quo.

Rosalind's problem now, of course, is that she does not take her own problems seriously enough to do the hard work necessary to begin to transform her approach to food. Even though she suffers from disordered eating, not a clinical eating disorder, it will take serious effort to develop the balanced approach to food she needs in order to feel healthier, happier, and more able to engage with the outside world. In fact, she will have to work as hard as any long-term bulimic or anorexic to develop new, healthy eating patterns.

Rosalind's story is in no way unusual or unique, and illustrates a type of disordered eating that begins in adolescence, and sometimes even in childhood.

And finally, another reason it is worth paying attention to disordered eating: while disordered eaters may have more control over their eating than those with full-blown eating disorders, researchers have found that disordered eating increases the risk of depression. For all of these reasons, and because your best chance of success when battling an eating disorder is the preemptive strike, disordered eating should not be ignored, but confronted as wholeheartedly as a full-blown disorder.

## How Prevalent Is Disordered Eating?

Since the mid-1980s, disordered eating has become so common that it affects the majority of adolescent girls. One researcher went so far as to call disordered eating and the body dissatisfaction that accompanies it "a normal discontent."

Recent studies have documented high rates of body dissatisfaction and dieting behavior in pre- and young adolescents, and shown that almost half of surveyed children as young as nine prefer thin bodies to more normal weight ones. In one study, 55 percent of the girls and 35 percent of the boys wanted to be thinner. What is surprising here is that so many boys felt this way.

## Disordered-Eating Subtypes

Here we will briefly explain the different forms of disordered eating, broadly separating them into three different subtypes, the disordered eater who restricts, binges, or purges.

### The Disordered Eater Who Restricts
The typical restricting-type disordered eater is on a diet, possibly one of the many fad diets that fall in and out of favor with the American public. She might also count calories or fat grams, and checks her weight often on a scale.

Sometimes restricting food and calorie intake is a way for college-aged students to work alcohol into their life.

## Dieting as Risky Behavior

It is difficult to think of something as ordinary and ubiquitous as dieting—restricting or changing food intake for the purpose of losing weight—as in any way "disordered" or abnormal. Dieting has become so much the norm in our society that, according to one study, somewhere between one-half and two-thirds of all girls are dieting at any given time. Yet dieting is the most common disordered-eating behavior, and one that clearly increases the risk of developing a full-blown eating disorder. Consider these facts:

- According to one study, dieters are eight times more likely to develop an eating disorder than non-dieters.
- Another study showed that the onset of an eating disorder is likely to be preceded by several years of abnormal eating attitudes and dieting behavior. Obviously not all dieters develop an eating disorder, but almost all of those who develop an eating disorder preceded their eating disorder with dieting.
- Several studies have shown that having other family members who suffer from an eating disorder, depression, alcoholism, or substance abuse increases the risk of developing an eating disorder. That risk is substantially increased if in addition to one or more of these risk factors, a parent is dieting. Parents should take heed of this finding because while you may not be able to control all of the risk factors your child is exposed to, you *can* put a stop to dieting behaviors.
- The simple fact that your child wants to weigh less, regardless of whether he has attempted to diet, creates significant risk for future eating problems.
- When an active child or teen diets, it is nearly impossible for them to get all the nutrients they need to maintain optimum health and to continue growing.
- Dieting causes fatigue, moodiness, irritability, and poor academic and athletic performance.
- Because dieting lowers metabolism and increases the likelihood of binge eating, in some cases it can lead to weight gain and even obesity.
- If a child is predisposed, through genetics, environmental factors (having a mother or friends who are either concerned about weight and dieting, or have eating disorders, for example), or personality characteristics (perfectionism or low self-esteem, for example) to an eating disorder, then simply going on a diet can be enough to trigger onset of the disorder.

For all of these reasons, many experts strongly believe that dieting behavior is risky, potentially unhealthy, and certainly not normal. The exceptions are children whose specific medical conditions make it necessary for them to stay on a specialized diet. For example, children with diabetes, food allergies, or gastrointestinal diseases may be put on special diets by their doctors. While some doctors may still prescribe weight-loss diets for obese children, a more current approach is to try to hold the child's weight steady and let her "grow out" of her obesity by eating normally. Doctors working with overweight children and other children requiring therapeutic diets should work hard to present dietary recommendations in a "non-diet" way (for example, eating normally, learning to listen and respond to the body's signals of hunger and fullness, and encouraging acceptance of the child's own size) because diets in general don't work. What they more often do is result in "dietary rebellion" on the part of the child who is put on the diet.

Sometimes simply making clear to your child at a young age that dieting will not be tolerated is enough to quash any ideas about experimenting with diets. Lynda's mother, Margaret, took a firm approach when Lynda declared her intention to lose ten pounds before next month's prom. "Lynda," Margaret said, "we don't diet in this family." Lynda told her friends that although she wanted to diet to lose weight, she couldn't because her mother wouldn't allow it.

## Restricting through Pseudo-Vegetarianism

Disordered eating may begin with what some call pseudo-vegetarianism. First the child eliminates red meat from the diet, and then gradually eliminates a whole host of foods because they are high in fat or perceived as unhealthy.

My patient, Trina, was thirteen when her eating problems began. At first her parents did not know what to make of her declaration one morning that she had decided to become a vegetarian. Trina claimed to be newly concerned about animal rights, and added, "Besides, meat isn't healthy to eat." Her family had always made meat, chicken, or fish the focal point of meals. Trina's father, Jerry, an avid hunter, had a particularly difficult time understanding this development. Carol, Trina's mother, wondered how she could make sure her meals were adequate. Trina assured her mother she had nothing to worry about since by talking to the clerks at the local health food store, she had collected some ideas for easy vegetarian dishes she could make herself. Initially, Trina's approach to vegetarianism sounded reasonable to Carol, who knew that Trina was more mature and thoughtful than other girls her age. "If anyone can pull this off, it's Trina," Carol reassured herself. At first Trina's family was in awe of Trina's developing proficiency in the kitchen. But her fussiness about any food that had come in contact with an animal product worried Jerry. Carol didn't start to worry until she noticed that Trina was becoming fat phobic. Several of Trina's friends shared this interest, but their diets seemed healthier to Carol because they would eat chicken, fish, and low-fat dairy products. Carol knew Trina was headed down a dangerous path when Trina told her, "No need to buy any more tofu for me, Mom. It's too high in fat."

Though Trina would deny it, her vegetarianism was a cover for an increasingly restrictive approach to eating.

### The Disordered Eater Who Purges

The disordered eater who purges may have some symptoms of bulimia, but perhaps does not engage in this behavior as frequently as a full-blown bulimic. He may, for example, only purge when he eats dessert or foods high in fat.

### The Disordered Eater Who Binges or Overeats

The disordered eater who overeats or binges may engage in this behavior more irregularly than the classic binge eater—for example, once a week instead of twice a week or more. Her binges may also be smaller than a full-fledged bulimic's.

Another variant is intentionally "banking" calories by undereating during the day, so in the evening those calories can be spent on party food, a big restaurant meal, or snacking freely while studying. This approach to eating is common among college-aged girls, who starve themselves all day so that they can feel free to indulge with their friends in the evening. In other cases, the disordered eater may skip breakfast and maybe even lunch, eat normally at dinner, and then before bed engage in a bona fide binge triggered by their undereating earlier in the day. Girls who regularly practice such behavior are at risk of developing an eating disorder.

Often disordered eaters at first feel their disordered behaviors are an effective method of weight control. They go through what I call the "honeymoon phase" of disordered eating, when the behaviors they have adopted are fairly new, and for the moment, at least, really seem to be working to control weight. Soon, however, they grow frustrated. They find that despite their efforts to reduce their food intake further, or to purge when they feel they have eaten too much, either they begin to gain weight, or at best can only maintain their higher-than-desired weight. On top of it all, they are stuck with a nasty disordered-eating habit that is extremely difficult to shake.

*Disorganized Eating*
Sometimes a child's bingeing problem is simply the result of disorganized eating patterns. If your child wakes up late and rushes off to school without eating breakfast and then skimps on lunch, she is likely to come home from school ravenous for a snack. The "snack" may turn into a binge, and this pattern may repeat itself periodically. If this description fits your child, she is suffering from a form of disordered eating that is easily remedied. (For more on normalizing eating, see chapters 10 and 11.)

## Risk Factors for Disordered Eating

Many of the risk factors for disordered eating, we should note, are the same as those for a full-blown eating disorder, which we discussed in chapter 1. In addition to these, however, researchers have recently isolated additional risk factors for developing disordered eating. Here we will first review some of the common risk factors for both disordered eating and full-blown eating disorders, and then describe those additional risk factors for disordered eating. (For specific preventive strategies targeted at reducing or eliminating these risk factors, see chapter 3.) The common risk factors are:

• **Low self-esteem.**  As we note in chapter 3, low self-esteem is one of the most powerful risk factors for both disordered eating and eating disorders. Children with low self-esteem hold their own personality, abilities, and general "likeability" in low regard. They find it hard to like and respect themselves, have little self-confidence, and take little or no pride in themselves or their accomplishments. Self-esteem is closely tied to body image, which means that improving your child's self-esteem will likely improve her body image, and vice versa. (For more on body image, see p. 131.) Self-esteem often declines in the face of difficult transitions and stressful situations. For girls, researchers have found that self-esteem takes a big dip between sixth and seventh grade, as they struggle to make the transition from grade school to junior high. Boys' self-esteem dips too during this period, but not as dramatically. Researchers think boys are protected by the fact that they mature later. For them, the transition from elementary school to middle school does not usually coincide with pubertal changes, and the stressful effect those changes often have on peer and family relationships. (See p. 73 for more information on boys and puberty.)

Meredith's leadership qualities were recognized by her teachers and peers at her rural grade school. An academic and social success in elementary school, she was excited to be taking the bus to the big junior high in the neighboring town. To her surprise, though, she found that she was not prepared for the highly stratified social scene she found there, the unspoken fashion rules, or the cliques. Formerly comfortable with and not overly concerned about her appearance, she came to realize over the course of her first frustrating year in junior high that the only thing she could change was her weight. Everyone knew "thin was in," so Meredith did everything she could to reduce her weight dramatically over the summer. Maybe, just maybe, Meredith hoped, becoming thin would make her more popular.

• **Depression.** While some research indicates that eating problems often precede or may cause depression, there is no doubt that depression can predispose a child to disordered eating. For the depressed child who perhaps has not yet learned healthier coping mechanisms, turning to binge eating or starvation is a simple and easy way of assuaging unpleasant emotions.

• **Perfectionism.** The tendency to live by unreasonably high standards is well known to increase risk of eating problems. Children who are perfectionists are often more eager than the average child to meet cultural, parental, or peer expectations to be thin. When a perfectionistic child is placed in a high-pressure environment, that risk is compounded. Nicole's perfectionistic personality made her a standout in ballet class. Her involvement in a high-powered ballet program, combined with her personality type, increased her risk of developing eating problems.

• **Skipping meals, fear of fat, or quirky food habits that restrict food choice and intake.** If your child saves her lunch money in order to buy the latest CD by her favorite recording artist, you should explore her motivation. Is it just an avid love of music, or fear of getting fat that has caused her to skip lunch? Fear of weight gain or extreme concern about the fat content of foods distinguishes disordered eating from more benign experiments with dieting. This is a clear sign that your child is at risk for disordered eating. "Quirky food habits" may simply be peculiar food preferences that your child will eventually outgrow, such as wanting to eat only white foods, or not wanting different foods on the same plate to touch each other. Sometimes, however, quirky habits can be the first clues to an impending eating disorder. If your child's quirky food habits consistently reduce fat and calorie intake, you should be more concerned. At first Colin's mother, Debra, didn't know what to make of her son's sudden interest in crisp green apples. It was not until Colin was eating five apples at a sitting that Debra finally realized that this was her son's way of filling himself up to avoid eating higher-calorie snack foods.

• **Weight concerns, picky eating, inhibited eating, slow eating, and food refusal in young children.** Weight concerns in a young child who is still growing and developing are in no way appropriate. Such concern can sometimes foreshadow both anorexia and bulimia.

A picky eater is one who has lots of food dislikes. An inhibited eater is a child who takes just a few bites, even of foods he likes. Although in most children the eating difficulties of childhood are transient, you should be aware that picky eating, inhibited eating, slow eating, or outright food refusal appear in some cases to foreshadow future anorexia. Researchers do not know if this is because these children are naturally inclined to have little interest in food and later find it easy to undereat, or if it is because they learn to hone these annoying habits into more extreme food behaviors as they grow older. They may decide that picky eating or food refusal worked so well to get their parents' attention when they were young, why not continue them as older children? You should be particularly concerned if your child's picky eating begins to inhibit normal growth, and you should make sure your picky eater's weight is checked regularly by her doctor.

Most doctors are not concerned about these eating styles if the child is growing normally, and most children outgrow their finicky approach to eating if parents are matter-of-fact about providing regular meals and snacks regardless of how much or how little the child eats. The challenge to you as parents is to meet your child's nutrient needs without catering to her too much, which will reinforce her pickiness. This may mean including simple foods that your child likes at meals, but not circumscribing the array of other foods offered at family meals. Children should not be forced to eat foods they do not like. Your pediatrician can advise you whether you need to seek professional nutritional help, for you or your child.

• **Secretive eating, overeating, and vomiting in young children.** These behaviors point with more certainty to a burgeoning eating problem than the behaviors listed in the previous item and are more likely to lead to disordered eating or bulimia. As with children who are picky, inhibited, or slow eaters, if your child exhibits any of these behaviors, you should see that she gets extra support to prevent the development of eating problems. If your child is exhibiting any of these behaviors, she is most likely feeling deprived in some way. If your attempt at changing these behaviors by changing your approach to food does not work, you should seek professional advice. (See chapter 14 for more information on how professionals can help.)

The following are additional risk factors for developing disordered eating that researchers have recently identified. As you will see, some of the most influential factors determining whether children develop eating problems come from parents and peers.

Keep in mind, however, that it is difficult to say with absolute certainty what the family-related risk factors for disordered eating are, since having a child who suffers from either disordered eating or an eating disorder causes such stress that family function is inevitably affected. Looking for causes or risk factors, in other words, is a classic chicken-and-egg situation. Having said that, the additional risk factors are:

• **Children who are encouraged by their parents to diet.**

• **Children whose parents are openly critical of their bodies.** Molly's mother Toni was, unlike her daughter, naturally thin. Toni was convinced Molly would have better self-esteem if she were thinner. When Molly tried on a pair of jeans recently, Toni commented, "I really hope those aren't size 13." Molly was devastated. Although she had wanted to buy the size 13 pants, faced with her mom's open disapproval, she bought the size 11 pants, which didn't fit comfortably and ended up being a constant reminder that she was bigger than her mother thought she should be.

Researchers have proven what Molly's story demonstrates: that parental comments, especially comments from mothers, have an effect on children's attitudes about their bodies and on their food behaviors.

• **Children who feel their father is not supportive.** Although Shelly knows her father loves her, he is so critical of everything she does, wears, and says that it is often easy for her to doubt this fact. "Would he love me more if I looked better?" she wonders.

Studies have shown that support from fathers has a surprisingly powerful effect on protecting children against developing eating problems.

• **Children from families who rarely eat together.** Children from families where parents do not regularly prepare meals for them often end up making food choices based on television ads, which push junk and fast foods, or what they read in their mothers' magazines, which encourage dieting. Parents who rarely share meals with their children are also likely to miss the early signs of eating problems simply because they don't see their child eat.

• **Families with an absolutist approach to food.** In my own practice, I have seen numerous cases in which a purist approach to food on the part of parents can lead to disordered eating. Parents who are vegetarian, or insist that only organic food or only low-fat foods be consumed are often surprised and baffled to find their child has become a disordered eater. Of course, in some families like this, children are able to negotiate their parents' eating edicts seemingly with ease and grow up to be perfectly balanced and carefree eaters.

• **Poor peer relationships.** As children mature, peers become increasingly important. By the time a child enters adolescence, peers are likely to be a major source of emotional support. When peer support is lacking, children may try to earn their peers' acceptance or at least their notice by attempting to lose weight. Some children react to peers competitively, including in the area of body size.

• **Being heavier than average.**

• **Early onset of menstrual periods.** This is a sign of early physical development, which is a well-established risk factor for disordered eating and eating disorders. Children who develop early usually feel bigger and fatter than their peers, and an early developing girl may have to deal with more attention from boys. As soon as girls begin dating they are likely to become more interested in and critical of their appearance.

• **Type 1 diabetes mellitus (juvenile diabetes).** The child or teenager with type 1 diabetes is at risk for both disordered eating and a full-blown eating disorder (usually binge eating) simply because she has had to think carefully about food and how to manage it from a very early age. If you are the parent of a diabetic child, doctors have no doubt checked your child's weight on a regular basis and emphasized the importance of dietary restraint and planning to help keep her blood sugar levels within a normal range. You have also probably been told that it is important that your child manage her exercise carefully. The danger inherent in these admonitions is that constant focus on what and how much is eaten increases the risk of developing eating problems. Children with diabetes face the additional challenge of coping with shifting weights caused by the onset of the disease itself and its treatment. Most young people with diabetes lose weight with the onset of the disease, then gain weight when insulin treatment begins. Researchers suspect that this change in weight can trigger disordered eating or an eating disorder.

All of these factors can make food issues stressful for both you and your child. Yet becoming overly concerned about eating habits and exercise can sometimes create a backlash, sending your child into an anxiety or rebellion-induced binge that in some cases will escalate into a full-blown case of binge-eating disorder or bulimia. (For more on diabetes and eating disorders, see chapter 6.)

## The Course of Disordered Eating

Predicting the course of disordered eating is as inexact a science as trying to determine how many people suffer from disordered eating. One study showed that about three-quarters of those who suffer from disordered eating go on to develop a full-blown eating disorder. While this figure may be debatable, what is more certain is that disordered eating creates the significant and real risk of developing a full-blown eating disorder.

**When Should You Take Action against Your Child's Disordered Eating?**
My advice to parents is to take the same approach as medical professionals and strive for early diagnosis and intervention. Both will improve your child's chances of recovery and lessen the possibility that your child will develop a full-blown eating disorder. You should take any complaints related to your child's eating seriously. A good time to intervene is when your child complains about her weight or expresses anxiety about food choices. Other concerns that should be taken seriously are menstrual irregularities, loss of hair, fatigue, weakness, dizziness, dental problems, abdominal pain, and constipation. This is not the time to minimize your child's concerns, but to show that you too are concerned, and want to help.

**How to Take Action against Your Child's Disordered Eating**
You are most likely to succeed at directly helping a child with disordered eating who is high school–aged or younger. If you are concerned that your college-aged child has disordered eating, the most productive route to take is to encourage her to take advantage of professional help either at college or during summers at home. (For more information, see chapter 9, p. 150.)

If your child is high school–aged or younger and insists he can improve his eating on his own, I advise giving him a month to turn things around. If he has not made improvements after a month, or there is any indication that his disordered-eating behaviors are continuing, you should intervene.

Alex, a serious cross-country runner just entering his junior year in high school, made an announcement one Saturday morning that surprised his parents: "From now on, I am going to eat healthier." The next weekend, he made another announcement: "I want to lose a few pounds so I am going to eat fewer calories." The alarm bells went off for Kris and Terry, Alex's parents. After a long discussion about their son, they expressed their concerns to him, saying, "Alex, we can't help but be worried about all these dietary goals of yours. We know that if you're not careful you can hurt your health."

"I know what I'm doing. You don't need to worry," Alex assured his parents.

"Let's see how the next month goes," Terry responded. "We'll need to talk again. Alex, you know we're not going to let you get into trouble with your eating," he added. "We'll do what it takes to keep you healthy."

Kris and Terry were relieved when, by the end of the month, Alex was again joining the family for meals when fish or chicken was served. To be sure he wasn't losing weight, Kris arranged for Alex to have his weight checked at his pediatrician's office. A year later, Alex has taken to expressing himself by dressing like a hippie, but he is healthy and eats balanced meals with his family. He even eats red meat once in a while.

Sometimes families do take action, but they find that they alone cannot do what it takes to get their child's eating back on track. Harriet's parents notice that over the past six months, twelve-year-old Harriet has shown a new interest in reading food labels, focusing in particular on the fat content of the foods she eats. Harriet has always liked dressing up, but her heightened awareness of the foods she eats coincides with an intensified interest in fashion. She begins studying fashion magazines, expressing a fear of dietary fat, and has a myriad of excuses to justify undereating. One morning Harriet declares she can't eat breakfast because she has a stomachache. Her parents, Glen and Vicki, feel frustrated and worried by her behavior, yet tell themselves they have done all they can to protect Harriet (who is anything but fat or even big-boned) from falling prey to food problems. When Harriet was seven her older sister teased her about being chubby. Her parents immediately put a stop to that. More recently, Harriet's friends commented on her weight during a piggyback race at school. Glen and Vicki were so concerned about Harriet's reaction to these comments that they made a point of speaking to the school counselor and protesting against activities that create an atmosphere where weight becomes an issue.

Although Vicki and Glen feel they have done their best to prevent eating problems in their daughter, some of their parenting approaches have in fact inadvertently fueled their daughter's problems. When Vicki tried to be more directive to Harriet about what she needed to eat to stay healthy, Harriet felt forced to eat. Harriet feels that Vicki has always been quite controlling about food, and she remembers not liking her mom's rule that she and her siblings had to wait for specific times to eat meals and snacks. Despite Glen and Vicki's best efforts, Harriet's problems seem to be getting worse, not better. They decide it is time to make an appointment with me.

In our first session, Harriet brings up some of the issues she has with her parents' approaches to food and eating. After some discussion, we all decide that Glen and Vicki's first task will be to try to be less controlling and more supportive.

You may find to your surprise, as did Glen and Vicki, that as you tackle your child's disordered eating, your own behaviors are implicated. (For more on the role of parents in eating problems, see chapter 8.) If this happens to you, remember that what is most important is that you get to the bottom of the problem and begin fixing it. Try to accept criticism of your own behaviors graciously and do what you can to make the changes that will improve your child's chances of recovery.

If your child is struggling with binge-eating behavior, it is best to tread lightly in this area. Because traditional weight loss methods such as strict dieting aggravate binge-eating behaviors, the best approach appears to be not to encourage dieting, and instead try to normalize your child's eating using the methods we outline in Part III.

## In Summary

The important messages of this chapter are that disordered eating can cause as much pain and anguish as a full-blown disorder, and that you as parents must do everything you can to correct a disordered-eating problem before it becomes full blown. Dieting is both the number-one form of disordered eating, and something which, despite its hallowed place in American life, should not be a family pursuit, or a topic of discussion within the family. Dieting should be *especially* forbidden among children, who are still growing and still developing everything from their bones to their brains. The nutritional well-being of your child, in short, should never be sacrificed for the sake of "slimming down," "shedding a few pounds," or "losing that baby fat."

Whether you decide to tackle your child's disordered-eating problem by yourselves or end up seeking professional help, we strongly encourage you to follow the guidelines for normalizing eating with a food plan, outlined in chapters 10 and 11.

# 3

# Prevention: The Power
# of the Preemptive Strike

In some cases, at the earliest signs of an eating disorder, parents can play an important part in ensuring that a child's eating habits and attitudes about food and body size veer back to healthier, rather than increasingly disordered, eating and thinking. In this chapter, we will outline some preventive strategies, which, if employed early enough, may be enough to turn your child's eating problem around.

## Prevention Means Reducing Risk

The most effective preventive measures you can take are to eliminate or reduce the risk factors that your child faces, or help her become immune to those risk factors. Because many factors have converged to set the stage for your child's eating disorder, identifying them all is no easy task. Yes, you may have set an unhealthy example by dieting yourself, or commented on your child's weight, but she may also have started getting her periods early, inherited a genetic predisposition toward depression or perfectionism, or fallen in love with a risky sport such as figure skating or gymnastics. At the same time, she is also surrounded by advertising for junk food and getting the message from her peers and from television, movies, and magazines that in order to be perfect, she must first be thin. With all of this going on, where should your preventive efforts begin?

The answer is "on all of these fronts." In this chapter, we will first discuss ways that you can arm your child emotionally and socially to help protect her from the specific personality traits, stressful life events, physical changes, and peer pressures that can put her at risk for eating problems. Next, we will turn to how you can arm your child with information and critical thinking abilities that will help protect her from the powerful and sometimes destructive cultural messages that saturate our modern-day lives. Finally, we will discuss ways in which you can arm your child with positive attitudes toward food, size, and shape. Taken as a whole, these strategies will form a kind of full-body armor against eating disorders for your child. No doubt some of these defenses will be stronger, and some weaker in your child. But your chances of success are greatest if you at least make an attempt to cover all these fronts.

If you know that your child is genetically susceptible to an eating disorder (either a parent or sibling suffers from an eating disorder, or inherited emotional or personality traits put your child at risk for one), then it is especially important that you practice these preventive measures. (See p. 126 for more information on inheritable risk factors.) By being careful to minimize the number of risk factors your child is exposed to, preventing an eating disorder even in a genetically susceptible child can be within your control.

## Arming Your Child Emotionally and Socially

The emotional and social risks that predispose your child to an eating disorder include depression, low self-esteem, perfectionism, lack of coping skills, and friends, siblings, or parents with eating issues. You can counter these risks by doing the following:

• **Work on building your child's self-esteem.** Low self-esteem is considered the most potent risk factor for disordered eating as well as full-blown eating disorders. For many adolescents, entering junior high heightens concerns about appearance, school performance, and social standing. These worries in turn put the child's self-esteem at risk and increase the risk of developing eating problems. To protect your child's self-esteem, try to foster in her a sense of autonomy, or the feeling that she has control over important aspects of her life. Other factors that researchers believe protect self-esteem include: confidence in some salient ability such as in academics or athletics, or even confidence in social standing or appearance.

You can help by letting your child know that her developing individuality is appreciated and giving her opportunities to succeed within the family, such as weighing in on important decisions that have to be made, or helping with at-home projects. These approaches will help your young adolescent child move confidently and safely into a complex world where peers and societal standards are powerful influences.

• **Seek help for your depressed child.** The depressed child is more vulnerable to disordered eating as well as to eating disorders. Children who are depressed may have a harder time letting an ill-timed comment from a friend about weight pass. Depressed children may turn to binge eating or starvation to distract themselves from their depressed feelings. Many of my patients have told me that binge eating is comforting when they are feeling down in the dumps, even though they know that later they will feel terribly guilty about bingeing.

If you notice your depressed child engaging in some of these negative behaviors, try to first teach her healthier ways of coping (see next guideline). If this does not work I advise seeking professional help, from a counselor or therapist. (For more on professional resources, see chapter 14.) Treating depression can protect your child from other problems as well as eating issues.

• **Teach healthier coping mechanisms.** Since eating disorders are a means of coping, show your child healthier ways to cope with anxiety, fear, anger, disappointment, or depression. Be careful not to encourage your child to use food to calm, soothe, or reward herself. For example, make it a point to give your upset child a hug instead of a cookie. Teach your child to identify her feelings and to understand that feelings, even unpleasant ones, are legitimate. Encouraging her to talk through and deal with problems instead of ignoring her feelings will help her develop strategies other than eating to cope with problems. It is not unusual for parents who have to be away when their children are home to suggest they pass the time by eating snack food. You will do better providing activities to help entertain your children. Not encouraging the pairing of snack food and television watching is another good practice.

The importance of teaching effective coping mechanisms becomes apparent when you understand that upsetting life events have the potential to affect your child's self-confidence and predispose her to eating problems. A move to a new town, changing schools, the death of an important family member, or parental or sibling illness are examples of an upsetting life event. Other stressors include going away to camp, a lack of friendships, siblings with problems, a breakup with a boyfriend or girlfriend, the loss of a friend (because of a fight or a move), death of a pet, and parents who have separated or divorced. Even events that might not seem significant to you, such as difficulty with a particular school subject, or disappointments in sports or other extracurricular activities, can be enough to trigger an eating disorder in a susceptible child. When a child experiences one of these life events and begins to slip into an eating disorder, healthy coping mechanisms and strong family support can be enough to turn the situation around.

• **Watch for early signs of perfectionism, compulsiveness, or obsessiveness.** Children who are perfectionists live by high, self-imposed standards of performance, and often appearance as well. For the perfectionist, each and every task must be executed flawlessly, including the task of meeting cultural or peer expectations of thinness. Perfectionists are especially at risk for eating problems if their ideas of perfect eating, exercise, and appearance are reinforced by the activities or sports they happen to be engaged in, whether wrestling or gymnastics or ballet.

While it may not be possible to change such a core personality trait, you should encourage your perfectionistic child to aim to achieve in more productive arenas than changing her body size, such as sports that are not size- or appearance-focused, academics, art, theater.

Juliet's parents knew that perfectionism ran in their family and saw early signs of this trait in their daughter when she did "extra-credit" work for her kindergarten teacher. From those early years, Juliet's parents instilled in her the message, "Bodies just are. They are not supposed to be changed or evaluated." At the same time, they provided Juliet with plenty of opportunities to challenge herself in other areas.

Obsessiveness is reflected in a preoccupation with orderliness at the expense of flexibility and spontaneity. Obsessive people often live by self-imposed "rules," including rules for eating and exercise. They are likely to pay painstaking attention to details and worry about making mistakes. Obsessiveness is evident, for instance, when a child becomes overly worried about performing his piano piece flawlessly at an upcoming recital. In an eating-disordered person, obsessiveness is often expressed as a constant worry that he has consumed too much fat or too many calories.

Compulsiveness is evident when children are so involved in tasks, for example a school project or even housework, that they do not have time for leisure. They may be involved in sports, which they are likely to take very seriously, but not in less organized play, such as hanging out with friends. In an eating-disordered individual, compulsiveness is often expressed in the form of counting calories and fat grams.

The "obsessive" component of obsessive-compulsive behavior, in other words, refers to a preoccupation with thoughts, while the "compulsive" component refers to a preoccupation with certain behaviors. An obsessive-compulsive child would have an *obsessive* personality and exhibit *compulsive* behavior. Obsessions and compulsions go together like peas in a pod and are often associated with anorexia.

Erica and Timothy's first clue to their daughter Tara's obsessive personality was her propensity to spend hours lining up her dolls in perfect formation and dressing them just so. Knowing that Tara's personality could put her at risk for eating problems, her parents vowed to adopt a relaxed approach toward Tara's eating habits and to model a casual, confident approach toward food issues, while remaining watchful that Tara's compulsiveness did not extend to her behaviors about food. Erica and Timothy were careful not to make any negative comments about food or body size, which could be easily misinterpreted by their observant child.

• **Be watchful if your child enjoys "living on the edge," has problems with impulse control, is moody, often overdoes things, or tends to get over-involved in fun activities.** A child with these characteristics may act without thinking through the consequences of his actions. He is also more apt than the average child to turn to food when he has had a bad day, and more likely to binge and to experiment with purging, especially if his friends are engaged in this behavior.

The child who always seems to be eating, drinking, or chewing gum to satisfy his constant need to have something in his mouth may also be at risk for bulimia or binge eating.

• **Be especially watchful with children who seem sensitive to peer and cultural messages.** (For more information, see chapter 9.)

• **Be watchful around the onset of puberty.** Hormonally induced changes in mood, body size and shape, and especially body fat can trigger eating problems among adolescents. First and foremost, you should make it clear that these changes are normal and expected. Then you should communicate in a respectful, nonintrusive way that you are happy that your child is experiencing this physical rite of passage. In our thinness-obsessed culture, parents need to be ready to counter the negative things adolescents often say about themselves and help them develop pride and joy in their changing bodies.

When Kimmy complained about her growing hips, her mother responded, "It's wonderful to know that your body is developing right on cue."

In some cases, you will find that the negative body talk your child adopts around the onset of puberty is tied to other issues that are causing her anxiety. Remember, at the same time that hormonal surges are causing your child's body to change in disconcerting ways, those hormones are also causing her moods and emotions to become more volatile as well. Raquel, getting ready for bed one night, complained to her mother, "I am so fat and ugly." Rose, Raquel's mother, quickly countered, "Raquel, that's just not true!"

Then she asked, "Why do you feel that way?" Rose learned that while Raquel was worried that her body changes would never stop, she was more upset about how difficult she was finding geometry. Not only was the subject matter difficult for her, Raquel added, "I just don't 'get' my geometry teacher."

Over the years, Raquel's parents had learned that she liked doing her homework on her own and had given up offering to help her. Nevertheless Rose said, "I am pretty good with math. Maybe I can be of help." "I doubt it, Mom," Raquel replied. Rose was not going to let this go. "Well, let's find out what I remember from my geometry days," she countered. "Tomorrow night I'll take a look at what you're studying."

Raquel later told me her mom's help made a big difference, and added proudly, "I am pretty sure I am getting a B-plus this quarter." Rose reported that though Raquel continued to overreact to disappointments, she knew these outbursts could be ascribed to "hormonal overload." By focusing less on these small meltdowns and more on remedying one of the sources of Raquel's anxiety, her lack of confidence in her geometry class, Rose found that Raquel's "bad body talk" stopped.

• **Provide warmth, attention, affection, empathy and acceptance, and strive for a close, communicative parent-child relationship.** All of these positive qualities in a parent-child relationship protect your child from any number of harmful influences and help make your child capable of loving and being loved. They are also particularly crucial in preventing eating disorders. Conversely, a chaotic, stressful home life where parents and/or children are disengaged adds to the risk of developing an eating disorder.

If family interactions in your home are marked by yelling, ridiculing, name-calling, or arguing over small points, try replacing those behaviors with positive communication. Instead of responding to your child's actions and opinions in anger or exasperation, try restating her opinion and making suggestions. Try replacing conflict with compromise.

Children, no matter what your circumstances are as parents, need to be able to count on you to listen to them when they want to talk, to love them and want them, and to provide opportunities for fun, laughter, and entertainment.

Let your child know you care about her, keep abreast of her activities and her current friendships, and strive to keep the lines of communication open. All of these will help your child develop a healthy body image, protect her from eating problems, and help give her the foundation she needs to live a happy, productive life.

• **Strive for positive father-child relationships.** Until recently researchers focused mostly on the role of the mother in the genesis of a child's eating disorder. This focus became so prevalent that experts in the field have been accused of "mother blaming." More recently, the impact of the father's style of parenting on the development of eating disorders has come under scrutiny. In one study, fathers of girls with eating disorders were found to be unavailable, critical, perfectionistic, and angry. Girls with eating disorders are likely to perceive their fathers as unloving, hostile, and aggressive. Researchers also found that girls who feel close to their fathers are less likely to have food and weight problems.

One carefully conducted study showed that the most influential factors in the development of eating problems among children relate to parents, especially supportiveness from fathers, and from peers.

Fathers are sometimes not quite sure how to react to their quickly developing daughters, and sometimes withdraw as a result. If you become more distant with a sexually maturing daughter the danger is that she may internalize this retreat and assume that her changing body is unacceptable. Ideally you as a father will continue a comfortable, appropriate relationship with your teenaged daughter. Both parents should remember that your young teen wants to grow up, but still needs much nurturing.

• **Eat together as a family as much as possible.** Frequent and harmonious family meals are protective because they are the exact opposite of the distant, acrimonious family relations that are often connected to eating-disordered children.

By preparing and enjoying healthy meals together as a family, you are helping to lay down a strong protective defense against eating problems. Try to stay involved with your child's eating choices until she is able to make healthy choices on her own. Young adolescents who eat most meals alone or with friends are more likely to diet, skip meals, and make unhealthy choices such as drinking soft drinks instead of milk or juice.

• **Provide extra support to a fast-maturing child.** Children who mature early, including girls who experience early onset of menstrual periods, seem to be at higher risk for developing an eating disorder. If your child is fast maturing, you should be particularly careful to provide extra support and to spend time with her. Making sure that your child has plenty of clothes she likes can help. Nothing makes a person feel too big the way clothes that are too small do. You should be willing to buy clothes as needed (within the limits of your budget, of course), without complaining, "Those perfectly good pants I bought you last month are barely worn!"

• **Make special efforts to counter the effects of divorce.** Researchers have noticed over the past ten years that in younger children with anorexia there is a relatively high rate of parental separation and divorce prior to the onset of the child's eating problems. If you are experiencing serious marital problems, no matter how worried you are about the effect of your problems on your child, you may find that a family rupture is inevitable.

If you find yourself in this situation and you know that your child may be at risk for developing an eating disorder, you should try to provide as much support as possible. Children often feel betrayed by the possibility of separation or divorce and need reassurance that parents will do what they can to provide the stability they need and crave. Spending time with them helps, and making time to talk with them about the changes divorce or separation will bring is essential. Some children may benefit from counseling, either individually or as a family.

• **Allow your child some privacy.** Striving for a warm, close-knit family environment does not mean that you should smother your child. Your child deserves privacy and the freedom to lead his own life. He should feel confident that you are going to respect closed doors, and are not going to snoop in his room, go through personal belongings, personal mail, e-mails, diaries, even trash, eavesdrop on telephone conversations, or try to keep tabs on his whereabouts every moment of the day.

The temptation to overstep boundaries and become overinvolved can be great if you suspect your child has an eating problem. But remember that in order to help him, you need to first show that you respect your child's privacy as well as his point of view. It helps to keep in mind that eating problems are not a sign of disobedience, but a sign that your child needs help, not more restrictive parenting.

Maintaining the ideal warm and affectionate relationship with your child can also be a challenge as he begins to draw away and strives to create an independent existence. Your goal during these years should be to remain nurturing and supportive while accepting the reality that your child is growing up and needs to create some distance from the family in order to do so.

• **Don't stray from your role as parent.** This means that mothers and fathers should avoid acting jealous of dates or boyfriends. Mothers should be careful not to compete with daughters for attention from their boyfriends. For example, you should not "dress up" for your daughter's date.

Fathers should be careful not to relate to daughters seductively or as a wife-surrogate. For example, you should be careful to give your daughter privacy in the bathroom and in dressing; you should avoid talking to your child about problems with her mother. You should not comment on the attractiveness of other women to your daughter, nor should you tell sexual jokes to your daughter. You should not confide your personal problems to your child, and you should avoid any physical contact that your child feels uncomfortable with. You should also not flirt with your daughter. Because children are easily confused by "flirting"-type interactions, parents should be careful not to stray into this territory.

• **Be careful not to foster a climate of shame.** Researchers have found that shame—a feeling of worthlessness and rejection—plays a central role in bulimia. Usually, this feeling is the result of children being told or made to feel that they are defective in some way. Within families, shame is internalized when children feel that their parents believe they need to be strictly controlled, or they are simply not worth their parents' attention.

You can counter or prevent such feelings by making sure that you do not indicate in your dealings with your child that she is in any way defective, not good enough, or inherently bad. While you must guide, correct, and at times even punish your child, you should make every effort not to embarrass or humiliate her. You should also be careful not to indicate that you are embarrassed by your child, and you should let your child know by word and deed that she is good enough just as she is. This is not to say that you should shield your child from making mistakes. She needs to learn to recognize her limitations, and to learn from her own mistakes. She also needs to learn to forgive herself, to "get over it," and to move on.

• **Strive to remain hopeful, with an optimistic vision for the future.** If you believe that your child's future is full of opportunities and you expect the best possible outcome for her you are likely to raise a child who is freer of food problems than the parent who is less hopeful and optimistic. This does not mean that you should turn into a Pollyanna, or that you should relentlessly push your child to excel in areas she is not interested in, or compare her unfavorably with peers in order to motivate her to do better. Strive for an optimism that is uncritical and meant to inspire a sunny feeling of hope, not the deadening pressure of too-high expectations.

• **Provide extra care to your child or children when you are bringing a new baby or an adopted child into the family.** As we have noted, any major stress creates risk in susceptible children, in part because parents may become less attentive to them. Certainly the arrival of a new child can create risk, particularly if you are not careful to provide enough attention to your older child or children.

Among families in my practice, I have noticed a significant number have recently adopted another child. This may be coincidental, and I am not suggesting that families who want to offer a home to an orphaned child should not do so. I do suggest, however, that when you are welcoming a new child into the family, that you try to provide extra support during this transition period to your other child or children, especially those who may be at risk for eating problems.

I also believe that it can be harder when parents adopt an older child rather than an infant. Older adopted children have more of an impact on other children because they are more interactive and often have more complex problems. In such situations you should be careful that your other child or children do not feel left out or deprived.

One of my patients, a twelve-year-old girl with an older biological brother, made it clear to her parents she did not want her parents to adopt a toddler from overseas. First my patient lost her role as the youngest in the family. Second, she was no longer the only girl. Third, her mother was now distracted trying to help her adopted sister (who also had emotional problems) fit into a new family, new schools, and a new culture.

## Arming Your Child with Knowledge and Information

In some cases, the risks that can predispose your child to eating problems or an eating disorder stem from the prevailing attitudes and beliefs that he or she encounters at school, among friends, or from society at large. Most experts believe that because these cultural messages are so pervasive and overwhelming, it would take wholesale changes at the national level to truly prevent eating disorders, a change in the cultural beauty ideal of extreme thinness, and the creation of a tolerance of diversity in body size and shape including large sizes.

Since this is not likely to happen any time soon, your best strategy is to arm your child with knowledge, information, and the ability to think critically about mass culture-promoted values. Following are steps you can take.

**Promote Media Literacy**
Like all of us, children today are bombarded with a ceaseless barrage of images and messages from our popular culture. Magazines targeted at young teens are increasingly read by even younger girls. Although these magazines do not usually push dieting these days, they do feature models and actresses who are extremely thin or super-fit-looking boys and men. To be attractive, we surmise, girls and women must be pencil-thin, and boys must be muscular yet devoid of even an ounce of fat. Young girls and, increasingly, boys, too, naturally want to emulate the culturally ordained ideal. On television and in the movies, fat jokes abound, and fat people are portrayed as unhealthy, unattractive, and incompetent.

So powerful is the effect of the media on our beliefs and values, in fact, that researchers have shown that when Hollywood and the fashion industry make it clear that "thin is in" there is an increase in disordered eating. This happened in the 1920s and again in recent years. Even new immigrants from countries in which eating disorders are virtually nonexistent, such as Vietnam and the former Soviet Union, become vulnerable to eating disorders once they are exposed to the social messages embedded in the prevailing culture. Researchers Mervat Nasser and Melanie Katzman call this the "Western toxin" effect, often spread through exposure to television and the Western emphasis on appearance and physical beauty. In one dramatic example of the Western toxin effect, a Harvard researcher reported a five-fold increase in eating disorders among teenage girls in Fiji just three years after television was widely introduced to the Pacific island nation in 1995. Favorite television programs on the island included *Melrose Place* and *ER.* Researcher Anne Becker told the Associated Press, "They're trying to emulate a lifestyle: Western-style clothes, haircuts and slim bodies," adding, "adolescents are particularly vulnerable." (For more on eating disorders in different cultures, see p. 80.)

It is our job as parents to teach our children to think critically about the influence of the media, to understand the power of magazines, movies, popular music, and television to influence the way we think and behave. To inoculate children from the potent negative power of these messages, it helps to show them these images are not meant to be prescriptions for body size but are simply designed to sell consumers certain products. Talking about these issues helps establish an important foundation for later lessons in critical thinking.

Although some schools work to sensitize students to how the media shapes our ideas about appearance and body size, these programs are usually aimed at teenagers. For the young child, hearing these messages at home will probably be the first time she is exposed to such ideas. Media literacy crusader Jean Kilbourne, author of *Can't Buy My Love: How Advertising Changes the Way We Think and Feel,* says, "Parents should start teaching children media literacy before kindergarten. Watch TV with your children and make comments during the programs and commercials. 'Why do you think the women in this program are so thin?' Brief, age-appropriate comments and questions are best."

Kilbourne notes that advertisers, by casting extremely thin young women and teenagers in a highly glamorous light, are contributing to the body hatred that many girls feel. To show your child how advertisers create and manipulate consumer demand, try asking your child, "Why is this product desirable to you?" "Is it the product itself, or the image of glamour associated with it?" "Is the glamorous image of the super-thin woman realistic?" "Is it healthy?" "How does the ad make you feel about your own body?" "What does it do to your self-esteem?"

By talking with our children about these subjects, we are teaching them to become more conscious of insidious advertising messages that contribute to poor body image and unfounded food fears. One of Kilbourne's ideas that we think has merit, and could also be fun for families, is her suggestion that parents make a point of exposing children to images from the past (take a field trip to a museum or rent some old films) and talking about how concepts of beauty change over time.

In addition to these suggested topics of discussion, you might discuss with your child:

- The inherent bias of "weightism," which glorifies thinness and insensitively denigrates the vast majority of people in our society who do not conform to that ideal.
- The limited picture of our world that she sees when she flips through a popular magazine. Is the diversity of size and shape that your child sees in her everyday life represented here?
- Whether or not he is as capable of being as happy, popular, or fulfilled as we are led to believe the waifish models and sculpted he-men in those magazines are. Children need to learn that thinness does not guarantee that one will be happy, successful, rich, smart, kind, or nice.

**Demonstrate That You Are Indifferent to the Cultural Ideal of Thinness**
It can be highly empowering to your child for you, through your words and actions, to demonstrate that you care little for the incessant messages our culture bombards us with promoting the thinness ideal.

When Lindsay comes home from school one day to tell her mother the latest locker room topic (how thin the actresses on the TV show *Friends* have become) she knows what her mother is going to say. Jo, Lindsay's mother, has told her repeatedly that being too thin can be unhealthy and that teenagers are supposed to be growing and slowly gaining weight, while adults' weight should be stable. Just as Lindsay predicted, Jo responds, "It's really too bad those accomplished women feel they need to lose weight. I really hope they don't damage their health or trigger an eating disorder."

Chloë is another example of the fortunate child whose family is careful to make their home environment a sanctuary from the destructive body-image messages of the outside world. Chloë, a naturally chubby child, is certain that her parents like how she looks just the way she is. They frequently compliment her on her appearance or her clothes, and turn a blind eye to the magazine and TV advertisements that push dieting and weight loss. This attitude helps Chloë negotiate the potentially difficult junior high social scene, where thinness is the epitome of physical attractiveness.

### Choose Your Child's Doctor with Care

Try to choose a primary care provider or pediatrician who appreciates children of all sizes and is informed about eating disorders. A good pediatrician can discuss with your child the natural changes that occur during puberty, and relieve some of the stress and anxiety that accompany these changes. A pediatrician who is knowledgeable about eating disorders will also be attuned to any early signs that your child may be exhibiting and can help you steer her back on track.

### Put Issues of Body Size, Shape, and Food in a Political Context

If you subscribe to a feminist interpretation of cultural issues you can help your child develop a broader understanding of weight, shape, size, and food issues by placing them in a political context. It can be helpful to explain to your child that according to the feminist perspective, a girl's developing body is a political issue. When girls are overly concerned with their appearance and are not accepting of the natural development of their bodies, they are unwittingly supporting deep-seated and long-standing inequities that have developed over the centuries, in part to keep women in the role of second-class citizen.

## Arming Your Child with Positive Attitudes toward Food, Size, and Shape

Instilling in your child from an early age healthy attitudes toward food, size, and shape can go a long way in preventing a future eating disorder. (For more detail on this topic, see chapter 8.) The following are suggestions on how to do that:

- Give your child the freedom to choose foods, while gently encouraging her to eat well.
- Provide regular meals and snacks.
- Encourage, but do not pressure, your picky eater, slow eater, or inhibited eater to eat a wide variety of foods.
- Model body self-acceptance by keeping disparaging remarks about your own body or plans to diet to yourself.
- Model healthy approaches to eating and exercise.
- Be watchful for age-inappropriate food and exercise behaviors.

For example, be watchful if your nine-year-old boy makes food choices based on calories and fat grams. Similarly, if your twelve-year-old girl worries when she does not get exercise every day, you should be on the lookout for concurrent signs of disordered eating. (Such a worry might be more appropriate for an adult tethered to a sedentary job.)

• **Explain at an early age that different kids have different body types; focus on body function over body shape and size.** Instead of criticism about her body shape or size, your child needs to hear that you care that her body is healthy and functional. Comments such as, "Isn't it great that your field hockey skills are improving?" communicate your interest in fostering skill development rather than a thinner, or differently shaped, body. The message you should strive to convey to your child through your words and actions is that you accept and love her "as is."

• **Limit the number of magazines you buy or subscribe to that glorify thinness.** If you enjoy these magazines, you might want to think twice about leaving many such magazines in easy view of your children. If these magazines are in your home, make a point of looking at them with your daughters and sons and discussing what you are seeing. Are the models shown too thin? Can they imagine those fashions looking good on a healthy-sized person? If not, what styles would be more flattering to a normal-weight person? Or, if you happen to be watching a television or movie starring an unhealthily thin favorite actress or singer, be sure to provide your child with commentary to that effect.

• **Ban all teasing about weight.** It is important not to tease, even in good humor, about your child's weight, body, or the changes that come with puberty. While it is sadly ironic that prior to puberty, girls are more likely to have bodies that match the cultural ideal for women, girls are more likely to see the sad part, but not the ironic part, of this truth.

Children need to learn from their parents that it is rude, wrong, harmful, and against the rules to make comments about other people's body size or to discriminate against them.

• **Avoid overly purist attitudes toward food.** When advising families about what they can do to protect their children from eating disorders, I tell them to limit food to normal serving sizes, but not to forbid consumption of junk and fast foods.

Forbidding or overly restricting your child's consumption of desserts, fast foods, and junk food will make these foods more attractive than they would be if she is allowed regular access to them as part of a healthy well-balanced diet.

• **Establish a family approach to eating that has no place for fear of fat, or counting calories or fat grams.**

• **Be wary of restricting your child's eating or access to food.** You should be very cautious if you feel you need to restrict your child's eating or access to food. You may have legitimate worries about your child developing eating problems or weight problems. Or, upon examination of your own motivations, you may find that your concerns stem from your own attitudes about weight gain and healthy eating. Because you yourself have trouble controlling your eating, you *assume,* perhaps incorrectly, that your child will have the same problem. Researchers have found that parents who worry about their own weight are more likely to worry about their child's weight and eating habits, to restrict their eating, and ultimately cause them to eat more of the foods that are restricted.

Although your worries may seem like rational concerns for your child's health, we remind you of two facts:

**Fact One:** Research has shown that the more overcontrolling parents are the less likely their child is to learn to regulate their own food intake. It seems that if parents control their child's food intake, the child does not develop the skills needed to do it for herself. This in turn can lead to overeating or the inability to make good food choices when the child has the chance to make her own decisions about food. This does not mean that eating should be a free-for-all. You should structure eating so your child eats meals and snacks at regular times and has a reasonable array of foods to choose from. (For more information, see chapter 10.)

**Fact Two:** Researchers Leann Birch and Jennifer Fisher have shown that the transfer of weight and food concerns and dieting behavior from parent to child can occur very early, as early as during the preschool period. By restricting your child's access to food the way you restrict your own, you are increasing the likelihood that you are transferring these concerns to your child. Even when your child is very young, within the boundaries of balanced food offerings, strive for an open, carefree attitude toward food and eating, instead of limiting and policing.

• **Avoid using food as a reward or punishment.** If you reward eating meals with dessert, reward behavior with food, or withhold food as a punishment, your child may become unable to view food and eating as pleasurable pursuits that help her grow. Instead, food will become a way to leverage power and to express emotions such as approval, disapproval, love, or anger.

By telling your child that in order to receive a reward such as dessert, or permission to watch television, she "has to" eat certain foods, she will learn to dislike those foods. She will learn to prefer foods used as rewards ("Clean up your room and you can have some cookies") or foods that are only allowed if paired with interactions with a friendly adult (going out for ice cream with a favorite aunt).

• **Avoid the "clean-plate" rule.** Another common strategy of parents, the clean-plate rule, telling a child she needs to clean her plate in order to get dessert, can also backfire. This practice teaches children to ignore bodily sensations signaling fullness and instead rely on eating what is available. Studies have shown that children whose parents exerted the most control over what, when, and how much they could eat showed the weakest ability to control their own food intake.

• **Don't label foods as "good" or "bad."** If you know a little bit about nutrition and are concerned that you raise a healthy, well-nourished child, you probably try to push fruits and vegetables and limit access to sugary foods. In fact, you are better off not labeling foods "good" or "bad."

Researchers have shown that well-educated parents tend to classify foods as either good or bad and restrict their children's access to "bad" foods and encourage consumption of "good" foods. Parents believe that restricting access to food will decrease the child's preference for that particular food. In fact, not only does restricting foods not result in a decreased desire for those foods on the part of the child, she will eat these foods when they become available even when she is not hungry.

## In Summary

Upon reading this chapter, you may be struck by how many of the prevention tips that we offer fall under the general heading of "Being a Good Parent." Foster good self-esteem, strive for positive parent-child relations, don't smother, provide regular meals and snacks, avoid being too strict with food—all of these hints might be found in any general book on parenting. Indeed, reading this chapter might make you feel that if your child has an eating disorder then you must have been a bad parent.

The point we make repeatedly in this book is that because a whole range of risk factors must be in alignment before your child develops an eating disorder, no one parenting lapse, or even several, is going to create an eating disorder. Our message instead is that shining up your parenting skills so that they are in peak form gives you maximum insurance against those risk factors over which you have no control: genetics, for instance, or to a lesser degree your child's peer group, her sports team, or the culture into which she was born.

Finally, we should note that all of the advice in this chapter is aimed at preventing eating problems, not at helping a child with a serious problem recover. While it is all good advice, if you are helping your underweight child gain weight or trying to protect a bulimic or binge-eating child from bingeing, you should turn to Part III of this book, the "Healthy Eating Guide," especially chapters 10 and 11.

# 4

# The Family on the Front Lines

While no two eating disorders are the same, and each disorder has a complicated history of genetic and environmental causes, there is no doubt that the family's role in recovery is crucial. Ideally, the family of the eating-disordered child will take action early on, swiftly, assertively, and effectively, without having to resort to expensive and stressful outpatient or inpatient treatment. In this chapter, we will outline the latest thinking in the area of the family's role in both the development of eating disorders and their treatment.

This chapter will also help you understand what you as parents can do to take charge of the situation, as well as give you the support you need in the often difficult battles of control that mark the early phases of recovery from an eating disorder.

Although you may find that you want and need an experienced professional or even a team of professionals to help you achieve some of the goals we will talk about here, the information that follows will help you understand your role as parents better, and how you can play a pivotal part in turning around your child's eating disorder.

## The Changing Role of Family in Eating Disorders

The role assigned to the family, both in precipitating an eating disorder and as a critical component of recovery, has changed as eating disorders themselves have become better understood. Early on, parents, especially the mother, were often blamed for causing anorexia, and experts advised a "parentectomy," or removal of the parents from the situation, in order for the child to recover.

This is a view that some professionals still hold. It was while Marlene, her husband, and three children were living in France that her daughter Annette, twelve, became anorexic. Annette's weight plummeted and she became so fearful of eating that she could not even brush her teeth for fear of swallowing toothpaste. Doctors told Marlene and her husband, Steve, that unless Annette was hospitalized and began tube feeding immediately, she would not live. "The French think that anorexia is the parents' fault," recalls Marlene, "so they allowed the bare minimum of visiting. We were allowed only half an hour a week. It was awful." Very soon after this the family realized they wanted to return to America to continue Annette's care in a setting where they could be more involved in her recovery. A year after her return to the United States, Annette, with the help of her family and a team of outpatient professionals that I was part of, had gained enough weight to try out for the lacrosse and hockey teams at her new school.

Perhaps earlier than in other countries, eating disorders treatment in America and Britain had by the 1980s begun to espouse family therapy as a way of treating adolescent eating disorders. Family therapy was founded on the belief that there are classic characteristics that the families of anorexics have in common: enmeshment, overprotectiveness, rigidity, and difficulty resolving conflict. Treatment consisted of figuring out how to change the patterns of interaction within the family thought to have caused the eating disorder.

Today some therapists still treat eating disorders by focusing primarily on resolving family dysfunction, with little direct therapeutic attention paid to the eating disorder itself. At the same time, however, an increasing number of experts are asserting that families are not to blame for the eating disorders of their children. Treatment approaches instead focus on the important role that families can play in the recovery of their child from an eating disorder. The best way to treat children with eating disorders, these researchers now believe, is to reinstill the confidence in their authority that many parents lose during their child's downward spiral into an eating disorder. Thus empowered, parents can once again take charge and help turn around the disorder, something that the child has secretly been all along hoping they will do. When this approach is adopted, traditional family therapy, focusing on improving family function, can be very helpful for the family as a whole once an eating disorder is resolved.

The younger the eating-disordered child is (clinical cases of eating disorders have been reported in children as young as seven), the more critical the role of family in helping turn the disorder around. Research, in fact, has shown that early direct involvement of the family promotes more consistent weight gain among anorexics.

## How Families Can Help

The approach that I use in my practice treating childhood eating disorders is to have parents highly involved in treatment, along with the pediatrician and psychologist who work closely with me. I consider hospitalization a last resort, when all else has failed.

What I most often see is parents who want to help but have no idea how to do so, and children who want to give up their eating disorder but are equally mystified as to how to go about it. I warn parents that while they must be prepared for recovery to take months of hard work, success is likely if they take the following suggestions and guidelines to heart.

### Stop Blaming, Move beyond Anger
Despite the trend among therapists to blame parents less for their children's eating disorders, in most families where a child is suffering from an eating disorder, parents *do* blame themselves for the problem. They worry that they have been too strict or not strict enough, too critical or too lax, too inattentive or too smothering.

Our advice is that rather than focusing on what you as parents have done wrong—an unproductive pursuit that ignores the complex tangle of genetic and environmental factors behind most eating disorders—let's talk about what you can do right. What can you do to help your child recover, or protect your child from engaging in an eating disorder at all? If you focus on blaming yourselves or each other for things you have done in the past, you will have neither the spirit nor the energy to make positive changes in the present.

Your focus as parents should not be, "What did we do to cause the eating disorder?" but instead, "What are the factors that are perpetuating it, and how can we change or eliminate them?"

It is important to remember that your child has not chosen to have an eating disorder, even though they may have set the stage for it by dieting. Remembering this will help you focus less on blaming yourself or the child for bringing on a seemingly frivolous disease (eating disorders are far from that) and help you focus your energy on quickly attacking and turning around the disorder.

You also need to move beyond the anger and exasperation that accompany blame. There is evidence that families in which parents make critical comments to their child during recovery have a reduced chance that recovery will occur. Supportive, noncritical parenting is a key factor in turning around an eating disorder.

### Establish a United Front

As parents you will be more effective at helping your child overcome an eating disorder if you have worked through conflict, poor communication, and any inconsistencies between yourselves. If you are divorced, separated, or struggling in your marriage, this may be difficult. Sometimes the best strategy in such situations is to put your own problems on hold and focus on your child's eating disorder first. As your child's disorder begins to improve, you can begin to address your own marital problems. This is not impossible; I have seen parents who have worked well together dealing with an eating-disordered child, despite their own marital problems.

As you work out a plan for solving the eating disorder, you may have to inform relatives or close friends so that they do not undo your hard work with a thoughtless comment or action.

### Don't Forget to Take Care of Yourselves

If you are depressed, exhausted, or feel guilty, you may not be the best parent to help your child recover. I know parents who have developed an effective "tag-team" approach in such situations. After a month of being on the front lines feeding her anorexic daughter, Jeri was feeling completely worn out and demoralized, as well as guilty that her daughter Kia was not making more progress. Jeri and her husband, James, decided that James would take over supervising Kia's eating, at least at dinnertime. Kia told me that though she loved her mom and felt she really understood her food issues, her dad's matter-of-fact approach was refreshing. "Dad doesn't take it personally like Mom does when I struggle," Kia told me.

Jeri, who was truly exhausted, benefited from seeing a counselor herself, who helped her sort out her feelings and develop a more productive outlook.

### Establish a Collaborative, Not Conflictive Relationship with Your Child

Once you have achieved a more positive frame of mind, you can turn to figuring out how you can collaborate with your child to devise an effective recovery plan. Parents can usually be most helpful at mealtimes at home. Is your child eating? Missing meals? Purging after them? (See chapter 11 for methods of monitoring these issues in a productive way.)

I have found that when I ask an eating-disordered child what her parents can do to help out, she often has definite ideas. She may suggest that they keep certain foods in or out of the house, fix her plate at dinner, ask if she is hungry when she reaches for thirds, or limit the amount of television she can watch if lack of exercise is a problem. What always surprises me is that even very independent children, when asked in a nonconfrontational way how parents can be helpful, can come up with practical and innovative methods.

I find that some children or adolescents initially insist they can solve their problems with little parental involvement. Although parents may be skeptical, I encourage them to give their child a chance to do this. Be ready, however, to step in if your child is not successful without saying, "I told you so."

**Collaborate, Don't Collude: You As Parents Are Ultimately in Charge**
While we have emphasized the collaborative nature of the ideal recovery, this is different from colluding with your child to keep the disorder going. It is important that you as parents are in charge of eating and food issues in the home. If you have not been before, you need to be in charge now. You should still take into account your child's likes, dislikes, even fears, but make it clear that you are ultimately in control of buying and preparing food.

The story of one of my patients, Marcy, illustrates what can happen when parents let a child's eating disorder dictate food choices. Marcy's eating disorder is one of the most medically serious types: anorexia complicated by bingeing and purging. Her agreement with her parents was that she would eat only food that she purchased with her father. At first she chose only healthy foods. As her eating disorder progressed, however, Marcy began buying more and more bread to binge on, and gallons of ice cream. Meanwhile, her purging increased, leaving her malnourished, worn out, and guilt-ridden by the endless cycle of bingeing and purging.

Her father had by then become so intimidated by the eating disorder, and so afraid his daughter wouldn't eat enough if he tried to restrict her purchases, that he looked the other way week after week. Marcy refused to let any other family member touch or eat the food she bought. Before she began working with me, Marcy's family had let her disorder get so out of hand that they had rented a separate apartment for Marcy and her father. The family's hope was that, isolated from the rest of the family, Marcy and her father could focus on her eating problems and bring them under control. Instead, the apartment became a storehouse for binge foods and a virtually private setting in which Marcy could binge, purge, and overexercise.

I advised Marcy's family to give up the apartment and get her room ready at home. Her parents began to insist that she eat with the family, allowing her some choice in what she ate as long as she had a balanced meal. An eating disorder as serious as Marcy's can take years to overcome, but she is slowly making progress with substantial professional help.

One caveat about establishing control: When it is necessary for you as parents to get involved in and even control your child's food intake, it is important that you take care that the controlling does not extend to other area's of your child's life, such as friends, clothes, and after-school activities. By interfering in those areas, you leave your child no room for self-expression or independence. Any credibility that you had in the area of food monitoring will be shattered as your child grows resentful and more rebellious at what she perceives as a gross breach of reasonable boundaries. She may, in fact, even turn with a vengeance to her disorder in part because she knows this is one way to really "get" to you, her parents.

Remember, the reason you have taken over food decisions is that the eating disorder has temporarily rendered your child incompetent in this aspect of her life, not in every aspect.

### Expect Rebellion

Having given you advice on one way to avoid eliciting a rebellious reaction from your child, I must now tell you that some amount of rebellion is almost inevitable. As you work on these concrete goals and actions, all designed to bring about a speedy recovery, it is important to remember that you are dealing with a child or an adolescent, which means that rebellion and testing limits is normal. Most children express their natural rebellion toward parents because we are handy. Although it is hard, I constantly remind parents that they need to remember this, and separate their child's natural rebelliousness from the eating-disordered behaviors that they are trying to eradicate. You should be quite surprised if your child does not rebel and resist your attempts to turn the eating disorder around.

When your child resists help, she is not deliberately being difficult, it is her fears that are causing her to act this way. The eating disorder has served as a coping mechanism, and you are threatening to take it away, a frightening prospect.

I try to help parents reframe their understanding of their child's resistance to change and rebelliousness, to see that it originates from their child's fears. Most parents find it easier to feel empathy for a child who is fearful than for a child who is rebellious. Addressing the fear rather than the rebellion can positively change the dynamic between you and your child, making you more clearly an ally of your child's rather than an enemy.

If you have agreed on a specific plan of action and your child strays from it, it is wrong to conclude that the child is disobedient. It means that the eating disorder is very strong. It may mean that the food or exercise plan you have agreed on is beyond what your child is capable of at this point. (See chapters 10, 11, and 12 for more on these plans.) If a second attempt at a renegotiated plan fails, you may want to reassess the situation and add professional help.

## Be Flexible

When parents take on the role of monitoring a child's eating, it is important to try to be flexible in your thinking about what "healthy food" is. I find that most people are far too rigid in what they find acceptable and what they find unacceptable. (See chapter 8 for more on how parents can improve their family's approach to food.)

It is especially important to be flexible in the area of fears that your child may have about specific nutrients and foods. The most common example is fear of high-fat or high-calorie foods. Here it is important not to be too rigid, but realize that your goal at first is to get your child to eat, not to quibble about the quality of the foods she eats. I often see parents who squander valuable negotiating capital by insisting, for instance, that their underweight child drink whole milk instead of skim milk. The frequent consequence is that the child refuses to drink any milk at all, thereby missing out on the calcium, protein, and other vitamins and minerals found in any kind of milk. Or the child will drink the whole milk, but feel misunderstood and bullied into doing something she doesn't want to do. A similar dilemma occurs when a child chooses diet sodas over regular sodas. Since skim milk and diet sodas are widely consumed by people without eating disorders, it usually is not productive to ban these products from a child's diet unless she grossly overconsumes these foods and is not making progress in her recovery.

My patient Cecilia is one example of an anorexic whose gross overconsumption of a diet product makes her an exception to the rule of flexibility. Cecilia was compulsively drinking six liters of Diet Coke per day and refusing to eat when her parents first called me. Her doctor was concerned about the stress that such an overconsumption of cold liquid placed on her already weakened body and worried that it would reduce her low body temperature to even more dangerous levels. Cecilia didn't feel hungry with so much fluid running through her body, which made changing her eating habits all the more difficult.

My advice to parents, in other words, is to let your child have as much control as possible within the framework of regular and healthy eating that you are trying to establish. Another example of this flexibility is not to insist that your child eat steak, but to insist that he have some protein for dinner. What kind will it be? The family is eating steak, but there is cheese and cottage cheese in the refrigerator, and tuna can easily be provided. It is important that you don't do too much catering, but that you provide food that meets your child's needs, and which he feels able to eat.

While some flexibility in thinking is necessary, you can also ask more of your child as his recovery progresses. At the beginning it is more important that he eats enough rather than what or where he eats. While your child may begin his recovery refusing any higher-fat foods, your eventual goal should be to help him achieve a confident, no-fuss approach to eating that includes a variety of foods, from high fat to low fat.

Progress in other areas, such as the settings in which your child is able to eat, should be similarly gradual. My patient Josie began to win her battle against anorexia by eating the meals her mother had prepared for her in the TV room. At the beginning of recovery, it is not uncommon for anorexic patients to feel hesitant to eat in front of others. Remembering the principle that early on eating enough was the goal, Josie's parents allowed her to eat where she chose. As she gained weight and felt better, they gently insisted that she eat one meal a day with the family, which she did. Over the course of a month, she went from eating no meals with her family to eating all of her meals with them once again.

### Fight the Disorder, Not Your Child

If you find that it is difficult to be firm, remind yourself that you are fighting the eating disorder, not your child. One technique, which may sound strange but is particularly helpful, is to think of the eating disorder as an outside force trying to lead the child astray, for example an evil twin.

Jane, one of my patients, named her eating disorder "Ed." At first, I didn't get the connection. "Why Ed?" I asked her. Jane replied, "Duh! Eating disorder—E, D." She felt she could hear Ed whispering things in her ear that made her afraid to eat certain foods and even to binge. A good portion of Jane's sessions were devoted to developing retorts she could use to put Ed in his place.

The goal for children who take to personifying their eating disorder is to first understand what thoughts and behaviors originate from the evil twin. Next they learn to counter these directives with healthier alternatives. Gillian's "evil twin" would tell her that she should never eat cheese because it was high in fat and would make her fat. She learned to respond, "But I know cheese is also high in protein and calcium." She knew she really had the upper hand when she could add, "And I know that some fat is good for me." The final step is for the child to evict the evil companion from their consciousness entirely.

It is also helpful to remember that as your child makes progress, control and management of eating should gradually be returned to her; this period of seemingly harsh prohibitions will end as the disorder resolves.

### Strive to Offer Compassion, Consistency, and Security

Research has shown that children who have formed secure attachments to their parents tend to show fewer weight concerns and a lower risk for eating disorders. In addition, children in families where parents behave consistently and are responsive to the child's needs have a lower risk of developing an eating disorder.

While it is of course not possible for you to undo early parenting, you can use these findings as a guide for dealing with problems you may be having now. Responsive parenting means responding constructively and compassionately to the distress signals emanating from your eating-disordered child, not waving them off as idle complaints, or ignoring them and hoping that they will go away. Ideally your children will come to view you as a safe haven or a secure base for helping them work through their problems.

Responsive parenting can also help in another important area: your child's self-esteem. While New Age concerns about self-esteem and "liking oneself" seem overworked and trite, it is something that is often overlooked when a child has an eating disorder. You can help by making it clear that you love your child and value her regardless of her achievements or performance. Parents cannot express their love and support too much. Don't be put off by your child's natural tendency to brush off your overtures; it is important that you express those emotions regardless of whether or not your child returns the affection.

As much as the eating disorder will seem to dominate your family life and your child's life, it is important to keep your eyes on the bigger picture. Try to remember what your child was like before the eating disorder. What did you enjoy talking about? What was your child interested in? Making an effort to engage your child around some of his interests and giving positive feedback for efforts in other areas can help him feel that you really care about him as a person, and counter the common feeling that he has been reduced to little more than his eating disorder. Acknowledge how hard your child is working at the challenge of overcoming his disorder, even though things may be at a very difficult stage at the moment.

## Andrea's Story

When Andrea's daughter Emma was twelve, she went away to summer camp a normal, healthy child. When she came home two weeks later, she had stopped eating. Where before she had relished eating pancakes with butter and syrup, now she panicked at the sight of butter and ate only a gradually diminishing list of "safe" foods. At camp, her family later discovered, several of Emma's friends had made a list of the characteristics of each girl in their group. Under Emma's name they wrote "Fatso."

At 107 pounds, Emma was hardly fat, but that did not matter; she became convinced that she was. On a subsequent family vacation Emma refused to eat at restaurants and exercised compulsively at every stop on the trip. Although Emma's weight was still normal, Andrea says, "the warning bells went off."

By the holidays, Emma's weight had dropped to 90 pounds and she was miserable. By the time they saw Emma's pediatrician in January, her weight had plummeted another 10 pounds.

"My husband and son and I were scared she was going to die," Andrea recalls. Meanwhile, Emma's behavior was nearly intolerable, making it hard for her family to respond sympathetically. "When someone is screaming at you and swearing at you because she's hungry and tired and malnourished," says Andrea, "it's really hard to take a step back and see the situation for what it is. Every time we had a meal, we were assaulted."

When the disorder was at its worst, in February, Andrea went through Emma's room after their cleaning lady complained that it was infested with ants. "I found all her lunches," recalls Andrea. "It was clear she wanted us to find them, they were all over the place."

The discovery of the lunches was the turning point in Emma's eating disorder. It was at this point that Andrea brought Emma to see me. I let Emma know that this incident was helpful to me in understanding the depths of her struggle. Then we went about the business of planning a simple lunch that she felt she would be able to manage.

This phase of recovery is never easy. The child feels she is giving up control by eating at all, while the parents feel that the child is being overly difficult by insisting on eating only certain foods.

On one family trip, Andrea called me from the airport to tell me that Emma was refusing to eat. Instead of arguing with Emma about the necessity of eating a healthy diet, I asked her what she thought she could eat. We decided that she could make a meal out of two protein bars and a glass of juice. The reasoning here was that it was better to eat two foods with lots of nutrients and a fair amount of calories, and which Emma was comfortable with, than nothing at all. Sometimes the help I or a parent offers simply has to be that pragmatic. Andrea ended up having a box of the bars sent overnight to her from home because they were not available locally.

As her mother, Andrea's job was to keep Emma's recovery on track. When Emma tried to fast after going out with a friend and eating what she considered too much, Andrea was the one who had to tell her she couldn't see her friend the next time unless she made better choices and decisions about food.

Sometimes Andrea's job as a parent was simply to leave the scene when the same old issues came up. "Whenever I tried to step in," Andrea says, "it backfired." Once when Emma was rebelling against eating, Andrea took her son out in her car, leaving Emma with her husband, Bill, who was less threatening to Emma. She and Bill found this type of tag-team approach effective because Bill had a more matter-of-fact and less emotional response to Emma. He was less likely to push her buttons and make her want to rebel by not eating.

Andrea also had to struggle with her own guilt over what had happened to her daughter. Two things helped Andrea get over these feelings. One was seeing her own therapist, who helped her stop being so hard on herself. The second was talking to her much younger sister, who confessed that she had overcome an eating disorder as an adolescent when Andrea was away at college. This helped Andrea see that, as research has shown, there is a strong hereditary component to anorexia. "My sister, who is a pediatrician, has been very helpful in saying, 'It's not your fault, and it wasn't Mama's fault,'" says Andrea.

Emma's anorexia was also extremely hard on her brother, Luke. Bill and Andrea bought Luke a mountain bike, so that when things got intolerable at home, he could simply get on his bike and ride away. They made it a point to have special nights out with Luke.

Just as Bill and Andrea had to work hard to make sure that Luke came through their family crisis intact, they also had to take special care that their marriage survived. Andrea and Bill tried to take an hour-and-a-half walk together every week. "Inevitably, we talked for an hour about Emma, but the last half hour, we would talk about us, and how it was affecting us. The couple also tried to make at least one date a month when they could go out to dinner. Once they told Emma and Luke they were going to dinner and to a movie and instead rented a hotel room for the evening. "It really bonded us," says Andrea. "It was like being a teenager and sneaking away from your parents; it got us through the next week, which was a really tough week."

Today a year after the summer camp experience that set Emma on the road to anorexia, her weight is much closer to normal. Yet the truth is that she is still struggling. When I last met with her, she told me she fought with her parents all weekend and refused to eat meals to convey how mad she was at them. She has gained enough weight that her doctor expects that the next three to six months will bring her first menstrual cycle.

Emma struggles now with needing to buy clothes that are bigger than size 0 at The Gap. And though she continues each week to tell me, "I would just rather be thinner," she seems to understand when I tell her, "Well, you can't. Your parents won't let you, I won't let you, your doctor won't let you, your therapist won't let you." The idea here is to outnumber and overpower the spirit of the eating disorder so that Emma's best option is to get better.

## The Maudsley Method for Anorexic Children

In Britain, a family-based approach known as the Maudsley method has been quite successful for adolescent anorexics under the age of nineteen who have been suffering from the disorder for less than three years.

We will devote some space to the Maudsley method here, because in its emphasis on family support as a means of overcoming an eating disorder, it is a close articulation of the style of treatment that my team and I have found successful for the past fifteen years.

If your child is just beginning to show signs of an eating disorder, this short primer will give you a framework within which to view her disorder and understand how you can help her.

Briefly summarized, the Maudsley method regards parents as an essential part of the anorexic child's recovery. Parents are urged to view the disorder as a crisis of the utmost urgency; everything else must be dropped so that they can concentrate on doing all that they can to halt the disorder as quickly as possible. Stopping your child's anorexia should be as urgent a priority, Maudsley practitioners assert, as halting an aggressive form of cancer. It has brought the child's natural development to a standstill, and in these important childhood and adolescent years, the patient cannot afford to have growth retarded. Secondly, research shows that the earlier anorexia is addressed, the better the chance of full recovery. Maudsley proponents believe that the disorder has made the child actually regress, emotionally and physically, to the level of a much younger child who needs far more help than is appropriate for her age. Parents, therefore, should interact with their child accordingly, while still treating the child with respect and trying to see things from the child's perspective.

In the view of Maudsley practitioners, parents have lost control over the situation because they blame themselves for the disorder. They are petrified at the way their child is wasting away before their eyes, yet they are afraid that if they act decisively they will only make the situation worse. After all, they believe they are the cause of the disorder in the first place.

The first step in the Maudsley method is to help parents understand that they are not the cause of their child's eating disorder, although they are crucial to helping them recover from it. Next, they are encouraged to take charge of their child's eating. Weight restoration is the goal that they must single-mindedly focus on. As the child begins to gain weight, control over eating and food issues is returned to the child.

We find the Maudsley method one of the most promising new approaches to treating eating disorders in part because it holds that the family is critical to reversing the anorexia of an adolescent or a child. The one thing the Maudsley method lacks, however, is specific direction to parents on how to get their child to begin eating normally again. Drs. Christopher Dare and Ivan Eisler, among the foremost proponents of the Maudsley method, say to parents, "Just do it." We hope that our practical tips, gleaned from families who have been successful in their efforts to intervene, and offered in this chapter and in Part III, will help you get started. (For more on the Maudsley method, see chapter 14, p. 259.)

## A Note about Bulimia

If your child suffers from bulimia, a slightly different approach than the one outlined above may be necessary, since overcontrol by parents is more likely to backfire unless the child is consulted about and involved in the plan. This is because while the typical anorexic is more compliant, perfectionistic, and strives to make others happy, the typical bulimic is more rebellious and independent. Most bulimics, after having suffered from their disorder for a while, hate it and are desperate to reverse the disorder, especially after it becomes clear to them that bulimia is not an effective long-term weight-loss method. This is a discovery that most bulimics eventually make, yet at the same time they feel "addicted" to their bulimic routines and to the feeling they are getting away with something that is done in secret.

When parents try to control their child's eating and purging behaviors, the bulimic feels a natural tendency to rebel even if she wants to stop bingeing and purging. Unlike anorexics, the bulimic's rebellion will not be obvious because she may not lose or fail to gain weight the way an anorexic would. Continued trouble with bulimia is harder for parents to assess because it can easily "go underground."

## Parenting Approaches for the Bulimic Child

For the reasons we have outlined above, consulting and involving your child in an effort to conquer bulimia is important. I advise parents to sit down with their child and discuss together how they will attack the problem.

Heather and her parents, Katharine and Hans, drew up a contract stating that Heather had to progressively decrease her bingeing and purging. When she got down to one episode per week and got into the habit of completely cleaning up after her binges, her parents would allow her to sign up for an after-school dance program she longed to enter. (See p. 67 for more on taking responsibility for one's own binge/purge episodes.) Heather had the summer to achieve her goals. By August, she was able to go two weeks between binges and purges. Katharine and Hans stuck to their part of the bargain by paying for the dance program, but reminded Heather that if she slipped into more frequent binge/purge behaviors she would have to miss class that week.

It is impossible to overemphasize that you as parents need to adhere to the contracts you have drawn up with your child. If you waver, you lose credibility. As hard as it may be to withhold something from your child, remember that you are doing it because you are desperate to help them overcome a destructive and dangerous disorder.

Contracts can also help by providing strict parameters that limit the size and nature of binges. Jackie found that she tended not to binge or purge at her grandparents' house. When she is feeling "bingey" she and her mom, Sarah, agree that she should spend the night at Grandma's. Sarah and Jackie also designate a special cupboard in the kitchen at home for Jackie's binge food, stocking it with the generic snack foods that Jackie finds less appealing than name-brand equivalents. Restricting binge foods to a certain cupboard like this and limiting their choices of binge foods can help a seriously bulimic child gain some control.

Roberto's family keeps binge foods locked in the trunk of their family car, making it more of an ordeal and a conscious choice to binge. Roberto also notices that he is less likely to binge on foods purchased in single-serving packages. He can eat a small box of animal crackers and drink a glass of milk and be satisfied, but confronted with an entire package of Oreos in the pantry, he is likely to eat them all. Roberto and his mother, Maria, decide to make their own single-serving snacks by dividing and storing them in individual plastic bags. At first, they keep only one bag at a time in the pantry. As Roberto gradually learns to control his portion sizes, they are able to loosen the rules of their contract.

Becki and her family decide that it is helpful for them not to keep ice cream and cookies, two of her favorite binge foods, in the house. They decide that if they want these things, they will go out for them. Becki finds that if she eats a good dinner and then goes out with her sister and mom for an ice-cream cone, she doesn't binge.

Often rewards such as Becki's are more effective than punishment for lapses in control. Allison's mom, Kate, at first is hesitant about rewarding Allison by driving her to the big mall in town when she goes a week without bingeing or purging. Until now, Kate has been grounding Allison, forbidding her to go out with friends or even using the telephone or computer after she binges. Although these tactics might be helpful for some bulimics, they are not for Allison. It is important that parents take an experimental approach. If a plan does not work, sit down with your child and try to figure out another strategy.

Allison explains to Kate that these restrictions make her feel that there's nothing left for her to do except binge and purge. The anger and resentment she feels toward her mother actually drive her to binge on larger and larger quantities of food. Gradually, Kate realizes that Allison is able to make progress when she has something positive to look forward to rather than a punishment.

One issue that parents find difficult to deal with is the mess that their bulimic child leaves behind when they binge and purge. I have seen parents whose worry about their child's health is overshadowed by anger at how messy their houses have become.

Kate tells me that Allison's room has gotten so bad that she has found maggots crawling in the vomit in the bedroom trash can. Kate and Allison decide that Allison has to confine her eating to the kitchen and the vomiting to the bathroom, and must also clean up after herself completely when she binges and purges. These rules, mutually agreed upon, help Allison gradually control her bingeing. She tells me that the rules help her to "stay conscious" instead of spacing out during a binge/purge episode, as she keeps in mind that she is responsible for cleaning up afterward. This rule provides a strong incentive for Allison to binge less.

Sometimes parents are surprised that I don't encourage a "cold turkey" approach to treating bulimia. I tell them that only one or two of my bulimia patients have ever been able to stop like this; most bulimics get better gradually. This is not what parents, who often find the idea that their child is purging horrifying, want to hear. I tell them that if my patients were capable of suddenly ceasing to binge and purge, I would be the first to advise them to do so. But the truth is that bulimia does not usually remit this way. (For more on food plans for bulimia, and parental monitoring strategies, see chapter 11, p. 200.)

## Parenting Styles: Anorexia vs. Bulimia

Having explained our belief that family structure and parenting styles should not be blamed for causing eating disorders, we must also note that researchers have found distinct differences between the families of anorexics and those of bulimics.

The families of anorexics tend to be more controlled and organized, while the families of bulimics tend to be more chaotic, conflicted, and critical. Yet it is not always clear whether the disorder has caused the family dysfunction, or the dysfunction has caused the disorder. As it bears repeating, we will say again: In order to successfully overcome an eating disorder in your family, you as parents have to stop blaming yourselves or your children. You may observe some of these family dynamics that researchers have described in your own family, but you must remember that family structure is only one component among many that can cause an eating disorder.

Because, however, it is one factor that you as a family can influence and turn from a negative to a positive influence, it can be highly constructive to engage in some non-blaming self-analysis in an effort to find some things that can be changed. So many of the factors that have caused your child's disorder: sociocultural factors, genetic factors, even economic class may be beyond your power to control. But family structure is dynamic—you can make a difference here.

## The Role of Siblings in Recovery

In families held hostage by an eating disorder, sibling relationships, like parent-child relationships, can suffer. My goal in working with families is to turn a negative or destructive sibling relationship into a positive, supportive one.

My patient Susan's older brother, Rob, believes that if Susan would just diet and exercise, she would lose the weight she has gained from her bulimia. Every time Rob delivers his "lecture" Susan feels devastated because those strategies are the very behaviors that triggered her eating disorder in the first place. Rob's mother has to intervene and tell him, "Stop. It is not okay to talk to Susan about these things. We are working on reversing her disorder in the most effective way possible and your comments are not helping. It will take time. What you need to do is just love and appreciate Susan as she is and keep quiet about her weight and appearance." Parents have to be particularly firm about sibling comments. It must be made absolutely clear that siblings are never ever allowed to tease a sibling about their weight.

The Maudsley method encourages siblings to take on the role of the anorexic child's noncritical confidant, the family member they can turn to for support and confide in about how hard it is to do what their parents are pushing them to do.

I, too, believe it is important to keep siblings away from policing food intake; that is the parents' job. I like to ask patients what individual members of their families can do to help. Sometimes they will suggest specific things a sibling can do, such as, "Sit with me and do your homework while I eat my evening snack, but don't you dare say a word about the fact that I have to eat the snack." One of my patients' siblings rearranged his eating so that he was hungry for an evening snack at the same time his anorexic sister needed to eat hers.

I never recommend, however, that siblings change their own eating to help another. This issue came up most recently with my patient Megan. She says her sister Alice has horrible eating habits, eats snack food all the time, then picks at her meals. Yet Alice's weight is within normal range and she is healthy, while Megan is the one with the eating disorder. While I always tell parents they need to prepare good meals with the expectation that all of the family will partake, and there is no question that good family food habits can only help everyone live a healthier life, I don't believe that other members of the family must change their eating to help the eating-disordered person. Doing so could in fact cause an eating disorder in a sibling. Megan simply had to accept that Alice, despite her poor eating habits, wasn't the one in serious medical trouble, Megan was. With patients such as Megan, I say, "Maybe some people can get away with sloppier eating habits and not get into trouble, but it looks like you can't, and I know that I can't either. I have to eat in a reasonably healthy way day-in and day-out to keep my eating disorder at a distance."

As Andrea's story illustrates, it is important that parents dealing with an eating-disordered child make sure to give other siblings enough attention. It is the lack of adequate attention that seems to most often stir up trouble for the other sibling, who subconsciously may think, "Maybe I'll get an eating disorder so I can get Mom's attention, too." Having a brother with cancer was a key factor in my own story, though I would never have recognized or admitted that fact.

I have worked with a number of sibling pairs, including several sets of identical twins. Many of these siblings tell me that though they know that it is "sick," they realize that part of what drives their eating-disordered behaviors is the desire to divert toward themselves some of the attention their sibling with the eating disorder is receiving.

Caitlin, at eleven years old, is candid in telling me that she is experimenting with dieting and purging because her older sister, Nora, now in her sixth month of residential treatment for an eating disorder, receives more than her fair share of attention from both Mom and Dad. Caitlin's mom, in particular, has recognized the danger and is proactive in providing Caitlin with several new activities to help distract her from the drama surrounding her sister's serious eating disorder. Nevertheless, Caitlin remains intrigued with and at risk for eating-disordered behaviors. I advise parents with one eating-disordered child to be watchful of their other children and to practice the preventive strategies we describe in chapter 3.

## In Summary

We have shown in this chapter that there are important and substantial ways in which you as parents can help your child overcome an eating disorder. In order to begin the process of recovery, however, you must stop blaming yourselves as parents for any role you may have played in causing the disorder (no parent has ever single-handedly triggered an eating disorder) and focus on what you can do to turn the problem around. Collaboration, flexibility, teamwork (instead of divisiveness), compassion, and perhaps most of all, patience and perseverance will be your best allies in this struggle. Turning around your child's eating disorder will likely be among the biggest challenges you will face as a family. It is not something to be taken lightly, but a supreme challenge that demands the entire family's early, wholehearted, and focused effort.

# 5

# Boys at Risk

Sixteen-year-old Travis and his family relocated to a rural college town several years ago from their home on a Montana Indian reservation. Travis seemed to make the transition with ease. He was well liked, was admired for his abilities on the baseball field, and had a number of close friends. With so much seemingly going for him, Travis's bulimia was easy to miss. He was a normal-weight, healthy-looking teenage boy who had spent his formative years in a culture that does not value thinness. Proud to call himself an Indian rather than the more politically correct Native American, Travis grew up riding horses, chasing cows, and going to powwows.

The first few times Travis's friends caught him in the bathroom throwing up they believed he had the flu or had eaten something that didn't agree with him. But after enough of these episodes, they finally put two and two together and came to the undeniable conclusion that Travis had an eating disorder. Bulimia was the last thing anyone thought he would struggle with, yet here he was, suffering from a case so severe that eventually he was regularly noticing blood in his vomit. When Travis's friends finally approached him with their concerns, he himself had become frightened and desperately wanted to turn his bulimia around. The intervention of his friends was the push he needed; he was ready to take their advice and confide in his parents.

As Travis's story illustrates, the face of eating disorders has changed, and is continuing to change. I have worked with many boys and men, as well as young people representing a diverse set of backgrounds. Eating disorders are now an equal-opportunity disease.

The rise in the number of boys suffering from eating disorders is especially striking. Because researchers only recently began to study the prevalence of eating disorders among boys, there are no statistics available to tell us how large that increase has been. Yet I, like all of my colleagues who treat eating disorders, have noticed a dramatic rise in the number of eating-disordered boys I am seeing.

The growing number of boys with both disordered eating and eating disorders does not come as a surprise when you consider the way that dieting and thinness are marketed with almost equal vigor to men as they are to women today. Neither does the corresponding rise in body dissatisfaction that researchers have documented among boys and young men.

In this chapter, we will discuss some of the reasons for this widely commented-on increase in male eating disorders, and how boys' disorders differ from those of girls'. We will also introduce some approaches that work best with boys.

Throughout this chapter, we will emphasize this point: When an eating disorder becomes full-blown, the issues you face as parents remain much the same, regardless of the gender of your child.

## Common Traits and Beliefs
## of the Eating-Disordered Boy

The boys I have seen as patients are likely to have taken their drive to improve sports performance too far, losing dangerous amounts of weight through overexercise and limited food intake. They are more often obsessed with altering their body shape rather than being focused on weight loss. Usually they are aiming for a highly muscled body without an ounce of fat. For some of them, their obsession with fitness and muscle building has been touched off by teasing about their weight and body shape from family members or peers. Other boy patients of mine have gone overboard trying to avoid the weight gain and diet-related health problems they see their fathers struggle with. A substantial number of the boys I have seen express concerns and beliefs identical to those of the typical eating-disordered girl: they believe wholeheartedly that losing weight will improve their appearance and self-esteem.

While their numbers are increasing, for boys the good news is that, in my experience at least, they are more open to getting treatment and seem less traumatized about having a "girl's" disease than in past years.

## How Are Boys' Eating Disorders Different from Girls'?

Although boys and girls appear to develop and experience eating disorders in much the same way, share a similar disease course, and respond to treatment in the same way, there are some important differences. It is rarer for boys to diet their way into an eating disorder, as girls usually do. When boys develop an eating disorder, they most often have additional risk factors that induce their eating disorder. (For a list of these risk factors, see below.)

While nonathletic boys are less likely to be at risk for an eating disorder, nonathletic girls face roughly as much risk as athletic girls. Another notable difference is that boys appear more often to have a later age of onset for eating disorders, which may be explained by the fact that the onset of puberty in boys is usually about two years later than in girls.

## Protective Factors in Boys

While puberty can make girls more prone to eating disorders, it seems to play an opposite, protective role against eating disorders for boys. Because boys reach puberty later than girls, they are better prepared emotionally to deal with the body changes associated with puberty. In addition, the pubertal changes boys experience give their bodies more muscle and less fat. These changes are more culturally acceptable than the increase in body fat that girls experience.

Another protective factor may be that because boys and men naturally have higher metabolic rates than girls and women, they usually find it easier to maintain a stable body weight than girls and women do. The fact that boys can more easily induce changes in body weight with modest changes in caloric intake may make them less tempted to try extreme eating-disordered behaviors.

Boys also tend to be less critical of their own bodies than girls. This characteristic seems to prevent normal weight boys from experimenting with eating-disordered behaviors.

## Factors That Put Boys at Risk for Eating Disorders

While we have some idea why girls are more susceptible to eating disorders than boys, a more perplexing question is why some boys are at risk for disordered eating and eating disorders, and others are not. The following are factors that are known to put boys at risk for eating disorders:

- Being chubby as children and/or experiencing more teasing about body size

- Having a higher-than-average body weight
- Body dissatisfaction
- Participation in high-risk sports that favor thinness or include weight classes, such as wrestling, boxing, crew, bodybuilding, weight-lifting, gymnastics, figure skating, or long-distance running
- Depression

### Shame and Invisibility: Obstacles to Treatment

One concern about boys who diet or engage in other behaviors that could foreshadow an eating disorder is that their problem may go unnoticed because parents, teachers, coaches, even doctors and other adults in the child's life may believe that eating disorders are a "girl problem." Although we have noted that this shame about male eating disorders seems to be diminishing somewhat, shame still keeps boys from admitting they have eating problems, and keeps others from detecting those problems, even very obvious ones.

## Anorexia among Boys

Connor, bright and inquisitive, was home-schooled until he was eleven, when he and his parents agreed he needed the stimulus of the local junior high. Connor was excited about finally joining his peers and was happy that a few of his friends from his rural neighborhood would be in his new class. Yet he was also nervous about this transition to a large junior high. Once there, he felt out of control and lost. Controlling his eating was his response to his distress, just as it is for young women who develop full-blown disorders when they enter high school or go away to college.

Today, looking back on this difficult period, Connor says that his interest in calories, fat grams, and losing weight made sense. He needed something he was certain he could master and there was no doubt that he was good at losing weight. Connor says he could see that his parents were worried, but it was not until his doctor told him in no uncertain terms that he was too thin and needed to gain weight that he understood the seriousness of his situation. Connor is an example of how an early intervention can be effective. His parents simply needed the doctor's help in getting Connor's attention; once that was done, they were able to help him gain weight.

Kent's story is more typical for a boy than for a girl, and illustrates the way that a susceptible boy will often get into trouble with food. Kent became aware that his naturally chubby physique was a "problem" when, at twelve, his track coach patted Kent's tummy and said, "Your times would be better if you got rid of that." "That should be easy to deal with," Kent thought. "I'll just skip dessert." Weight loss was easy for Kent, who, just by giving up dessert, lost enough weight for his coach to notice. Boys usually lose weight quickly because of their naturally fast metabolisms. Pleased with the positive feedback his weight loss generated, Kent decided to give up snacking. Although missing his afternoon snack left him feeling a little light-headed at track practice, he really didn't mind, and besides, he was able to lose another five pounds. Soon losing weight felt like a game: if Kent didn't lose at least a little when he checked his weight before bed, he promised himself that he would eat a little less the following day. Fortunately, Kent's parents, aware that distance running was a sport that could spawn an eating disorder, were keeping an eye on him. They intervened before Kent had done any real damage to his health. "Sorry, Kent," they told him matter-of-factly when he protested, "we are not going to allow you to lose any more weight." Kent's parents let the coach know of their concerns, making it clear that Kent's health depended on preventing even an ounce of further weight loss. Since young athletes rarely complain to coaches about weight-loss induced symptoms, such as dizziness or fatigue, the coach often remains in the dark.

## Bulimia among Boys

Rod was in his last year of high school when he fell prey to bulimia. He told me he first learned about self-induced vomiting as a method of weight loss from his teammates on the crew team. When the season was over, the other boys stopped their disordered behaviors, but Rod, to his dismay, found that he could not.

Bulimic boys tend to be less concerned with strict weight control than eating-disordered girls and are less likely to use laxatives and more likely to engage in excessive exercise than girls. You should be suspicious, therefore, if your son dramatically increases his exercise or begins to restrict food choices. All are symptoms that can indicate either bulimia or anorexia.

While there has not been enough research done yet in this area to be able to say with certainty whether or not bulimia among boys is increasing, clinicians, including myself, report that they are seeing more boys and men with eating disorders of all types.

I came to know Dylan, who had been bulimic since ninth grade, when he was a college student. Dylan told me that his shame about having an eating disorder kept him from confiding in his parents when he lived at home. Even now, with access to confidential counseling, he had difficulty accepting treatment for his "girl's disorder." My own experience with parents of boys is that they are likely to take bulimic and anorexic behaviors in their sons appropriately seriously. Ironically, this is not always true of parents of girls, who may look at these behaviors as simply a rite of passage that most girls these days experience. When parents are matter-of-fact about their son's eating disorder and are careful not to repeat gender-based stereotypes, boys can quickly grasp that cultural pressures on boys and girls in this day and age are becoming increasingly similar.

## Binge Eating among Boys

The higher percentage of boys and men who binge eat (they account for 40 percent of all binge eaters) compared to other eating-disordered behaviors can probably be explained by several reasons:

- It is more culturally acceptable for boys and men to eat large quantities of food than it is for girls and women.
- Boys and men, with their faster metabolisms, are less likely to gain weight if they occasionally binge. This makes them less likely to worry about binge eating affecting their weight and more likely that bingeing becomes habitual, albeit without the guilt that most girls who binge experience.

These cultural, attitudinal, and physiological factors may protect boys from bulimia, and also may explain why binge eating is the only eating disorder category in which the incidence among boys and men almost reaches parity with women.

## Disordered Eating among Boys

As with disordered eating among the general population, it is hard to come by consistent figures for the number of boys who suffer from disordered eating. What we do know is that a substantial number of boys are clearly dieting, and therefore at risk for developing eating problems. Several recent studies have documented an increase in men and boys who admit they have dieted to lose weight.

Compared to non-eating-disordered boys, boys with disordered eating have been found to be more dissatisfied with their bodies even if they are normal weight, restrained in their eating, perfectionistic, more depressed, and have more difficulty distinguishing between emotions and physical sensations. An example of the latter symptom would be that they might confuse disappointment with hunger, which could lead to bingeing when disappointed, angry, or depressed. These findings replicate the symptoms of body dissatisfaction and eating-disordered behavior found in girls who suffer from disordered eating, a fact that has led researchers to conclude that boys and girls with eating disorders share remarkably similar characteristics.

## Boys and the "Adonis Complex"

A variation on male body-image and eating problems is that of boys who show increased interest in fitness, sports, and muscle building. Instead of feeling too large, they consistently underestimate their own size and feel ashamed of being too small and puny. To remedy this perceived fault, they may overexercise, compulsively lift weights, and use diets and supplements that purport to build muscle. This commonly seen syndrome (known to experts as muscle dysmorphia) has been dubbed the "Adonis complex" by Harrison Pope, Katherine Phillips, and Roberto Olivardia, researchers at Harvard and Brown Universities who have written a book by the same title.

Boys who suffer from the Adonis complex have an obsession with appearance that leads to what Dr. Pope terms a kind of "reverse anorexia." Usually, they use muscle building and fitness magazines or other weight lifters (who are convinced that their own special diet explains their success) as their guides on how to restrict their diets. Their disordered eating often takes the form of extreme diets, either high in protein or low in fat, or both. They may also restrict other foods they believe are unhealthy. Currently, the high-protein diets that are popular with muscle builders are those that advise almost total abstinence from breads, cereals, and other high-carbohydrate foods, and sometimes abstinence from fats.

Most of the protein supplements favored by body-building boys, while no better than high-protein foods, are safe if used properly. If they are overused they can cause kidney damage. Several of my patients who have overused protein supplements have had abnormal kidney function tests. Fortunately, in each case kidney function returned to normal as soon as the boy stopped using the protein supplements. Another popular supplement among male athletes is creatine. Makers of this product advertise creatine for its ability to increase muscle mass. Creatine is extracted from the protein found in meats and is probably safe, although the effects of long-term use of creatine pills are unknown. Use of this supplement is of concern to researchers who worry about young people taking large doses of a concentrated substance that has not been tested for long-term side effects.

Ephedrine, a form of amphetamine derived from the Chinese herb ma huang, is touted as a quick weight-loss aid. It is also far from safe: it may be addictive and can lead to heart problems and even death. Despite widespread evidence of the danger of ephedrine, surprisingly, it remains available over-the-counter, and is widely used by boys and girls for weight loss.

Boys may also use any of the many hormonal preparations (DHEA and other adrenal hormones are popular) available by mail order or at health food stores. Often these products are marketed as "legal steroids," with promises that they will increase muscle mass. Yet so far, supplemental adrenal hormones have not lived up to those promises. One concern among researchers is that supplemental adrenal hormones may increase blood cholesterol levels.

Some boys may even use illegal and dangerous anabolic steroids. Steroids are dangerous in the short term mostly because of the mood changes, aggressiveness, and even violence they can cause. The most serious long-term health consequences are high cholesterol and possibly prostate and liver cancer. Boys who diet are more likely to use steroids than boys who do not diet, researchers have found.

When I first met sixteen-year-old Morgan, he described himself as a "gym rat" who spent all his free time at the local gym, even though he was well aware that the gym atmosphere, with its focus on weight loss and physical appearance, was not helping him in his yearlong battle with bulimia. When we met again a month later, Morgan confessed that he had been using ephedrine on the recommendation of one of his college-age friends at the gym. He described how on the ephedrine he could binge and still lose weight, but admitted that he was worried about how "spacey and hyper" ephedrine made him feel. I asked about the other common complaints of ephedrine users: headaches, insomnia, and racing heart. Yes, he replied, he had them all. Morgan said that the most disappointing part of his experience with the supplement was that when he stopped taking ephedrine a week or so ago, he gained back all the weight and five pounds more.

## Boys and Bone Mineral Density

Surprisingly, new studies indicate that eating-disordered boys may be at even higher risk of developing low bone mineral density than girls. While explanations are still speculative, it appears that testosterone levels, which are lowered in boys with eating disorders, are a key factor in producing this higher risk. Another surprise is that among eating-disordered boys, those with bulimia seem to be at as high a risk of losing bone density as those with anorexia. In this respect, eating-disordered boys differ from eating-disordered girls, who are more likely to suffer from low bone density if they are anorexic rather than bulimic. Arnold Andersen, the respected expert on eating disorders in males, advises that boys with eating disorders have bone-density tests done. If bone mineral density is found to be low, he also advises that contact sports and other high-impact activities be limited until bone density improves.

## Treatment Approaches That Work with Boys

As we noted earlier, the treatment approaches for eating-disordered girls work equally well with boys. I would also add that you should be careful not to tease your son about having a girl's disease and make sure his siblings do not do so, either. You should make sure your child knows that eating disorders do occur among boys and are in fact not uncommon. You should be aware that your son may be likely to abuse exercise and you should be watchful about use of dangerous supplements. You should also remember that although your son may not be trying to lose weight, he may be trying to alter his body shape, which can also lead to eating problems.

## Homosexual Boys and Eating Disorders

Homosexual boys may be at higher risk for eating disorders for the same reason that homosexual men are, namely the high value gay culture places on thinness and physical attractiveness. Researchers have also concluded that homosexuality in boys may exacerbate an eating disorder.

Parents should remember that heterosexual boys get eating disorders, too. You should be careful not to assume that the fact that your son is struggling with an eating problem means he is gay.

## In Summary

In this chapter, we have tried to shatter the myth of eating disorders as an affluent young woman's disease, to explain how boys' eating disorders differ from those of girls', and to provide some advice on treating eating disorders among boys. If your son is suffering from an eating disorder, you should now be well beyond any notion that there is anything unusual or shameful about a male eating disorder. You have been alerted to the fact that bone mineral loss may be a serious threat to your son, and know how to spot a boy suffering from the Adonis complex. Most of all, you now understand that while there may be small differences in the way that eating disorders manifest themselves in boys and girls, the vast majority of the problems and issues they face are identical, regardless of gender.

# No One Is Immune:
# The Toxic Spread of Eating Disorders

Just as the incidence of eating disorders has risen dramatically among boys and men, so has their prevalence among people of virtually every race, ethnicity, sexuality, and socioeconomic class. The common denominator, the universal thread linking all of these trends is the way that "white" American beauty standards—and their toxic effect on body image and attitudes toward food—have permeated our society and much of the world. Ethnic minorities and races that once seemed immune to eating problems because of their acceptance, even celebration, of larger body sizes and shapes are now falling prey to a disease that was once thought exclusively the problem of upper-middle-class white girls and women.

I have worked not only with a number of boys and men, both gay and straight, but with lesbian girls and women, African Americans, Hispanics, Native Americans, and Asian Americans of widely differing backgrounds, as well as college students from all over the world.

My patient Crystal, for instance, was afflicted with the sense of internal conflict that can result among eating-disordered lesbians. As a member of a subculture that deemphasizes thinness and dieting and emphasizes body acceptance and carefree eating, she explained her dilemma to me: "Gay girls just aren't supposed to have poor body image or eating disorders."

Among minority groups in this country, it is the most acculturated girls and boys who are most at risk for eating disorders, while minority children and adolescents who have a strong cultural identity still seem to be protected from eating problems. New young immigrants who are attempting to integrate into American society are at high risk for developing food problems. In fact, researchers have shown that dieting and adopting the preference for thinness is viewed by some immigrants as a way to fit into their new society.

I recall meeting Tom, a Cambodian refugee who was about to graduate from college and start his job on Wall Street, and being taken aback by his matter-of-fact acceptance of the need to diet. The surprising thing about Tom was how unperturbed he was about his likely anorexia, and how uninterested he seemed in treatment. His drive to acculturate and to succeed in this country was so strong that he was willfully blinding himself to the dangers inherent in his adopted culture.

In short, if you are minority parents who have assumed your child will be protected from an eating disorder by your culture's acceptance of a wide range of body size and shapes, be forewarned: many of those protections lose their power as your children struggle to integrate into mainstream society.

# 6

# Understanding the Medical Consequences
# of an Eating Disorder

In this chapter, we will help you recognize and understand the medical complications and laboratory findings often seen with eating disorders. Before we get into what can be a long and sometimes frightening list of eating disorder–related medical problems however, we want to issue one caveat: Keep in mind that for the most part these symptoms and conditions are reversible upon refeeding or restoration of normal weight, or when a child stops purging. You should therefore not become unduly alarmed at reading the following compendium of possible complications, but realize that if you direct your efforts at implementing the food and exercise plans we outline in Part III of this book, most if not all of these symptoms can be either avoided or reversed with weight restoration or cessation of purging.

You should also realize that because the conditions we describe are for the most part fully reversible, it is rarely crucial to do an intensive medical investigation on a child or adolescent known to be suffering from an eating disorder. When a patient is not forthcoming about her eating problems or weight loss, or parents have not shared their suspicions, doctors will often order a complete medical workup, subjecting the patient to a whole array of X rays and tests for endocrine, gastrointestinal, thyroid, and liver function as they search for possible explanations for the child's weight loss and other symptoms. It is important, therefore, that parents give doctors their impressions of the extent of their child's undereating, overexercising, or purging. By quickly arriving at the diagnosis of an eating disorder that you suspect, you may be able to save a substantial amount of anxiety, time, and money. Your first priority should be to reverse the eating disorder as quickly as possible before it becomes entrenched and to restore your child's healthy relationship with food, not to waste valuable time and energy searching for a medical diagnosis that might explain away the eating disorder.

## What to Expect on Your First Visit to a Medical Doctor

When you first inform your doctor that you suspect your child is suffering from an eating disorder, he or she will probably want to talk to you about your concerns and observations. The doctor should then meet with your child alone (unless your child is very young or shy) and will likely ask your child about her food and exercise habits and her weight history. The doctor will also take a social history, conduct a complete physical exam and psychological assessment, and order general blood work, urinalysis, and possibly a stool sample. If your child has sustained serious weight loss, the doctor may also order an EKG (electrocardiogram) to test heart function, chest X rays to measure heart size, MRI (magnetic resonance imaging) or CT (computed tomography) scans to measure brain size, and bone-density tests to help identify signs of malnutrition.

You should not be alarmed about or object to these tests; your doctor has ordered them to help attain a clearer picture of your child's condition. If you have been fully forthcoming about your child's behaviors and symptoms and any suspicions you may have of an eating disorder, you have done all you can to prevent unnecessary tests. You must now rely on your doctor's judgment.

## Medical Symptoms and Complications Associated with Anorexia

Any child who undereats is at risk for the conditions we will describe. The longer the undereating goes on, the more likely it is that it will turn into full-blown anorexia. We use the term "anorexic" here, recognizing that bulimics and binge eaters can also experience the same medical complications and symptoms from bouts of undereating.

Anorexia, in severe cases, can affect almost all the major organ systems. In this section, we will discuss the symptoms of anorexia, which we have organized by the different functions and areas of the body that are affected.

### Growth

In children, the effects of anorexia are particularly devastating because the child has not yet finished growing and maturing. Height, for instance, can be compromised among anorexic children. While most children are expected to be as tall or taller than their parents, children whose anorexia has become chronic will likely be shorter than would have been predicted without the illness.

### Sexual Development

Anorexia can also delay sexual development. Anorexic girls may stop getting their menstrual periods, a change that gives rise to mixed feelings in most girls. At first they are glad not to have to bother with a monthly cycle. They may have heard that athletic girls are not likely to have periods, so their condition seems even somewhat desirable. On this point, you can inform your child that doctors today believe that loss of menstrual periods among athletes is almost always the result of undereating, not overexercise, as was once believed.

Anorexics may also admire the way anorexia delays the development of hips and breasts, physical features they associate with being fat. Girls whose anorexia predates menarche (the beginning of menstruation), on the other hand, will usually not realize that their starvation has delayed its onset. By substantially delaying puberty and permanently interfering with height and breast development, anorexia at this young age has an even more detrimental effect on health and development than does anorexia in adolescents. One reason that children are thought to be at increased medical risk from anorexia is that they naturally have smaller fat stores than do adolescents and so lose vital tissues more quickly with weight loss.

Boys and young men with anorexia may also experience delayed sexual development. The primary symptom of this is decreased levels of serum testosterone, a condition that can be determined by blood tests.

### Gastrointestinal Symptoms

Anorexics may experience a variety of gastrointestinal symptoms, all of which are believed to be caused by malnutrition and underuse of the gastrointestinal tract. Chronic undereating actually causes the musculature of the small and large intestine, which churns and digests food, to atrophy. The anorexic may experience stomachaches and bloating as food sits in the stomach longer than usual. The constipation anorexics often suffer from is frequently confused with fullness, a feeling they use to rationalize not eating.

This delayed emptying of the stomach, and the bloating that accompanies it, can lead to yet another uncomfortable symptom, reflux. Slightly different than the "acid reflux" caused by eating too much spicy food that many over-the-counter medications claim to eliminate, this type of reflux causes food to rise up into the esophagus or sometimes even into the mouth, and can increase the likelihood of developing bulimia.

All of these problems reverse relatively quickly with weight gain.

## Low Blood Pressure, Dizziness, Hypothermia, and Poor Concentration

Anorexics also often experience dizziness and low blood pressure, which can lead to fainting spells. Although Olivia's coach noticed she was thinner, he didn't suspect a problem until Olivia fainted two weeks in a row at soccer practice. Parents should be alert to complaints by their children of feeling faint; this is not a common occurrence in healthy children, but can be an early symptom of an eating disorder.

Fainting spells can show up even before the child has lost a significant amount of weight and can be dangerous. Maggie, an accomplished young horsewoman, was lucky she was not seriously hurt when undereating led her to lose consciousness while atop her jumping horse. Maggie had a hard time believing that just skipping breakfast and lunch could result in passing out. She had only lost a few pounds that month and was still technically within normal weight ranges.

Another frequently seen symptom, loss of too much of the body's essential fat stores, causes hypothermia, or low body temperature, which in turn will cause the anorexic child to feel cold when everyone else is comfortable, and require layers and layers of clothing to feel warm. The anorexic's surprisingly cold hands are another tip-off to a developing eating disorder. Other common symptoms are lethargy, apathy, and poor concentration. For reasons that are not well understood, most anorexics are able to concentrate on academic schoolwork, but may have difficulty following a simple conversation.

Natalie's parents were falsely reassured about some of the symptoms they were seeing because she continued to get straight A's even as she struggled to remember what plans she had made for after-school transportation, or to engage in a casual chat. Although she had clearly become more absent-minded, it was hard for her parents to point to any clear sign of illness since all the changes were so gradual and subtle.

## Adaptations to Starvation: Hair, Nails, Skin, and Muscle Changes

The anorexic's body adapts to starvation by focusing on maintaining the most essential major organ functions, while withholding nourishment from more superficial parts of the body, such as hair and nails. Brittle nails and extreme dryness of the skin caused by lack of protein and fat in the diet are common signs of anorexia, as well as loss of scalp, body, and even pubic hair.

Sarah's response to the realization that the thinning of her beautiful, flaxen hair was due to her weight loss was to break down into wrenching sobs. As superficial as it may seem, the loss of hair is often the only symptom anorexics worry about. I have seen a number of patients who were motivated to change their eating-disordered behavior solely for the sake of saving or restoring their hair. Because anorexics will often worry more about such minor symptoms rather than the more life-threatening aspects of the disorder, I often tell parents to explore what it is about the disorder that scares their child most, and help them understand that improving their eating will help solve that problem.

With more extreme weight loss, patients may develop lanugo, a fine, downy body hair on their back, arms, and legs (and sometimes faces and necks) that is characteristic of the human fetus while it is still in the womb. On the bodies of anorexics, lanugo is thought to be a primitive attempt by the body to maintain body temperature, as this type of hair takes fewer calories to produce than normal hair. Anorexics may also experience bone pain when exercising, and, despite the fact that they are exercising, muscle wasting. Muscle loss is particularly noticeable in the arms and legs, a change that at first thrills many anorexics.

### Cardiac Symptoms

Although the following information may be frightening to you as parents, it is important to remember that the body is capable of making a remarkable recovery once food intake is improved and eating-disordered behaviors are discontinued. Because cardiac symptoms are among the most serious complications associated with eating disorders, however, it is important to be able to recognize them if and when they occur in your child. Early signs that anorexia may be affecting the heart are fatigue, light-headedness (feeling dizzy upon standing or sitting up from a sitting or prone position), or cold, bluish, splotchy hands and feet. More serious symptoms, which warrant calling your doctor immediately, include slowed or irregular heartbeat, shortness of breath, chest pain, leg pain, and rapid breathing.

Heart palpitations (the subjective awareness of one's own irregular heartbeat) and chest pains are often experienced at night in bed, causing anorexics to fear they may be dying. Often these symptoms go hand-in-hand with bradycardia (slow heart rate indicated by a slow pulse) and low blood pressure. Although bradycardia is quickly resolved by adequate nutrition, unless it is rectified it can, in the most serious cases, put the anorexic at risk for congestive heart failure. An electrocardiogram (EKG) can confirm slowed heart rate and/or arrhythmias. Because the malnutrition of anorexia can reduce the size of the heart to a dangerous degree, chest X rays are used to detect changes in heart size.

Some patients, keenly aware of their slow heart rate, become obsessed with measuring it. Heather was sure as she counted heartbeats per minute at night as she lay in bed that her heart had stopped between beats. Amy, noticing the same phenomenon, became hysterical and had her parents call an ambulance to take her to the emergency room.

Victoria told me that as scary as some of these physical signs are, she found them oddly reassuring. In her case, constantly feeling cold, a slowed heart rate, even her brittle nails and hair all meant she could not be eating too much.

In rare cases, anorexics experience edema, or fluid retention, in their abdomen or legs, especially when they have entered a period of weight gain or have stopped abusing laxatives or diuretics. Edema is an early sign that the heart is not functioning well enough to handle the increases in fluid that naturally result when weight is gained or laxatives and diuretics are discontinued. If your child does experience such edema, close monitoring by your doctor can ensure that your child is not in acute danger. Again, while this symptom and others we describe are potentially dangerous, good, close medical supervision and a wholehearted effort to reverse the disorder is the approach that will get your child out of medical danger most quickly and safely.

As the anorexic body wastes away, so does the heart. Some researchers have noted that even a week or two of severe dieting can lead to substantial loss of heart muscle.

One example of a rare cardiac complication associated with severe anorexia is mitral valve prolapse. This type of heart-valve prolapse occurs because although the malnourished heart muscle shrinks, the valves inside the heart chamber do not. The result is a set of misshapen valves that do not close properly. The faulty valves cause blood to leak back into the heart chamber, which in turn causes palpitations and chest pain. Although mitral valve prolapse is a potentially fatal condition, it appears to be reversible with weight gain.

In the most extreme cases of anorexia, the cumulative effects of long-term starvation (an irregular heartbeat, edema, bradycardia, to name a few possible contributing factors) can cause sudden heart failure. Malnutrition has caused the heart to shrink, resulting in decreased cardiac output and low blood pressure. Finally, the heart simply gives out.

Most often, this type of sudden death occurs while the anorexic is asleep. Such is the insidious nature of anorexia, a disease in which slow starvation can coexist with a surprising degree of functional well-being, that sometimes an autopsy will show no obvious heart problems. Though the thought of chronic anorexia leading to sudden death is an extremely frightening one, this tragedy does occasionally happen. Those most at risk are severe anorexics who have suffered a long period of extreme emaciation. By intervening early, you can be assured that you are protecting your child from this, the most devastating consequence of an eating disorder.

## Bone Problems

Osteoporosis is among the most dangerous and common results of anorexia. When starvation causes the body to stop menstruating, the body's supply of naturally circulating estrogen is reduced, which in turn can lead to significant bone loss. Severe bone loss has been documented in as many as half of patients with anorexia-related amenorrhea (cessation of menstrual periods).

Adolescent anorexia is particularly devastating because adolescence is a time when children should be building bone to last a lifetime, not losing it. Over half of bone mineral density is acquired from age ten through puberty. Once a person reaches their middle to late twenties they lose the ability to improve bone density. For this reason, any disruption in hormone levels should be taken seriously.

Furthermore, researchers have found that anorexic adolescent patients lose more bone than adults with anorexia. Adolescents with eating disorders can exhibit delayed maturation of bone, and anorexics of any age are at risk for bone fractures. Usually, fractures will occur as the anorexic ages, or engages in high-impact exercises such as running on hard pavement. Having an eating disorder for as little as one year can reduce an adolescent's bone density to that of an eighty-year-old woman.

## Testing Bone Density

A bone density test commonly known as a "DEXA" (dual-energy X-ray absorptiometry) is the state-of-the art method for measuring bone mineral density. For anorexic adolescents whose disorder is a long-standing problem, having your doctor order a DEXA (also known as a densitometry) can sometimes be helpful in breaking through the anorexic's denial that her eating behaviors are having an effect on her health.

After two years of maintaining a below-normal weight, first-year graduate student Selena finally agrees to have a DEXA. Her results came back comparing her bones to those of someone four times her age. "But I feel fine!" was her first response. Over the course of time, she was able to motivate herself to gain some much-needed weight by focusing on doing everything she could to protect her bones from more damage.

As with Selena, bone density tests are compared to a statistical norm, and do not measure actual bone loss unless they are repeated periodically. Only by doing a baseline test and then repeating it six months or a year later will you be able to tell if your child's bone density has improved or deteriorated.

Because it can take six months to a year of restricted eating before any measurable bone loss occurs, DEXAs are not currently advised unless the anorexic is either older or has a long-term eating disorder.

For anorexics who fit this description, the test can be quite helpful. Most major hospitals offer this relatively inexpensive (under $200 in most facilities) and accurate test. The exposure to radiation is one-tenth of that of a chest X ray.

### Recovering Bone Density

Most experts believe that once it is lost, bone density cannot be improved without weight gain. Even with weight gain, only partial recovery of bone density is likely. The latest research indicates that supplemental estrogen, which in the past was routinely prescribed for anorexics (usually in the form of birth control pills) to improve bone health, is of little help. Estrogen also induces periods in patients whose self-starvation has caused amenorrhea, making it impossible for doctors to tell whether an eating-disordered patient has gained enough weight to protect her bones. For both these reasons, many physicians no longer prescribe estrogen to anorexics.

Osteoporosis medications (Fosamax is one) show some promise in helping restore bones in anorexic patients. Although these drugs are currently being tested for anorexics, they are not yet routinely prescribed for them. Only weight gain, and the better nutrition it requires, can reliably improve the bone density of eating-disorder sufferers. Your goal as parents of an anorexic child should be to improve nutrition and restore weight as quickly as possible.

### Fertility Issues

Researchers have still not determined to what extent a bout of anorexia during childhood or adolescence will affect future fertility. Although ample research has shown that adult anorexia, if not reversed, is likely to lead to infertility, there are numerous reports of severely low-weight, even chronic, anorexics becoming pregnant.

Because of these contradictory data, little is gained by telling young anorexics (who often worry that they might not be able to have children) that they will face infertility as adults. Instead, they should be assured that if their disorder is treated and resolved, they can expect to bear children if they want to.

My patient Nellie was not assured of this, but instead was told by a school nurse that she was ruining her chance of ever having a family, thanks to her eating disorder. In response, Nellie's eating became even more self-destructive. When we discussed the issue, she told me, "If I can't have kids, I might as well be really thin."

Huron County Library

--- Currently checked out ---

Title: Massive manga : techniques for drawing, inking an
Date due: 24 July 2015 23:59

Library name: HCGODE
User ID: 06492001699241

Title: The parent's guide to childhood eating disorders
Date due: 07 August 2015 23:59

Handled sensitively, however, the question of an eating disorder's effect on future fertility can sometimes be used as motivation to turn around the disorder.

Katrina has suffered from anorexia for all of her teenage years and as a result has never had a period. Now, as a senior in high school, she is acutely aware that she eventually wants children, but she worries that her disorder may affect her chances of doing so. She and I are focusing on the natural desire to someday have healthy children to help her get motivated to increase her weight.

Another fact that can be used as motivation to end a course of anorexia before a teenager reaches adulthood is that there is evidence of higher rates of prematurity and low birth weight among babies born to mothers with a long history of anorexia.

It is important to guard against giving a sexually active anorexic teen the impression that her present condition, including lack of periods, is a guarantee that she will not get pregnant. Even amenorrheic girls with anorexia can become pregnant if they do not practice birth control. Despite the lack of periods, the bodies of these girls will occasionally and unpredictably create a hormonal environment that allows pregnancy.

**Blood Values**

The most common blood work findings are leukopenia (low white blood cell count) and mild anemia (low iron count), and in rare cases, thrombocytopenia (low platelet count).

Usually, when lab tests reveal these abnormal blood values, the anorexic feels no symptoms. Yet almost immediately upon resumption of adequate food intake, and even before she necessarily begins gaining weight, she feels noticeably warmer, much more energetic, and exhibits improved skin color. Tonya was thrilled to have me feel how warm her hands had become since she started improving her diet. Warm hands are a good sign your child is moving in the right direction.

As an anorexic's condition worsens, her daily life is more likely to be affected by these hematologic changes and the cardiac symptoms we have described. She will most likely notice fatigue, weakness, dizziness, and inability to exercise at former levels. Jill was a dancer who also liked to jog and play tennis. As her anorexia worsened, she increased her exercise in an attempt to burn off more and more calories and fat. She recognized how serious her problem was when eventually she didn't want to go to dance class, turned down offers to play Frisbee, and had to walk instead of run her usual jogging route.

I notice regularly the difficulty my anorexic patients have with even mild exercise. My office is on the third floor of an old turn-of-the-century building. Though my anorexic patients usually decline to use the elevator, these formerly athletic girls are exhausted and out of breath after climbing three flights of stairs.

Jill was delighted when her nutrition and weight recovery allowed her to climb those stairs with ease. Soon she was back to a fairly rigorous, but now not excessive, exercise schedule of no more than an hour a day.

As in Jill's case, these changes in blood values and cardiac function that we have described are secondary to malnutrition, and improve almost immediately with improved nutrition and weight gain.

Parents should also be aware, however, that even in severe cases of anorexia, blood values can be normal and cannot, therefore, be used as a proof of adequate nutrition. Sometimes lab values improve before your child has reached a safe, healthy weight. This is often confusing to parents, whose eating-disordered child may point to improved lab findings as proof that they need not continue to gain weight. I remind parents that though their child looks and reports feeling energetic, if she remains too thin, she is still not cured and remains at risk for anorexia-related health problems. This can be a difficult juncture for some parents because their child seems to have regained her health while remaining fashionably thin. Your child's pediatrician or your family doctor can help you assess whether your child is at a truly healthy weight, as can the charts we provide in Appendix B.

### Fluid and Cholesterol Imbalances

Anorexics are often dehydrated from restricting their fluid intake, undereating, and sometimes misusing diuretics, all of which are reflected in an elevated blood urea nitrogen (BUN) reading.

Although anorexics usually have low cholesterol levels, abnormally high levels are not uncommon. Some researchers suspect these abnormally high cholesterol levels are related to the effects of starvation on the liver. Without adequate nutrition, the liver, which both makes and metabolizes cholesterol, is unable to break down cholesterol properly. High cholesterol levels are also thought to be caused by starvation-induced abnormalities in estrogen, thyroid, and other hormones.

Whatever the cause, high cholesterol is most likely to occur in acute anorexia and disappears either with weight restoration or if the anorexia becomes chronic. High cholesterol associated with anorexia is much more common in children and adolescents with anorexia than in adult patients.

What is important to know is that anorexics should not be treated for high cholesterol levels with standard low-fat and low-calorie diets, an approach that would only worsen the patient's malnutrition and likely raise her cholesterol levels even higher. Like other findings associated with anorexia, as the patient recovers, abnormally high cholesterol levels, along with the abnormal liver function tests that often accompany them, return to normal.

If your very thin child is found to have high cholesterol, anorexia is a likely cause, particularly if previous tests have found cholesterol to be normal, and there is no family history of high cholesterol. You should be careful how this information is passed on to your child, since it may trigger even more stringent restricting. It is helpful to tell your child that the heart problems anorexics face are unlike the kinds of heart problems some adults have; malnutrition can dangerously shrink and weaken her heart, but she is certainly not suffering from the hardening of the arteries some adults develop on long-term, high-fat diets.

Instead of reducing dietary fat to lower cholesterol, as an adult might be advised, the anorexic child needs to increase fat intake and actually reduce consumption of fruits and vegetables (which fill their stomachs and make it difficult to eat anything else) to achieve a lower cholesterol level.

One of my patients, Allison, was advised by her psychiatrist of her high cholesterol level. The doctor did not say anything more than, "I think you should know that your cholesterol is above normal." Allison, whom I was treating for severe anorexia, immediately removed the little bit of fat that remained in her diet and proceeded to lose more weight, ever more certain that this was the healthy thing to do. I had to inform Allison, her doctor, and her parents about the anorexia and cholesterol connection and reassure them that fat was not only okay, it was necessary to add to her diet before she could start to make progress. Allison has made a hard-won recovery and is now in graduate school.

**Nutrient Imbalances**

Low levels of magnesium, zinc, and phosphate are sometimes found among malnourished anorexics. Low levels of magnesium contribute to osteoporosis and can sometimes lead to cardiac arrhythmias, and low phosphate can contribute to weakness and fatigue. One of the unfortunate consequences of low zinc is a decrease in taste sensitivity. Anorexics often complain that food just does not have any taste to them, which further reinforces their unwillingness to eat. Though the anorexic may be losing calcium from her bones, calcium blood levels are usually normal.

The elevated serum carotene levels, or hypercarotenemia, found in many anorexics, often results in a yellowish cast to the patient's skin. This is thought to be a consequence of the malnourished liver's inability to metabolize vegetable pigments.

## Hormonal Imbalances

Anorexia affects the body's hormonal balance in profound ways. Some hormone levels are lowered, others are elevated. Hormones are necessary for development of healthy bones, growth, and the onset of puberty and maintaining a healthy energy level and mood. Many of these changes are not well understood, but they are all reversible with refeeding.

Hormones responsible for adolescent sexual maturation—estrogen in girls, testosterone in boys, and LH (luteinizing hormone) and FSH (follicle-stimulating hormone) in both girls and boys—tend to be lowered in anorexics. These neuroendocrine findings show how, hormonally, the anorexic adolescent regresses to the level of a prepubescent girl or boy.

Cassie is now graduating from high school, yet she has never had a period. Her anorexia began just as she was about to go through puberty, and she has only recently sought treatment for it. Because the anorexia has prevented normal maturation, her body looks like that of a young girl's—she is barely five feet tall, and shows very little breast development. Her doctors are worried about the health of her bones and her ability to have children.

Thyroid function tests are occasionally abnormal in anorexics, a finding that confirms researchers' observation that starvation sets the body's basal, or resting, metabolism at a lower level to conserve energy. Lowered thyroid hormone levels, like slowed heart rate and cold intolerance, dry skin and constipation, are part of the body's effort to keep functioning even as it is vastly undernourished.

The malnutrition of anorexia can cause metabolic changes that may be picked up on standard thyroid function tests. These lab findings are sometimes misinterpreted as a condition known as Euthyroid Sick Syndrome, when in fact the changes are due to starvation. The thyroid hormone treatment usually prescribed for Euthyroid Sick Syndrome will not correct an anorexic's abnormally functioning thyroid, only weight restoration will. Hormone replacement, in fact, may cause further weight loss because it raises metabolism.

Another reason not to give anorexics thyroid hormones is that they are well known to abuse such hormones in an effort to lose even more weight.

## Brain Abnormalities

Anorexic patients sometimes suffer impairments in their ability to think clearly, known as "cognitive deficits." Examples of these deficits include attention/concentration difficulties, impaired automatic processing, difficulty problem solving, inflexibility, poor planning, and lack of insight.

These characteristics account in part for the difficulty of treating entrenched anorexia. Erin, thirteen, is quite young to have serious anorexia. She has a vacant, spacey look and difficulty carrying on a coherent conversation. She seems unable to summon the energy even to project her voice, which makes her responses to my questions bare whispers. Many of my patients are exceptionally bright, and Erin is no exception. So it is surprising that she cannot remember simple statements made just minutes before in our sessions. She seems immobilized by her eating disorder, unable to make use of any of the strategies that I or her therapist suggest. She remains focused on only one thing: not eating. She refuses to let her parents watch her eat, and drinks so much diet soda that her doctor is worried she is washing critical electrolytes (minerals essential to maintaining the body's water and pH balance) from her body. Erin also has a harder time being honest than most of my patients. After several sessions, she confesses that she has been flushing her meals down the toilet.

The inflexibility of the anorexic is often striking to parents. Their formerly easygoing child now has to have everything just so, and flies into a rage if minor things don't go right.

Kelsey's mother is being run ragged by her increasingly persnickety daughter. Kelsey complains and obsesses about everything from her clothes, the noise level in the house, to of course the food that her mother makes and serves.

Kelsey's mom also notices how her daughter falls apart if plans have to be changed unexpectedly. All of these are things she used to handle with ease before she lost weight. Now Kelsey, who once had time to help her younger siblings in the morning, has trouble just getting herself ready for school.

In severe cases of anorexia, brain changes can place patients in danger of harming themselves. My patient Elizabeth, at twelve years old, weighs only 60 pounds. During our first session, she staged a tantrum, locked herself in the rest room, and would not come out, despite the pleading of her mother. Finally, we had to call a security guard to get her out of the rest room. Elizabeth's condition has made tantrums like this a common behavior of hers. Her parents have had to lock up all toxic cleaning supplies because Elizabeth regularly feels suicidal enough to drink these dangerous liquids.

Most experts believe that cognitive impairments such as those of Erin, Kelsey, and Elizabeth are related to metabolic and endocrine abnormalities associated with malnutrition, and that they improve with refeeding and weight gain. These patients may also be suffering from obsessive-compulsive or other psychiatric disorders that the emotional stress of the eating disorder has brought to the fore. If the types of problems we describe in these three cases do not begin to resolve with weight gain, you should see that your child gets a psychological evaluation; your child may benefit from counseling and/or medication.

It is also possible, however, that some of these cognitive deficits seen in anorexics may be connected to the structural changes in the brains of anorexics that have been detected by researchers in recent years, although there is no clear scientific proof of this link so far.

---

## Critical Areas

The need for swift and aggressive treatment of an eating disorder is underscored by the two areas we have described in which the ravages of eating disorders may not be completely reversible: bone mass changes and brain abnormalities. Though there is some recovery in these areas with weight gain, recent research casts doubt on any guarantee of a full recovery. Bone loss due to anorexia can occur in as little as one year and even bouts of anorexia as brief as three months have been associated with brain changes.

These findings on bone mass changes and brain abnormalities make early recognition and aggressive treatment essential for young people.

---

### Refeeding Complications

The relatively brief but dangerous period when an anorexic first begins to eat or be fed again is known as "refeeding." Before we go further, we want to stress that only severely malnourished and underweight anorexics who are refed rapidly are at risk for the refeeding problems we describe. Our hope is that your child's eating disorders will be turned around well before any of these complications become an issue. We discuss them here largely because they illustrate how dangerous serious anorexia can become.

Because rapid refeeding is almost impossible to achieve without tube feeding (liquid meals fed through a tube, which runs through the nose and into the stomach) or TPN (total parenteral nutrition; that is, liquid nutrition given directly into a large vein), refeeding complications are generally only seen in the hospital settings where tube feeding or TPN are administered to save a severely emaciated anorexic's life.

Tube feeding, moreover, which was once routinely used to treat anorexia, and TPN (a more medically complicated method of refeeding) are now rarely used for eating-disordered patients, and instead are reserved for life-threatening cases of chronic food refusal. Today, treatment is more focused on getting the anorexic to choose to eat, not simply ensuring she is receiving adequate nutrition.

In the rare instances when refeeding complications do occur, they can lead to severe myocardial dysfunction (heart muscle problems) and sometimes seizures. The severely malnourished heart, weakened and reduced in size, can also have difficulty managing the sudden increase in blood flow caused by refeeding. Although the health of the heart quickly improves with adequate nutrition, if refeeding is done too quickly, the heart can fail.

Refeeding can also result in acute dilation of the stomach, characterized by the sudden onset of abdominal pain, nausea, vomiting, and persistent abdominal distention. Often this phenomenon can be treated by inserting a nasogastric tube, which allows the removal of foods and fluids. In rare cases, surgical intervention is called for to prevent a rupture of the stomach, which is nearly always fatal.

Anorexia in the refeeding stages has also been associated with acute pancreatitis (see p. 102, for more information).

### Are Your Child's Lab Findings Too Good to Be True?

Often the need for such aggressive treatment is masked initially by the time it takes for lab findings to reflect the serious ways in which the body is being hurt by anorexia. The lowered metabolic rate of anorexics that we have described is thought to be one reason that laboratory assessments of anorexics, despite the fact that they are starving, often will appear normal in many respects. It is important, however, that you as parents not be lulled into thinking your child is fine because lab tests are normal despite the eating-disordered behavior or weight loss you have noticed. Laboratory values may be normal for quite some time and then suddenly take a dramatic turn for the worse. Children and teens with anorexia should have regular medical monitoring (routine screening blood tests, measures of heart rate and blood pressure) because, as we have said, anorexia can cause physical complications in every organ system in the body.

### Medical Monitoring vs. Full Workups

Regular medical monitoring should not be confused with the excessive medical tests that we discouraged at the beginning of this chapter, which aims to find a medical reason to explain the eating-disordered child's symptoms. Ongoing medical monitoring alerts parents and professionals to serious impending problems, and is most important when the anorexic is not making at least slow steady progress or is recovering quickly and so might be at risk for the refeeding problems we mention above.

# Medical Symptoms and Complications
## Associated with Bulimia

We have already explained that many of the symptoms of bulimia and anorexia overlap, especially among anorexics who purge, a subgroup described earlier. For ease of reading, we have separated the symptoms of bulimia from those of anorexia. But readers should understand that the following symptoms and lab findings described for bulimics also apply to purging anorexics. Extremely low-weight patients are more likely to experience the most dire consequences outlined here than those whose weight remains within normal ranges.

### Electrolyte and Mineral Imbalances

As we have said, in many ways the physiology of eating disorders is still a mystery to experts. Electrolyte imbalances, which can be detected by blood tests, are a case in point. Electrolyte imbalances are common among bulimics, since vomiting can cause them to lose valuable minerals. Yet for unknown reasons, not all bulimics develop these imbalances.

Electrolyte disturbances, most often in the form of severely low potassium levels, can cause a wide range of symptoms ranging from muscle weakness (bulimic patients may notice that they feel weak and tired), constipation, cloudy thinking, and, in severe cases, cardiac arrhythmias that can cause sudden death. Often, however, eating-disorder patients report feeling fine despite dangerously low potassium levels, a sense of well-being that can be misleading.

In cases of dangerously low potassium levels, oral supplements or intravenous solutions are often prescribed to protect heart function, although these measures are short-term fixes that cannot solve the problems caused by repeated purging. Although over-the-counter potassium supplements are available, we urge you not to attempt independently to correct your child's potassium imbalance, because supplemental potassium can easily reach toxic levels. Restoring potassium levels must be undertaken under the supervision of a medical professional who can do frequent lab tests. If potassium is not restored properly, the patient is at high risk for potentially fatal heart problems. One practical solution available to you at home is to encourage your child to eat potassium-rich foods. Almost all foods contain some potassium; fruits and vegetables are particularly good sources. Just helping your child to stop purging and to begin to eat a normal array of foods in normal amounts will go a long way in maintaining healthy potassium levels.

Even when potassium levels are normal, however, you cannot assume that a child is not purging. Many patients manage to maintain normal potassium levels despite significant purging. If, however, potassium is low and there is no other medical explanation, it is almost certain the patient is purging, either by vomiting or by abusing laxatives or diuretics.

Purging also throws the body's acid-base balance off-kilter, which is reflected in another type of electrolyte disturbance, elevated bicarbonate levels in the blood. To the unsuspecting or inexperienced doctor, these laboratory values, low potassium and elevated bicarbonate levels, could incorrectly indicate a kidney problem instead of surreptitious vomiting.

Although elevated serum bicarbonate is not so serious as the low potassium that can accompany purging behaviors, it is something that can be tested for, and is a much more reliable marker than potassium for purging behaviors. For this reason, some doctors order this test when they suspect purging, even though potassium levels are normal.

The important point to remember about purging is that lab and physical changes and serious medical problems are more likely to occur when a child or adolescent is at a very low weight. (See Appendix B for more on how to determine if your child is at a dangerously low weight.) The normal or overweight child is protected to a certain extent, simply because their bodies are healthier and stronger than the malnourished anorexic's.

### Glandular Abnormalities

Sometimes the salivary glands, located below the ear and along the lower jawbone, may become visibly swollen, leading to the "chipmunk" cheeks of the bulimic. Parents may recognize this look, since these parotid glands are those that are affected by mumps. The exact cause of this symptom is somewhat of a mystery. One theory is that the glands become irritated by regurgitated stomach acid that leaks through a duct in the throat. Another is that they are overstimulated to produce enzymes to digest binged foods. It is likely that both theories are true.

The swollen parotid glands of bulimics may secrete abnormally high levels of amylase, an enzyme that digests carbohydrates. Elevated amylase levels, however, may also indicate a problem with the pancreas, such as pancreatitis or pancreatic gallstones. Blood tests can determine whether the high blood levels are from the salivary glands or the pancreas. Although it is rare, acute pancreatitis has been reported in connection with bulimia as well as in anorexia in the refeeding stage.

### Dental Problems

Repeated vomiting among bulimics and purging anorexics will eventually lead to serious dental problems. An increase in cavities is often the first dental complication, or extreme sensitivity of the teeth to heat and cold. The teeth may become chipped and ragged looking (especially if a spoon is used to induce vomiting) and the front teeth can lose their natural shine as the enamel, battered by repeated exposure to gastric acid, softens. The lingual, or back side of the front teeth, which faces the tongue, and the occlusal, or the flat top of molars, also lose their enamel and begin to take on a yellowish hue. As the enamel becomes thinner and thinner, you can see through it to the dentin, or core of the tooth. In severe cases, even the dentin is eroded as well, and the pulp of the tooth is exposed. This is extremely painful and the tooth usually dies as a result.

The gums of bulimics are often sore and may even bleed, usually the result of "toothbrush trauma." In their efforts to clean their teeth and mouths after vomiting, bulimics will often brush their teeth vigorously immediately after purging, adding significantly to existing dental damage.

Some bulimics have such naturally resilient teeth that despite significant purging it takes longer than usual for damage to occur. At first, my patient Kerrie would tell me how odd it would make her feel to hear her dentist compliment her on her wonderful teeth and their apparent health. She and I knew that she was throwing up regularly, yet even her own dentist saw no dental signs of bulimia. A good report from your child's dentist doesn't necessarily mean that your child is not purging.

In bulimics who have been vomiting for about four years or longer, dental fillings, which are more resistant to the effects of gastric acid than dental enamel, are likely to project above the surface of the teeth as the enamel around them erodes. Dental cavities may increase, probably because of the increased exposure to sugary binge food combined with the softening effect vomiting has on tooth enamel.

If you suspect your child has an eating disorder, you should alert your child's dentist at the earliest opportunity. The dentist can look for any telltale signs of purging and, if such signs are present, can discuss preventive measures available to protect the teeth. Protective measures include using a fluoride or a baking soda rinse, or rinsing with water after purging rather than brushing (which can damage teeth softened by stomach acid). Your child can also minimize erosion of their dental enamel by avoiding acidic foods such as citrus fruits or juices and even diet or regular colas.

If your child is having difficulty giving up purging, talk to your dentist about the possibility of dental sealants to protect her teeth from stomach acids. Sealants, which were developed to protect the teeth of children prone to cavities, are clear coatings that dentists bond into the grooves of teeth that are particularly subject to decay. While sealants clearly are protective, some dentists are reluctant to use them as they may reduce the bulimic's incentive to recover. Another problem is that sealants are difficult to apply well on the teeth that need them the most. If they are poorly applied, they can make dental hygiene more difficult for the patient.

An alternative to sealants that dentists prefer to use is custom-made, fluoride-filled dental trays that actually protect the teeth from direct contact with purged stomach fluids and improve the resistance of the enamel to acid dissolution.

Another advantage of enlisting your dentist in your cause is that your child may be more willing to listen to him or her talk about the high risk of future dental problems than you. Hearing from a dental authority that the appearance and health of their teeth may be permanently affected by purging can have quite a positive impact on the child who is just starting to experiment with purging.

## Throat and Esophageal Problems

Chronic, self-induced vomiting leads to a number of problems that result from the sensitive tissues of the throat coming in contact with harsh stomach acid. Swallowing may become painful or difficult. Hoarseness and a chronic sore throat are common.

Bulimics who frequently self-induce vomiting will experience a diminished gag reflex. Because of this, or because in some cases bulimics are not able to "learn" to self-induce vomiting easily, they may resort to forcefully stimulating their throats to induce vomiting. They may use elongated objects in increasingly vigorous efforts to self-induce vomiting. I have had several patients who after accidentally swallowing either a toothbrush or a spoon have had to have the "instrument" surgically removed. Behaviors such as this can sometimes lead to injuries to the surfaces of the back of the throat, which can in turn become infected.

Libby, a college student, told me how embarrassed and scared she was to tell her roommate that she needed to go to the emergency room because she had swallowed her toothbrush. Once there, she was chagrined to overhear a doctor asking a group of interns if they could identify the object in her X rays. None of them could; they had never heard of bulimics going to such lengths to purge.

Bulimics run the added risks of rare but potentially fatal complications such as tears in the esophagus from frequent vomiting. Tears are indicated when there is blood in the vomit. Although it is only in rare cases that the presence of blood indicates a life-threatening esophageal rupture or a tear serious enough to require immediate medical attention, any blood in the vomit should be taken seriously, and the child should be seen promptly by a medical professional. At the very least, the presence of blood in the vomit indicates significant purging.

Most bulimics find the presence of blood disturbing, something of a wake-up call telling them of the seriousness of their situation. Parents can use this opportunity to open a dialogue about the gravity of future problems if the bulimia is not addressed. Marta was sure she was dying when she first noticed traces of blood in the toilet bowl after she had vomited. Her parents made sure she was evaluated by a physician known for her work with eating-disordered patients. Bess's doctor, on the other hand, minimized the blood, saying, "It just looks like a lot of blood because it is diluted in water," and noted that Bess had only microscopic abrasions in her throat that were nothing to worry about. Though this is often true in such situations, this physician missed a golden opportunity to get her to see the seriousness of her eating disorder.

### Hand and Eye Problems

Bulimics who vomit by manually stimulating the gag reflex may develop calluses or scars on the backs of the fingers and across their knuckles from repeated contact with the teeth. Experienced doctors will recognize these marks as "Russell's sign," named after the researcher, Gerald Russell, who first described it in 1979.

Eight months after she stopped purging, Sophie told me that one of the best things about her recovery was that she no longer had to make sure to keep her hands out of view. While she was bulimic Sophie worried that eventually someone would figure out she was bulimic from how red and inflamed the back of her hands had become.

Vomiting, and the increased pressure on the eyes that it causes, is the likely cause of burst blood vessels in the eyes of bulimics and purging anorexics. Known as conjunctival hemorrhages, this reddening of the eye is usually transient, and although scary-looking, is not dangerous. As with esophageal tears, such hemorrhages can present an opportunity for you to discuss the disorder with your child, sometimes even providing the excuse your child has been looking for to accept help from you.

One of my patients suffered another, more serious, consequence from forcible vomiting: a retinal detachment, which required laser surgery to repair.

Another eye-area symptom is petechiae. These small red dots are caused by minute amounts of blood that escape into the skin around the eyes when vomiting is forcefully induced.

Lucy's reddened eyes were the first clue her parents had that she was engaged in self-induced vomiting. They knew that she was anorexic, but Lucy told me she was a master at hiding the evidence of her purging and had successfully kept that part of her disorder a secret. Then her mother confronted her about her hemorrhages and wondered "out loud" if Lucy could possibly be vomiting. Lucy confessed immediately, relieved she could finally allow her parents to help her with her purging habit.

## Gastrointestinal Problems

Vomiting or chronic abuse of laxatives can result in gastrointestinal bleeding. Persistent vomiting can also cause the problem of spontaneous regurgitation, or reflux. Frequent purging causes the lower esophagus to relax, making it easy for the contents of the stomach to rise up into the throat or even mouth. When the bulimic leans over after eating or burps, for example, sometimes for no apparent reason, she will spontaneously vomit.

Many bulimics experience this reflux as extreme heartburn. The esophagus becomes inflamed, which can in serious chronic cases progress to precancerous changes in the esophagus.

Another complication that requires immediate attention is gastric rupture, when the stomach becomes so full it literally bursts. Sometimes an extremely large binge cannot be purged because it changes the pressure in the gut, making it impossible to vomit. Lisa had to be rushed to the emergency room one weekend after bingeing on a big bowl of chocolate chip cookie dough. The dough expanded in her stomach, causing it to rupture. (See p. 105 for more information.)

## Bowel Problems

Bulimics who chronically abuse laxatives may become dependent on them to stimulate bowel movements. As the colon stretches and loses its muscle tone, sufferers may experience chronic and severe constipation and an uncomfortable sense of fullness and even pain. In severe cases of long-standing laxative abuse, adult patients have been known to permanently lose bowel function and be doomed to life with a colostomy bag.

## Fluid Imbalances

The feeling of emptiness and even the changes in body weight patients experience after self-induced vomiting and/or laxative or diuretic abuse convinces them that they have rid their bodies of binge calories. In fact, however, their main achievement is a temporary reduction in body fluid. Researchers have proven that the stomach and intestines retain significant calories in spite of self-induced vomiting. Laxatives rid the body of only about 10 percent of calories consumed, and diuretics have no effect whatsoever on caloric retention. The chronic purger, however, is often convinced that she is losing weight because she feels lighter after purging. She eventually discovers that purging does not rid her body of all the calories consumed during bingeing, and that the sad fate of most bulimics is weight gain.

Purging can sometimes even cause the exact opposite effect that the anorexic or bulimic desires. Chronic vomiting and laxative or diuretic abuse leads to dehydration. Dehydration in turn stimulates the body's renin-aldosterone system, which helps the kidneys regulate the body's fluid and electrolyte balance. The result is "rebound water retention," in which the kidneys begin to reabsorb fluid to make up for what was lost by purging. A vicious cycle begins in which the fluid and electrolyte losses of purging cause the body to hold on to even more water and electrolytes. The bulimic feels as if she is "retaining" water, which in fact she is. This is a situation that might tempt the bulimic to try a different form of purging, such as diuretics, when previously she may have used self-induced vomiting or laxatives. The dehydration continues or worsens, and the cycle starts over again.

Diuretics are rarely used by children and young adolescents because they are less likely to be aware that diuretics can dramatically affect body weight by causing loss of fluid. Younger patients, just by virtue of being younger, are also less likely to have access to prescription diuretics. Most young patients who do abuse diuretics take over-the-counter brands such as Aqua-Ban and Diurex, which their mothers may have on hand for premenstrual water retention. I advise parents not to keep diuretics and laxatives in easy view in the family medicine cabinet.

Abusing diuretics signals a serious problem that should be addressed immediately. Nonprescription pills in and of themselves are not very effective and consequently rarely cause health problems; what they can do, however, is confound the doctor's assessment of a patient's urinalysis by masking indicators of chronic vomiting. Doctors often routinely check the urine of bulimic patients. Simple tests can show if the patient is chronically vomiting. If the patient is using diuretics, however, the diuretics change urine chemistry, resulting in false normal readings. If you or your child's doctor suspects diuretic abuse, urine can be tested for this.

Prescription diuretics are far more dangerous than over-the-counter brands, sometimes causing weakness, nausea, heart palpitations, frequent urination, constipation, and abdominal pain. Chronic use can permanently damage the kidneys, potentially leading to a lifetime of dialysis.

### Kidney and Pancreatic Problems
Purging can lead to impaired kidney function caused by chronic dehydration and low potassium levels associated with purging or the abuse of diuretics. As we note above, chronic abuse of diuretics has caused some patients to require dialysis.

Acute pancreatitis has been reported in connection with bulimia as well as in anorexia in the refeeding stage. With bulimia, pancreatitis is thought to be caused by the irritation of the pancreas by repeated bingeing and chronic diuretic abuse. With anorexia, pancreatitis is associated with malnutrition, although why it sometimes occurs during the refeeding stage is not well understood.

### Menstrual Irregularities, Fertility, and Pregnancy

Menstrual irregularities or amenorrhea (cessation of menstrual periods) can occur among girls with bulimia, although it is unclear whether these symptoms are due to malnourishment, weight fluctuations, or emotional stress. Underweight bulimics are most likely to have menstrual irregularities.

If untreated, bulimia, like anorexia, may result in infertility for women of childbearing ages. Eating-disorder expert Fred Hofeldt, M.D., reports that a high percentage of women seeking help through infertility clinics are suffering from either chronic, long-standing anorexia or bulimia. Remarkably, most recovered anorexics and bulimics are able to have healthy children.

For former eating-disordered patients who do become pregnant, pregnancy itself can stir up old eating-disordered behaviors, particularly bingeing and purging.

Paula came to see me years after I had treated her teenage anorexia and bulimia. She had recovered, finished college, and now was married and pregnant with her first child. Paula felt at risk for a relapse after a serious bout of morning sickness landed her in the hospital. She and I decided to return to a food plan tailored to meet the increased nutrient needs of pregnancy. Paula delivered a beautiful baby girl, and I saw her several more times after that because she just wanted to be sure she was on the right track.

Eating-disordered patients who, unlike Paula, have not been able to shake their disorder before pregnancy have higher than average rates of miscarriages, premature births, and low birth weight infants.

### A Word about Ipecac

Although bulimics rarely make regular use of syrup of ipecac, experimentation with this common, nonprescription emetic (which many families have in their medicine cabinets as a precaution in case a toddler accidentally ingests a poison) is not unusual. As many as 28 percent of bulimics have experimented with ipecac, which is believed to have contributed to singer Karen Carpenter's untimely death from an eating disorder in 1983.

Progressive weakening of skeletal muscles and heart problems have resulted from abuse of ipecac. The cardiac problems are the most serious, in some cases resulting in sudden death. Cardiac involvement, which can be detected by an electrocardiogram (EKG), is indicated by difficult breathing, rapid heart rate, low blood pressure, and arrhythmias. Early signs of ipecac toxicity are weakness, aching, chest pain, gait abnormalities, tenderness, and stiffness, especially in the neck. Ipecac is particularly dangerous because it builds up in the body; doctors warn patients that taking it regularly or even with some frequency means they are building up a lifetime cumulative dose.

We advise parents who no longer have toddlers in the house to get rid of their supply of ipecac. As little as three standard one-ounce-sized (30 ml) bottles of ipecac, even if taken in small doses over a long period of time, are toxic enough to be fatal. If you suspect your child has used ipecac, an electrocardiogram, an echocardiogram, and a thorough medical evaluation are in order.

### Brain Abnormalities

There has been far less research done among bulimics than among anorexics on the subject of cognitive impairment. One research group did, however, find impaired cognitive performance in chronic bulimics. Brain-imaging studies have also shown some structural changes in some but not all tested bulimics.

### Insulin Refusal: A Dangerous Temptation for the Type 1 Diabetic

Although insulin-dependent type 1 diabetes is much less common than type 2 diabetes, those that it does affect are primarily children, adolescents, and young adults. Unfortunately, eating disorders are becoming increasingly common among insulin-dependent diabetic adolescents who have figured out that when they stop using insulin or reduce their dose, they lose weight. If a diabetic does not take insulin, then sugar, the basic cellular fuel, cannot enter the body's cells and is excreted into the urine. Although the diabetic may continue to eat normally, her cells in effect starve, and weight loss results. Most children before they are diagnosed with diabetes lose weight for this very reason.

The diabetic who fails to take insulin can suffer serious long-term consequences, including vision and heart and related circulation problems. In the short term, avoiding insulin can result in abdominal pain, nausea, blurred vision, headache, and general malaise. Diabetics with eating disorders have been found to have a higher rate of early eye, kidney, and nerve damage than do diabetics without eating disorders.

## Medical Complications Associated with Binge-Eating Disorder

### Obesity

Binge eating alone is not associated with many immediate health problems. Approximately half of those suffering from binge-eating disorder eventually become obese. Long-term obesity is associated with a variety of well-known physical complications such as high blood pressure, high cholesterol, type 2 diabetes, and heart disease. Obesity is also associated with degenerative arthritis, gallbladder disease, and a risk of cancer, especially increased breast, prostate, and colon cancers. For those whose obesity persists into adulthood, the risk of developing any of these conditions rises as body weight increases. Lab tests that can indicate health risk associated with body weight are blood pressure, cholesterol, lipids, and blood sugar. It is important to remember that these well-known complications arise only after obesity has been an issue for years, and can be prevented by addressing a binge-eating problem early on.

## Type 2 Diabetes

The biggest risk for children and teens who binge eat their way into obesity is type 2, non-insulin dependent diabetes. As obesity among American children has increased, so has type 2 diabetes. Until recently, this form of diabetes was almost exclusively a health risk to genetically susceptible, obese adults. Obesity is thought to make cells "insulin resistant" so the pancreas must produce increasing amounts of insulin. Eventually, the overstressed pancreas cannot produce enough. Type 2 diabetes is treated with a regular eating plan and weight loss. Because the high levels of blood sugar in type 2 diabetics increase risk of heart disease along with a host of other serious medical problems, medical experts are quite concerned about the recent increase in type 2 diabetes in children and adolescents.

## Gastrointestinal and Bowel Problems

Children who engage in binge eating will be troubled by abdominal pain, bloating, and constipation, symptoms that usually are not of any serious health consequence. More serious are symptoms of stomach dilatation, caused by binge eating in the extreme. These include abdominal pain accompanied by nausea, vomiting, and abdominal distention. Because these symptoms may indicate impending stomach rupture, it is important to seek immediate medical attention. When stomach rupture occurs, the results are often fatal.

# In Summary

A serious eating disorder has the potential to affect and disrupt virtually every system of a person's body. When the body so affected belongs to a child or an adolescent who is still growing, the results can be particularly heartbreaking to witness. We hope that this chapter will serve first to inform you and your child of the dangerous potential consequences of a serious eating disorder, and second, to deter your child from engaging in such behaviors. Remember, almost all of the conditions and lab findings discussed in this chapter are reversible with weight gain or the cessation of bingeing and purging. It is your job as parents to see that your child gets the medical attention that she or he needs, and that you do everything in your power to reverse the disorder as quickly as possible.

# PART TWO

# TAKING

# ACTION

Now that you are familiar with the different types of eating disorders and disordered eating, as well as their various causes, risk factors, and medical consequences, we can begin to discuss how to take action to begin combating your child's disorder. In this part of the book we will offer suggestions on how to broach the first difficult conversation with your child about his or her eating issues, and how to help a friend who is struggling with food problems. We will also look at parental body image and the influences of school, friends, and summer camp on a child's eating disorder.

# 7

# Breaking the Ice:
# How to Open the Discussion

Few things are harder than confronting an eating-disordered child for the first time and offering help. You are afraid you will encounter resistance, anger, even outright hostility. How can you negotiate this difficult conversation without losing your temper, widening the communication gap between you and your child, or making her retreat even further into her eating-disordered behavior? In my practice, I have been struck by the number of times parents of patients have told me that what they need are actual words to say to their child. This chapter responds to those requests, drawing on the latest research in problem solving and communication, as well as on my own clinical repertoire, to compile our collection of "words that work." We also owe a large debt of gratitude in this chapter to Douglas Stone, Bruce Patton, and Sheila Heen of the Harvard Negotiation Project, whose excellent and useful book, *Difficult Conversations* (Penguin Books, 1999), I have recommended to many parents.

We will first start with a sample dialogue to show how the difficult initial confrontation with your child might unfold. Then we will deconstruct the dialogue, showing you how you can tailor this conversation to fit your needs, and point out critical junctures and turning points to look for.

It is a normal reaction for teens, especially, to feel judged and attacked when their parents raise any topic that could possibly be interpreted as critical. In order to keep the conversation on the right track, you will have to work hard to reassure your child that being critical is not your intention. If the conversation becomes heated, your child will focus on how they have been wronged by you instead of on their eating problems. This can serve as a subconscious (or sometimes conscious) diversionary tactic that keeps parents at bay while the eating disorder remains unexamined.

## Karen and Monica's Difficult Conversation

Monica's mom, Karen, waits for a quiet moment to begin the conversation she has been dreading, the conversation in which she plans to confront her daughter about her increasingly alarming eating behaviors. Over the summer Karen and her husband, John, noticed that Monica's food intake had diminished. She was not only eating less, she was also careful to avoid high-fat foods, she ran every day, and Karen suspected that Monica might be throwing up. Monica, who had just completed her freshman year of high school, was spending a lot of time in the bathroom after meals. It was suspicious, Karen thought, how Monica always seemed to run the water when she was in the bathroom and how when she emerged she often looked as if she had been crying, with reddened eyes and flushed face.

Karen is so nervous about the conversation that she has even gone as far as role-playing the conversation with Monica's older sister, Pam, who is also concerned about Monica, and rereading her favorite passages in *Difficult Conversations.*

Karen and Pam talk about how Karen needs to remember to listen for and acknowledge Monica's feelings and point of view, to try not to blame Monica for her eating problems but instead focus on what she herself can do differently to be of help. Karen reminds herself to be calm, to avoid being accusatory, and above all, give Monica an opportunity to talk about what is going on.

Unfortunately, Karen's husband is away on a monthlong business trip. Karen feels this is too urgent to put on hold, however; every day that passes, Monica seems to be sinking further into her disorder.

Karen takes a deep breath and knocks on Monica's door. "Hi, honey. Can I talk to you for a moment? This is hard for me to say, but I am really worried about you. I know that you are losing weight and you never eat with us anymore." Monica protests that she has been busy with school and sports activities and then says emphatically, "I am *not* losing weight!" In a calmer tone, she adds, "Mom, you really don't need to worry about me. I am fine, just fine."

Karen plunges on, hoping she can stay calm. "I appreciate that you don't want me to worry, honey, but it's my job to. If it's your activities that make it impossible for you to eat with us, we'd better do something about your schedule or figure out another way for you to get the food you need." They talk a few minutes about how hectic high school is compared to middle school. Monica seems almost relieved to be discussing scheduling issues.

Karen guides the conversation back to the topic she has rehearsed. "Have you been feeling okay? I've noticed that you complain about how cold you are. I think this is often a sign you aren't getting enough to eat."

"Mom, like I said, I'm fine, you don't need to worry," Monica says.

"I know you don't like to hear this, but I *am* worried that you aren't doing a good enough job with eating, and that it's affecting your health. Pam is worried about you, too, especially since Beth (Monica's best friend since grade school) asked her what was going on with you."

Monica is teary now, slowly shaking her head. "Mom, I can take care of this." Karen, also in tears, but able to speak, responds first by putting her arms around her daughter. "I hope you can, but I want you to know that I am here to help in any way I can. We all are. Dad is worried, too. He and I have been talking about this for a while now. I know enough about these problems to know that often seeing a doctor is helpful. Monica, you are going to have to let me know how I can help. Do I need to fix a plate of food for you and leave it in the fridge? Are there foods I can get for you at the store that could help? Do we need to get you in to see a nutritionist or therapist soon?"

"Mom, please don't, I'll be fine," Monica insists through her tears.

"Okay, okay, honey, but I'm here, don't you forget, ready and willing to talk about any of this stuff at any time, day or night. And if you need some professional help we can make that happen, too."

Karen leaves a few minutes later, hoping she didn't take this first conversation too far. Often it takes a number of talks to figure out what to do next. Karen suspects that her daughter is in serious trouble and will likely need professional help. As she replays the conversation for her husband over the phone, she realizes that she has made a good start. She talked specifically about her major concerns and observations, and she let Monica know that professional help is available. Karen wished Monica had been less defensive and that she had taken a little more time to ask Monica what she thought was going on, but all in all it was a good start.

## Plan Your Conversation in Advance

Here are some things to keep in mind as you prepare to confront your child about a suspected eating disorder:

- Be calm, and do your best to stay calm.
- Avoid accusations.
- Don't alienate your child by monopolizing the conversation. Simply explain how your child's eating problems make you feel, how you are afraid, upset, worried.

- Give your child an opportunity to talk about her own feelings and concerns. What is it about her eating-disordered behaviors that works for her? Recognize that the eating disorder probably has some positive aspects for your child.
- Avoid unproductive arguments about how harmful or dangerous your child's behavior is; ask instead how you can help.
- Try role-playing in advance.

## Put Yourself in Your Child's Shoes

A mistake parents often make is that they are so consumed with worry about their child's disorder and fear about what will happen to them because of it that they become incapable of listening to and understanding their child's point of view. Though it can be hard to be curious about your child's motivations, fears, and insecurities when you are in a state of panic about his health, you must try to calm down and return to that point of curiosity. If you do, you may learn how you can truly, constructively, be of help, instead of simply standing by, wringing your hands, and haranguing your child for his poor judgment in developing an eating disorder. Your child must feel heard, must feel that you understand what he is saying and what he is feeling. Your child must feel cared for. Ask questions, paraphrase to make sure you understand. Tell him, "Help me understand."

## Avoid the Blame Game

Notice that Karen scrupulously avoided blaming or accusing Monica, which would have been a surefire way to ensure an unproductive conversation. When you focus on blame, it becomes difficult to get a clear picture of each person's point of view, and how to fix the problem. Blame only engenders defensiveness and a "tuning out" of parental input.

Avoiding anger goes hand in hand with avoiding blame. Do not approach your child when you are seething with anger, or even feeling annoyed or put out, but when you are feeling calm and able to think rationally.

Remember that your child's intentions were probably good: She wanted to improve herself, she wanted to eat more healthily, she wanted to be in control, she wanted to be more popular. It is easy for you to take your child's eating disorder personally ("she is trying to defy me, worry me, embarrass me"), but an eating disorder rarely starts out with this motivation.

Remember also that if your child is not asking for your help, as in the case of Karen and Monica, you need to tread lightly as you broach the topic of your concerns.

## Words That Work

The following is a selection of "words that work," opening lines, phrases, and responses that can help set a conversation that is careening out of control back on track, defuse tense situations, and in general come to your aid when you are floundering in a difficult conversation. Keep in mind that these are just suggestions to get the conversation going. By internalizing the rationale behind these lines, you will feel free to improvise and come up with the most appropriate words for your particular situation.

**Opening Lines**

First, think about things that you might say to open the conversation. Try to ask questions instead of making statements, and seek answers instead of dispensing advice.

Focus on one or two of the most pressing issues that concern you, and don't recite a litany of concerns that will overwhelm your child. Remember, your aim is to understand what is going on and to jointly come up with remedies.

Possible opening lines are:

- "I'm worried about your _____ [eating habits, weight loss, the amount of time you spend exercising], are you concerned?"
- "I've noticed that you aren't eating much at dinner."
- "I know this is hard for me to talk about and for you to hear, but I am pretty sure you've been throwing up, and that worries me."

This last statement illustrates how to be specific about both your concerns and your feelings about your concerns. Of course, if your child says, as she might, "I don't want to talk about it," you will be tempted to comply and drop the subject for fear of making things worse. You will probably be worried that your child will feel criticized and hurt if you elaborate on your concerns. It is normal for you to worry that she will get angry at you.

As a concerned parent, you know that you are addressing these issues because you love your child. The topic must be pursued, and the situation must be discussed for the sake of your child's health and well-being. If you are tentative yet sincere, not authoritarian and hysterical, your words are more likely to be heard.

You will have to be the judge, as Karen was, about how far to take the first conversation. As long as you are committed to bringing up the issue again, you should trust your intuition about how far to push a difficult conversation.

## Exploring Your Child's Concerns

Once you have opened the conversation (probably the most difficult part), you can move on to an exploration of your child's concerns. Remember, try not to open by airing a laundry list of your own worries and concerns. What matters here is what your child is feeling and how you can better understand those feelings. From there you have a shot at coming up with some creative solutions.

Here are some suggested exploratory statements. Instead of bombarding your child with all of the below, try picking one or two and making them your own:

- "Are you happy with your eating patterns or food behaviors?"
- "What would you say your major eating problems are?"
- "Which of your eating problems or symptoms bother you the most?"

Because eating-disordered behaviors are almost always an attempt to solve another problem, you should be respectfully curious about what the underlying problem is. Try saying:

- "I know enough about eating problems to know that they are often a way of dealing with other worries. Is there anything that is bothering you?"
- "I am trying to understand how the eating disorder helps you cope with _____ [depression, anxiety, boredom]. If it helps, I can understand why it would be hard to give up."
- "So it is not that you think this is the right or the best way to live, but rather that it beats the other alternatives that seem available to you right now."

Remember that it is not productive to argue with someone about how they feel. They feel how they feel, period. You want to aim to understand *why* your child is feeling the way she is and to give her a chance, without criticizing her, to explain these thoughts and emotions.

It is not unusual by this point to have hit a nerve. In Karen and Monica's conversation, both of them get teary-eyed, yet Karen keeps her head and carries on, making it to the most important part of the conversation, her expression of concern and her offer to help.

Your child might get misty-eyed, or even cry or sob. Your natural tendency will be to say, "Please don't cry, everything is going to be all right, I didn't mean to upset you." While all of this may be true and you may want to say these very words (or give your child a hug, as Karen does with Monica), don't let comforting or reassuring your child distract you from your purpose of beginning to talk constructively about solutions. Give your child a moment to collect herself and then move ahead by focusing on acknowledging that she is upset and that this is a normal reaction.

Remember that an important goal in these early conversations is for your child to feel understood and that her point of view is important. We do this by letting her know that what she is saying has made an impression on us, that how she is feeling matters to us, and that we are trying our best to understand her.

### Sharing Your Feelings

The authors of *Difficult Conversations* remind us that being able to describe your feelings is necessary before you can both productively solve the problem at hand. They explain that beginning sentences with the simple phrase "I feel . . ." is extremely effective. You want to take a few moments to talk about how you feel, but be careful not to overwhelm your child with your feelings, especially in preliminary conversations.

Naturally, your child may feel very differently than you do about her situation. The key to successfully sharing your feelings is that while you do this, you also work hard to let your child know that her feelings matter, that this is not a one-way street.

### Sharing Information

Once you have given your child a chance to express her point of view and her concerns and you have shared your feelings, this is where you can begin to share more factual information from your point of view. It is important to be honest, to describe what you are seeing and why you are concerned.

Remember also to keep it tentative, in an information-seeking mode, and curious, not didactic or preachy. When children are first confronted about an eating disorder, even as gently as we advocate in this chapter, the most common first reaction is denial. The following approaches can help you keep the conversation going in spite of your child's vigorous assertion that everything is fine.

You might say:

- "I don't know if this fits you, but . . ."

Karen uses this approach when she says during a later conversation with Monica, "I had a friend who had eating problems. She told me that it wasn't that she didn't want to eat, but that she was afraid to eat." Karen is able to use what she knows about her friend's eating to explore Monica's problems, yet without sounding as if she is confronting her.

- "Everyone is different, I wonder what it is like for you _____ [when your friends/siblings/coaches are so concerned, or when you have so little energy you fall asleep every night after dinner]."
- "I don't know if this will concern you, but _____ [weight loss reduces brain and heart size and saps the natural strength of bones]."

Beware of too much information sharing. When confidences are broken, the effect on a dialogue can be more negative than positive. Karen let Monica know that she was worried that her eating was affecting her health. She also let Monica know that her sister, father, and best friend were concerned, too. It is tempting to do this because it corroborates your concerns. But as is often the case, Monica felt uncomfortable knowing that she had been the topic of conversations held behind her back. She felt betrayed by her friend and sister because they had not come directly to her with their concerns. These issues dominate Karen's next conversation with Monica and distract from the points Karen wants to make. In retrospect, Karen wished she had stuck to her own concerns.

### Problem Solving

Let's say the conversation up until this point has gone as smoothly as can be expected and both you and your child have had a chance to describe how you are feeling. Now you are ready to brainstorm, to come up with some solutions to the eating-disordered behavior you are finally beginning to discuss.

The key once again is collaboration, letting your child know that her opinions and feelings matter, and that you want to help. You want to guard against blaming your child if things do not go as you hoped. Instead you should take some more time to listen to and understand the nature of her difficulty. (For more on collaborative problem solving see chapter 4, p. 56.)

Some suggested problem-solving openers:

- "Let's see if together we can figure out how to solve your difficulties."
- "What can you do this week to improve your eating?"
- "Is there anything I can do to be of help?"
- "How can we keep your doctor happy?" This is quite effective if your child's doctor has outlined some goals, such as gaining a certain amount of weight, decreasing exercise, or decreasing purging.
- "Let's experiment . . ."
- "Let's figure out what went wrong."
- "Can I fix a plate for you?" or "Can I sit with you at snack time?"

Sometimes, when a child seems overwhelmed, parents have to be proactive and suggest, as Karen did, some practical help. If your child declines your help, however, you need to accept the denial and let the issue drop.

**Play the Role of Cheerleader**
Once you have openly addressed the issue and you and your child agree that you are going to help them lick their eating disorder, a large part of your role as parents will be as cheerleader and morale booster. When the going gets tough, you must be there for your child with gumption-filled words that encourage and inspire confidence. Even corny analogies like "Let's work on this like a fear of heights" or "Let's get back on the horse" are surprisingly helpful. (For more information, see chapter 11, p. 187.) A nonthreatening and hopeful way to review how your child is doing is to ask, "So what has improved since we last talked?"

**Be the Voice of Reason**
Keep in mind that recovery from an eating disorder is usually slow and that there will be ups and downs, progress offset by regressions in eating-disordered behaviors. Once your child can see and admit that she has a problem, the natural tendency of wishful thinkers (meaning all of us, to varying degrees) is to expect more rapid changes than can be reasonably achieved. The discouragement that can result can lead to a relapse instead of recovery.

Like most parents, Karen secretly hoped that after her success at opening the conversation about Monica's eating disorder, Monica would miraculously be cured. Yet Monica continued to undereat and lose weight, and Karen had to come to grips with her disappointment and anger at what she perceived as their lack of results. Over time, Karen realized that eating problems are rarely solved overnight and that she needed to measure success one step at a time.

Try to temper the expectations of both your child and yourself by saying:

- "Let's be really sure you can _____ [eat a bigger dinner, add a slice of cheese to your sandwich, or add a bagel to your breakfast]. If you aren't sure, what can you be sure you can do?"

Try turning the focus on yourself, and how you can make your child's difficult situation easier by saying:

- "Do you need more or different help than you are getting from me or us?"

Karen had several good ideas about how she could help Monica, including offering to shop for foods Monica was comfortable eating. Although she shared her ideas before Monica was ready to hear them, Monica eventually accepted Karen's offer. Karen, meanwhile, learned a valuable lesson in patience.

### Be Prepared to Discuss Weight Issues

Because weight issues are likely at the center of your child's problem, you need to be prepared with ready answers when the topic arises. If your child is underweight and needs to gain weight, he will need your help in accepting and achieving this. (See chapter 11, p. 196, for tips on how to do this.) The following are some responses to common weight-related issues that can arise when you talk to your child with eating disorders. Chapters 10 and 11 will give you the background you need to confidently make and defend the following statements:

- "The fact that your weight is going up as you eat more might mean that your metabolism is healthy." (If your anorexic child is upset by her success in achieving a healthier weight.)
- "People gain weight from bingeing, not from normal eating." (If your child is a binge eater or bulimic and is worried that normal eating will cause weight gain.)
- "Breakfast followed by regular eating throughout the day will calibrate your hunger and fullness."
- "No food in and of itself is fattening."
- "Eating enough protein will keep you from overeating."
- "I wonder why, since you understand that _____ [purging, skipping breakfast, avoiding fat] doesn't help you lose weight, you continue to do it?" (This comment should be delivered with a heartfelt sense of curiosity, otherwise it might be taken as being critical or sarcastic.)

### Countering Denials

If your child is like most, he will at first try to deny the problem, just as Monica did with Karen. Or he may tell you it is none of your business. Some sample responses to this denial are:

- "It's my job to worry about you."
- "I'm worried that you are not doing a good enough job of eating."

### Lay the Groundwork for Your Next Conversation

You can take a page out of the professional's handbook here by, at the end of your conversation, building in a check-in time to revisit the issue and see what has changed.

At the end of your conversation, try saying:

- "Let's talk again in a week." (Or, if you are really worried, in several days.)
- "Let's see where you are in a week."

**Keep the Dialogue Open over the Course of Your Child's Recovery**
Because recovery from an eating disorder is often a long and arduous process, it is important to adopt the conversational tools and techniques we describe in this chapter for the long haul. Our approach is not about a short fix, but a fundamental shift in the way your child approaches food, eating, and exercise, which takes time to achieve.

Since you will be having many conversations over the course of your child's recovery, think about what worked and what did not work in previous conversations.

If your child has responded in anger, this is a sign that you need to learn more about her feelings and thoughts on the issues under discussion. The typically slow pace of recovery from an eating disorder often frustrates parents, who can become so impatient that they say things they regret such as, "I give up," or "I don't care." While ill advised, such comments are not irredeemable sins. Remember that you can always fix interpersonal snafus by being willing to discuss them, even when some time has elapsed since your initial comment.

**When Your First Effort Fails**
If the conversation goes wrong, when things cool off you can, as *Difficult Conversations* advises, talk about how to talk about the difficult subject in a way that is helpful. What if, for instance, during Karen and Monica's conversation, Monica had rejected Karen's opening conversational gambit outright? Karen might a few days later make as the topic of their conversation the fact that they are not able to discuss Monica's eating:

"Monica, I know when I've tried to bring this up before, it's just exasperated you. Can we talk about how we can begin to address this issue more comfortably? I'm worried about your eating, but I don't know how to talk to you about it. Can you give me any advice about how to talk about these issues without upsetting you?" The trick here is that Karen must really listen and make a sincere effort to alter her approach as Monica suggests.

## Words That Work for Friends

While this book is primarily addressed to parents of children struggling with eating problems, we would like to diverge here for a moment to speak to the concerned friends of an eating-disordered child or adolescent. By "friends" we mean not only peers but adult friends, coaches, and teachers.

Because friends are often the first to detect an eating problem, we feel it is important to talk about what they can do to help. Parents may also find this section helpful if your child is trying to help a troubled friend through an eating disorder, or even for words to use in approaching your own child.

### How Friends Can Help

Here are a few tips on how you can help your struggling friend:

• **Tell an adult.** A good place to start is with your school's nurse or guidance counselor or a trusted teacher. Your friend may have a serious problem. She may need help from a therapist, a nutritionist, and/or a medical professional. If so, her parents will need to be informed about your concerns. Try offering to go with her to an appointment to see the school nurse or guidance counselor. Offer to be with her when she talks to her parents, but be willing to let your friend go it alone if she chooses.

• **Be supportive but don't overwhelm your friend.** Though it may be tempting to seek moral support by asking your other friends to join you in confronting your friend, resist this impulse. Rather than trying to outnumber your friend, it is usually best to either talk to your friend one-on-one or with another equally concerned person.

If you are one of a group of friends who are concerned, first decide who is best suited to approach your friend. This might be the person who is closest to the friend, or someone who has overcome an eating disorder herself.

• **Be honest.** Tell your friend what you are seeing. Tell her why you are concerned, and be specific. For example, rather than saying, "I think you have an eating disorder," try saying, "I am worried about your health because you never eat lunch."

• **Be tentative.** If you are working up your courage to confront a friend about her eating disorder, you may be afraid that you will say the wrong thing, make things worse, or destroy the friendship.

The best way to approach difficult conversations is to be tentative and to give your friend a chance to respond, remembering always that you are not an expert and it is possible you have come to the wrong conclusion. I suggest starting with something along these lines:

• "I can't help noticing you've seemed unhappy lately. Is everything okay?" If your friend claims she is fine, as she is likely to do, you should proceed cautiously. You might say:

- "I could be totally wrong here, but I am worried that _____ [you aren't eating enough, you're exercising too much, you're throwing up your food, or you seem overly focused on your weight]."

During these difficult conversations, voice your concern that you may have said the wrong thing; you may have inadvertently made things worse or even said something that could affect your friendship. The truth, you may want to add, is that you are so worried and feel so committed to your friend that you feel compelled to risk making her angry to share your concerns.

Again, remember, you are not an expert; your objective is to get your friend to talk to an adult—a parent, school nurse, or guidance counselor.

- **Don't approach your friend in anger.** If you feel anger toward your friend (which is not uncommon), wait until those feelings subside to open the discussion, or ask someone else to be involved as well. Remember, your friend is struggling with a disorder that is not her fault, she deserves your sympathy not your anger.

- **Know your limits.** It is important to set limits on how involved you become with your friend's problem. Setting reasonable limits will help keep your involvement a positive one, not one that turns destructive to both of you. One example of setting limits is to avoid agreeing to "always" eat lunch with your friend. This can easily evolve into "I won't eat unless you eat with me," or "It's your fault I am not eating," which is not helpful for either you or your friend.

- **Beware of secrets.** A corollary to "Know your limits" is to be careful about secrets when it comes to eating disorders. Though it is natural for those with eating problems to want to swear their confidants to secrecy, be careful about promising to keep secrets if it becomes apparent your friend's health is in danger.

It is okay to agree to keep something secret for a limited amount of time, or if the friend is getting better on her own. But remember, it is better to break a promise than to ignore the fact that your friend needs more help than you can give her.

- **Don't judge her on her behaviors.** Her problems may seem puzzling to you, but as we have stressed, eating disorders are complicated conditions with more than one cause. Your friend likely does not completely understand what is happening to her.

• **Share your feelings.** People with eating disorders may have trouble expressing their feelings or may find it hard to be honest about their feelings. By being honest about your own emotions you set a good example.

• **Make sure to listen.** If you are nervous, it will be tempting to do all the talking or even to lecture your friend. The best way to show your friend that you are empathetic is to listen. Remember, you don't need to express every last thing on your mind in your first conversation.

• **Acknowledge your friend's inner turmoil.** It can be hard for your friend to fix her eating problems if she has emotional and psychological issues that she is not facing. You can help your friend consider counseling for these issues by letting her know that you won't think less of her if she sees a counselor. If you yourself have had counseling and you feel comfortable talking about it, you might share this information with your friend. Keep in mind, however, that if your friend is a minor, her parents will have to be informed in order for her to get professional help. Her parents will have to either pay for the visit or arrange for insurance coverage. Most professionals require that a parent or guardian call to make the appointment.

• **Ask what you can do to help.** Perhaps there is some kind of support she would especially like from you, such as sitting with her while she eats, standing next to her in line at the cafeteria, or giving her a call or sending an e-mail in the evening.

• **Don't be a police officer.** Avoid getting involved in ways that are not productive, such as food and bathroom monitoring. Keeping a careful watch on your friend's food and purging behaviors is not likely to be helpful to either one of you. Once your friend realizes you are monitoring her, she is likely to become more secretive. The last thing she needs is a friend telling her what to do. Her recovery needs to be between her and her parents and whatever professional help she might need eventually.

This is not to say that you should turn a blind eye to obvious signs that your friend is in trouble.

• **Acknowledge that you can't change her.** Only she can do this; it is not your responsibility to cure your friend.

• **Don't blame yourself.** You may, especially if you have had your own problems, feel blame for your friend's eating problems and feel that somehow you infected your friend. Or you may feel responsible if your efforts to help appear to fail. It is important to remember, as we have said before, that eating disorders are caused by a constellation of factors. No one person can cause another person's eating problems. Since most children and adolescents need the support of their families and sometimes a team of professionals to recover, you should not hold yourself responsible for your friend's recovery.

• **Take care of yourself.** You need to put yourself first in order to be healthy. If you can help your friend at the same time, that is fine. Taking care of yourself first makes sense because the best thing you can do for a friend is be a good example. Strive to respect yourself and love your body no matter what size it is. Show your friend that it is possible. Anything you are doing to help your friend that weakens your resolve to keep your own eating on track isn't of real help to either one of you.

### When Should You Approach Your Friend's Parents or Another Adult?

You may find yourself in the common scenario where you and your friends are the first to notice that someone in your circle is struggling with an eating disorder. You must grapple with this difficult situation, deciding whether or not to say something to an adult, and if so, who. Jennifer really wanted to speak directly to her best friend Cheryl about Cheryl's obvious eating problems, but Jennifer, a naturally quiet, shy girl, just couldn't get the words out. She decided it was better to say something to Cheryl's parents than not to say anything at all. Although Cheryl was frosty to Jennifer the next day at school, Jennifer felt redeemed when several days later Cheryl gave her hand a squeeze and said, "Thank you." They both knew what Cheryl meant.

### Strategies for Dealing with a Friend's Denial

Often, friends deny their eating problems by insisting that everything is fine, that there is no need to worry. When this happens, your best strategy is to stick to the facts and be specific. Your job as a concerned friend is to explain exactly what you are worried about: missed meals, lack of energy during sports, noticing that your friend seems only to want to talk about food or weight. It is a good strategy to present your concerns but to avoid a long drawn-out conversation in which you try to convince your friend to admit she has a problem. A better approach when your friend is in denial is to explain why you are concerned and leave it at that for the time being. If your friend does not make progress, try bringing up your concerns again in a week or two. It may take a series of conversations before your friend sees the legitimacy of your worry and is willing to do something to protect her health.

Some experts advise against any talk about weight. They worry that comments about weight loss may encourage troubled girls to lose even more weight. My advice, however, is that if your friend's weight loss is what worries you the most, you should mention it. I have seen friends pussyfoot around this issue, asking, "Have you been sick? You don't look good." Or they may even make a severely misguided comment such as, "It looks like your diet is going well." Rarely are such roundabout approaches successful at getting to the heart of the matter.

### When You Worry That Being Honest Will Affect Your Friendship

The worry that bringing up one's concern about a friend's eating disorder will harm a friendship is one that I hear often from high school–age girls. My advice is always the same: Friends should not feel obligated to confront their friends, but they may choose to when it becomes obvious the friend is suffering or is at risk for serious problems. It is realistic to expect that a friend may react negatively when confronted. You can soften the impact of the confrontation by making it clear that you are concerned, not angry, and that you could be wrong since you are not an expert. Nevertheless, as a good friend you can no longer keep your concerns to yourself. Most concerned friends tell me that *not* talking about these issues can have a greater negative impact on friendships than taking the bull by the horns and addressing the problem.

## In Summary

Confronting someone about an eating problem, whether it is a child or a friend, is hard work, and something that most of us would rather avoid. We hope that this chapter has helped give you the confidence you need to tackle such conversations, and provided you with some conversational strategies to rely on when the going gets tough.

Remember that your emotional stance is everything. If you are open, receptive, curious, honest, tentative, and work hard at understanding your child's or friend's point of view (really *listening* is crucial), no matter what words you use, your chances of success will be greater.

# 8

# Avoiding Parent Traps:
# How Improving Your Relationship to Food
# and Your Body Can Help Your Child

Having a child with an eating disorder often leads parents to wonder how they may have contributed to its onset. In this chapter we will discuss what is known about genetics and eating disorders, and more important, how your own eating habits and body image help shape your child's attitudes toward food. There is no doubt that genetics play a role in susceptibility to an eating disorder. Yet even if your child has inherited traits that make him vulnerable to an eating disorder, there is much that you can do to promote healthy eating and inoculate him against eating problems.

If you as a parent have ever struggled with diets and/or body-image issues in the past, or are still wrestling with them, you are probably concerned about how those struggles may affect your child. Some of you may worry that your occasional dieting or your worries about weight and appearance may send the wrong message to him. Some of you may be struggling with your own eating disorder as you attempt to raise your child free of the disorders that have plagued you.

As you will see, children from families where fat is taboo, where dieting is a way of life, or where weight is a source of discussion are more prone to eating disorders than children from families with more positive attitudes toward food. In this chapter we will explain how to examine the overt and covert messages your family is passing on about food. For those of you who realize that those messages have been negative and destructive ones, we will discuss how to change them and better your child's chances for an eating disorder–free future.

## Genetics and Eating Disorders

Genetic influences help explain why when a whole society is exposed to the same cultural ideal of thinness not everyone develops eating or body-image problems. Your daughter may watch the same shows on MTV and the WB network as your neighbor's daughter, and they both may read *Seventeen* magazine and admire the same fashion models, but your daughter develops an eating disorder, and your neighbor's daughter does not.

Researchers believe these differences can be explained in part by the fact that some people inherit a brain chemistry that makes them more prone to food problems. Several studies have shown that eating disorders seem to be transmitted among female family members. While researchers have not yet conclusively proven that these familial eating-disorder patterns are caused by genetics, there is enough evidence to lead most experts to believe that it is certainly part of the picture.

Researchers have also detected a genetic link between eating disorders, anxiety, and depression. Disordered eaters and those suffering from eating disorders are not only more likely to have relatives with disordered eating or eating disorders, they are also more likely to have relatives with depression or anxiety. Conversely, children and adolescents who suffer from depression or anxiety are at higher risk for eating disorders.

In some cases, specific psychological disorders or personality traits have been linked to particular types of eating disorders. If your family shares a history of obsessive-compulsive disorders or a tendency toward perfectionism, for example, you should be particularly watchful for signs of anorexia in your children, even if there is no history of eating disorders in your family. Similarly, if your family shares a history of substance abuse, you should be especially watchful for bulimia in your children, as this behavior indicates an inherited personality type that can lead to bulimia (again, even if there is no history of eating disorders in your family). Conversely, parents of children with eating problems should be on the lookout for depression, anxiety, and other psychological problems.

## More Important Than Genes: What You Do and What You Say

If your child has inherited a genetic susceptibility toward eating problems, there is not much, at least at this point in the evolution of gene therapy, that you can do to change that. More important than your child's genetic makeup are the attitudes about food, eating, and body image that you as parents pass on to him or her through both your words and your actions.

The rest of this chapter is devoted to the large, influential, and nongenetic legacy that you leave your child.

## A Word about Self-Blame

Before we launch into more detail about the effects of your own body image, food attitudes, and behaviors on your child, a word of explanation. The purpose of the following information is not to make you feel like the world's worst parents, but to illuminate an area you may have not given much thought to before. Feeling guilty and blaming yourself for past parenting behaviors is useless for the following reasons:

- First, because the causes of eating disorders are multifactorial, meaning that many factors converged to produce your child's disorder. Parenting alone is rarely to blame.
- Second, as we have said before, no good comes out of blaming yourself for causing the disorder. Feeling guilty will only render you less capable of helping your child recover and more likely to get angry at your child for not making quick progress. Parents who are unencumbered by guilt will be more capable of providing the support you will need to stay on the front lines in the battle against your child's disorder.

Our point here is that instead of wasting psychic energy on feeling guilty, it is more productive to focus on what you can do now to help your child recover. If you have younger children, you may want to do some gentle self-assessment and, if necessary, make some changes to avoid making the same mistakes in the future.

## Assess Your Food and Body-Image Attitudes

Let's first figure out if you need to do work in the area of body image and food attitudes and behaviors. If you check one or more of the following items, which indicate behaviors or attitudes shown by researchers to increase a child's risk of developing an eating problem, we suggest reading on for more on how you can adopt healthier attitudes about eating, body shape, and size. If you check none of the following items, you are setting a good example where food and body-image issues are concerned, and can skip this chapter entirely.

## Parental Attitudes Checklist

---

❑ Are you engaged in dieting or obsessive exercise? Do you worry about fat grams or calories?

❑ Do you overeat, use food to cope, eat in secret, or purge by self-inducing vomiting or by using laxatives or diuretics?

❑ Does your family discuss the weight, shape, and appearance of others in a judgmental fashion?

❑ Do you accept without criticism the dictates of the fashion industry and the ways in which the diet industry promotes a body size that is impossible (without severe dietary restriction) for normal-size people to attain?

❑ Do you show excessive concern for or interest in your child's weight, shape, and appearance? Are you critical of your child in these areas?

❑ Are you overinvolved or underinvolved in your child's "food business?"

❑ Do you respond negatively or critically to the changes in your daughter's body as she goes through puberty and develops a woman's body?

## How Your Attitudes Shape Your Child's Body Image and Eating Habits

Marla called me for advice when she could no longer ignore the now-obvious fact that her five-year-old daughter, Franki, was dieting to lose weight. Perplexed about Franki's sudden and serious interest in weight loss, Marla, in the course of our conversation casually mentioned that her husband, Bill, was dieting. Bill was following a popular high-protein diet in an effort to lose the 20 pounds he had gained over the past year. I followed up with a few questions about Franki's awareness of Bill's weight-loss efforts. Suddenly making the connection, Marla had to talk through tears to tell me that Bill had for the past year complained vocally, though always with self-deprecating humor, about his hated "love handles" and his efforts to get rid of them by eating less. Like magic, Franki dropped her interest in dieting when Bill vowed to keep his weight-loss efforts between himself and Marla. This family is lucky that their quick correction was so effective.

As parents, most of us are aware of the enormous influence that we wield over our children. And yet when it comes to certain areas, we drop the ball. Sometimes our behaviors or attitudes are so ingrained, so much a part of us, that we have difficulty seeing them as in any way threatening to our children. Dieting and food attitudes are among those "blind spots" for many parents.

Experts believe that the following factors have a direct impact on the eating attitudes and habits of children.

## Your Own Eating Attitudes and Behaviors

As psychotherapist Steven Levenkron, author of *Anatomy of Anorexia* and *The Best Little Girl in the World,* has noted, children absorb everything they hear their parents saying and observe them doing, even when it appears they are not paying attention. "Kids are listening and watching all the time," he says. "I've had anorexic patients say, 'I've watched my mother for years staring into the mirror and asking my father and me, "Do you think I'm too fat, do you think my dress is too tight, my arms are too big?"' We live in a society that doesn't let women feel adequate about their bodies."

It is true that our society makes it difficult for most women to feel good about their natural body size and shape, and that this dissatisfaction can affect our own children negatively. In my own practice, I have too often seen how a dieting child's behavior is reinforced by his or her immediate family. Before you decide to go on another diet, or begin another week on your current diet, consider these facts about the effects of parental dieting on children:

- Studies have found that if one or both parents diet, their children are more likely to have eating problems. Even hearing their parents talk about their own efforts to diet, or their desire to lose weight, increases the likelihood that children will take up dieting themselves.
- When mothers are very concerned about their own weight, their daughters are more likely to have eating problems. In particular, maternal eating attitudes and dieting have been connected to high school girls' bulimic symptoms.
- Dieting parents are more likely to be overconcerned with their child's appearance.

## Parental Criticism about Weight, Body Shape, or Size

When a child feels uncomfortable eating in front of parents because parents tease or make comments about the child's weight or body shape or size, the child is at higher risk for developing eating problems. For girls, these issues often come to the fore as they enter puberty. They develop hips and fat stores, physical changes that can make girls feel insecure and more sensitive to comments that could be construed as negative.

## Monitoring or Critiquing Your Child's Food Intake

If you critique, monitor, or limit your child's food choices, conflicts are likely to arise around food consumption. All of these behaviors are associated with eating problems. Your young teenage child naturally desires more independence at this stage, a chance to make more of his own decisions, including decisions about food and diet. Stepping up your monitoring or controlling of his food intake is an invitation to disordered eating or eating-disordered behavior.

## Encouraging Your Child to Diet

Putting your child on a special diet, pressuring your child to exercise or "get in shape," or bribing your child to lose weight or exercise with clothes, money, or activities are all dangerous behaviors. When you overtly encourage dieting, your child is more likely to have eating problems.

Leigh's parents had high hopes for their bright, pretty daughter. When Leigh gained 10 pounds the spring she turned twelve, Sandra, Leigh's mother, suggested she think about losing some weight. Maybe they could go on the latest *Good Housekeeping* diet together. "You know, Leigh," Sandra, meaning well, advised, "learning how to manage your weight will serve you well in the future. I am afraid you've inherited my hips. You won't look good in your new swimsuit unless you really watch it." Leigh was devastated. She knew that the people Sandra thought were attractive were slender and that her mom was quick to make a derisive comment when a Hollywood personality or a friend gained weight. But to hear her mom criticize her body was more than she could take. Leigh herself was hardly comfortable with the changes her body was going through and wondered if she would ever stop gaining weight.

## How You Are Influenced by Cultural Norms

Even if you do not overtly encourage your child to diet or lose weight, but send more covert messages promoting such behavior, you are still putting your child at risk for eating problems. Children are quick to deduce where parents stand on culturally influenced issues. If you know that your views on attractiveness have been irreconcilably influenced by constant exposure to media messages about the importance of being thin, you can make a conscious effort not to pass these attitudes on to your children. Hearing from parents a critical rather than accepting response to such media messages can help children begin to identify and question the wisdom of valuing thinness. (See chapter 3, p. 47, for more on this.) Even telling your child that she looks thin or trim can cause harm. Children who know their bodies are changing or are about to change may worry that they will lose their parents' approval if they gain weight. They may also conclude that Mom or Dad may like them even more if they are thinner or trimmer.

Emily's story illustrates how parents can unwittingly become complicit in their child's eating disorder. The twelve-year-old's parents take her for a checkup when she begins having "fainting spells." The "fainting" turns out to be the result of woefully inadequate calorie intake and Emily's 10-pound weight loss over the past two months. She has been restricting, counting calories, skipping breakfast, eating little or no lunch. Often she makes a show of packing her lunch in front of her mom, but then drops it into the garbage can on her way to school.

Emily's mother, Marion, is slow to recognize how her acceptance of cultural norms about weight and dieting have subtly encouraged Emily's eating disorder. Although Marion is unaware of the extent of her daughter's increasingly restrictive eating, and has said nothing to directly encourage it, she has been supportive of her "dieting," hoping that the loss of a few pounds would improve Emily's self-esteem. Marion sent other subtle messages as well, such as her quiet substitution of Diet Coke over regular Coke in their home refrigerator. The most telling episode, according to Emily, occurred on a family trip to Los Angeles. Emily, her two brothers and her parents, Marion and Nick, were enjoying themselves at a Hard Rock Cafe. Nick's meal happened to come with a brownie for dessert. As Nick was about to take a bite, Marion, with a look of disapproval and disgust on her face, grabbed the offending brownie and gave it to a passing waiter, saying, "Nick, you know you shouldn't be eating junk like that!" Marion's far-from-subtle, vigilante approach to her husband's eating led Emily to make a mental note about watching her own dessert intake.

Emily's case demonstrates how children absorb and are influenced by their parents' attitudes and beliefs, no matter how covert (or in this case, overt) they may be. By catching it early, Emily's parents, who had no idea how dangerous dieting can be for a child, are able to help her turn her eating disorder around. Nick, with a touch of irony, says they are all better off now that they all know that dieting can be trouble, especially for vulnerable teenagers like Emily.

**Menopause Coupled with Increased Worries about Weight and Size**
One group of researchers looked at the relationship of menopause in mothers to their daughters' eating behavior. The profound physical transition of menopause is often associated with weight gain, which can provoke increased concern about body weight, size, and dieting in adult women. It appears that some girls, especially girls who are going through puberty, are negatively affected when their menopausal mother diets or expresses dissatisfaction about how her own body shape is changing.

## Body Image: What Is It, and What Does It Have to Do with Eating Disorders?

Body image is both the mental picture one has of one's body and the feelings one has about his or her own body. Although body image is based on the body's actual characteristics, it can be affected by past experiences, moods, or feedback from others. In other words, while a person's body image to some degree reflects objective truth, there is also a subjective element to it, often revealing how happy the person is with herself in general. The more disordered a person's eating is, the less objective her view of her body.

People with good body image usually see themselves accurately, but do not tie their sense of self-esteem to their body weight. Some may be happy with their appearance, others may be accepting, and still others may be resigned to what they feel they cannot change. Whatever their feeling about their own weight or shape, they keep their assessment of their body separate from their sense of self-esteem.

People with poor body image have negative and critical thoughts about their bodies and often are unable to perceive their bodies' size and shape accurately. Body-image issues, or "body-image disturbances," as they are known, are a common thread that links the various eating disorders. Classic anorexics nearly always suffer from body-image disturbances, characterized by an exaggerated view of the size and shape of their own bodies. They may feel overweight or even obese, even though actually they are underweight. Or the anorexic may be convinced that certain body parts are too fat or big. Although this gross distortion in the perception of body size, or in the size of specific body parts, can happen among bulimics and binge eaters as well, it is much more common among anorexics.

For those who suffer from body-image disturbance, body image becomes inextricably linked to self-esteem; the eating-disordered person bases her self-esteem almost entirely on her evaluation of her body shape and weight, so that poor body image leads to poor self-esteem. Whereas people without eating disorders have a variety of ways to feel good about themselves, the eating-disordered person has just one: self-evaluation of her own body.

For anorexics, losing weight seems ironically to magnify body-image disturbances. Fortunately, the anorexic's ability to accurately assess her own body size and shape is usually restored with weight gain.

## Your Own Body Image and How It Affects Your Child's Body Image

As parents, examining your own body image and seeing how it has affected your child's body image is another way of understanding the profound influence you have on your child's attitudes about food, weight, and shape.

Liz, only nine, is perplexed about her mom's complaints about her own weight. After hearing these complaints over and over, Liz is likely to learn that the female body is something that must be watched, dieted, and exercised in order to keep it acceptable.

Poor body image can also develop when you teach your child that her own body is changeable, susceptible to manipulation. Nikita, naturally chubby and a bookworm at fifteen, was taken aback when her mother offered to "set her up" with a personal trainer to help her get in shape for the summer. "It made me feel like Mom thought I should do something about my body," she sadly told me. To her credit, Nikita did not internalize her mother's judgment and spiral into a bout of shame and self-loathing, as she once might have. Instead, Nikita, who after five years of working with me had grown self-assured enough to know her body was just fine as it was, stood her ground. Later, Nikita proudly repeated to me what she had told her mom that day: "Mom, I like my body just fine, so thanks but no thanks." It was stories like this that gave me insight into why overcoming her body-image problems was so difficult for Nikita.

When your child internalizes the thought that you find her body unacceptable, the risk is that when she experiences negative feelings or disappointments, she will project those onto her body, and may unconsciously turn to dieting and overexercise as a way to compensate for her negative feelings. For example, the high school student who is disappointed in her SAT scores and has poor body image may feel that though she cannot fix those scores, she can change the body she believes (and which she believes her parents believe) is fat and out of shape. She plans to diet, embarks on a strict regimen of exercise, begins to feel better and temporarily in control. Instead of learning how to employ healthy coping mechanisms, this child has turned to eating-disordered behavior to assuage disappointment. The danger is that these habits will become habitual, to the point that any disappointment, even a minor one, will trigger disordered behaviors.

## Body Image among Children

While high rates of body dissatisfaction and dieting behavior have been well documented among pre- and young adolescents, a recent surprise has been that these attitudes have been identified even among young children. Children as young as kindergarten age already have negative attitudes toward fatness in themselves and others, and children as young as third-graders are knowledgeable about dieting. In one study, one-half of children between third and sixth grade said they wanted to weigh less, and over a third wanted a thinner body shape.

## Boys and Body Image

It is important to note that boys are not immune to body-image concerns. In one study, close to half of the younger boys surveyed said they had tried either to lose or gain weight. Graham, a husky twelve-year-old, wants to trim down for the upcoming soccer season. Graham has always been on the pudgy side; it is likely that he inherited the tendency toward chubbiness from his mother and father, who themselves were larger-than-average children. Commenting on how things have changed, Graham's dad, David, said, "When I was a boy, I was told I would 'grow out of it.' And you know what? I did." Then he added, "It worries me that Graham wants to do something about his weight."

## Early Adolescence as an Assault on Body Image

Psychologist Marsha H. Levy-Warren has perceptively described the changes that occur in early adolescence: the way children become hyper-aware of how their body is becoming bigger and more adultlike, and the way they gain the ability to see themselves, their families, and the world more accurately than they did as children. Where as children they felt they were beautiful, strong, and smart, as adolescents they may be disappointed to find that in reality they are less gifted in these ways than they supposed. Levy-Warren writes, "Adolescents become acutely, self-consciously aware of their bodily changes, the social and cultural significance of those changes, and their parents' (and others') reactions to those changes."

The adolescent may also feel overwhelmed by her new role. Inside, she feels too young and not yet competent enough to shoulder the responsibilities of adulthood. Levy-Warren believes that an eating disorder at this stage can be a "secret announcement" that the girl does not feel ready to grow up.

Because this turbulent and vulnerable period is a time of heightened sensitivity about their own bodies and the changes they are going through, young adolescents can be deeply hurt by negative comments from parents or peers. You should therefore work hard during your child's early adolescence (which may begin as early as 10½ in girls and 12½ in boys) to help cultivate a strong, positive body image. You can:

- Teach your child to respect a variety of body sizes and shapes and understand that size and shape are primarily genetically predetermined.
- Foster in your child a sense of wonder about the bodily changes that come with growing up.

Gaining some insight into the biological and physiological changes that are occurring within young adolescents may help offset their newly acquired feelings of awkwardness, insecurity, and moodiness.

- Help your young teen achieve a sense of self-worth that is not based primarily on appearance.

Families that work hard to help their children develop a self-concept based on personal qualities (patience or kindness, for example) and on achievements rather than on appearance seem to do better at protecting their children from developing eating problems. Being part of a larger social community that does not make thinness a criterion for beauty is also protective. Researchers believe this is one reason that African-American girls raised in families with strong racial identities are more resilient when it comes to eating problems.

As these suggestions illustrate, even though many middle-school and teenaged children, especially girls, live in a subculture of intense weight and body-shape concerns, there are concrete, positive lessons you can teach your child that will help her emerge from the trials and tribulations of adolescence with a good body image. By fostering your child's positive body image, you are also protecting your child from eating problems and unhealthy attitudes toward food and their bodies.

Now that we have described what body image is, why it is important, and how you can strengthen your child's body image, you may be thinking that this is all pretty straightforward and obvious. Where it gets more difficult is when we turn to your own food attitudes and behaviors, namely dieting. You may talk all you want about the wonders of biology, your child's changing body, and your child's inherent good qualities. But if at the same time you diet or complain about your own weight, you are undercutting all the positive parenting messages you have so carefully passed on to your child. To begin remedying this, you can stop dieting and work at accepting your own body.

## Accepting Your Own Body Shape and Size

The best evidence available tells us that if you as parents are comfortable and accepting of your own bodies, and care for yourselves through food and exercise in a natural, healthy, relaxed, and carefree way, those attitudes and behaviors will be protective against eating disorders for your child.

We realize that these approaches may be somewhat or even quite different from your own. But both because they are healthier for you, and because of the great benefit they can be to your child, we urge you to at least be aware of them. None of us are perfect, but making your goal an attitude of acceptance and naturalness toward food, weight, and shape can take you a long way.

For those of you who cannot possibly imagine life without a diet to keep you in line and at a comfortable weight, consider the findings on p. 129, as well as these facts:

- When you diet, you are modeling restricted eating, which can set the stage for an eating disorder.
- When you diet, especially if you feel your diet has been successful, you are covertly encouraging your child to diet, and sending the message that body shape and size can and should be controlled.

**What If You Can't Stop Dieting?**
Sometimes, despite being confronted with these facts, parents find it too difficult to change what in some cases is a lifelong habit of dieting. The most realistic approach in such cases is to figure out ways to minimize the effect of your dieting on your child.

Here are some tips on how to do that.

• **Keep your own battle with weight to yourself.** Although you may be engaged in a hard-fought battle against weight gain and devote a significant amount of time to thinking about dieting, or planning your diet and exercise regimen, none of this is anything that you need to share with your child.

• **Let your child know that the dieting behavior they see among adults is in no way appropriate for them as children.** If you yourself happen to have lost weight, make sure your child knows weight loss is not what growing children should be aiming for.

• **Make sure that your child knows what to expect about her body's development as she matures.** It can help to assure your child that the body changes she is experiencing are normal. Again, you should take care not to signal to your child, through your actions or words, that being thin is important.

The following story illustrates how, if the family is grappling with a serious disorder that requires the family's full attention, it is especially important that you as parents do not start a new diet or make casual remarks about how you would like to lose weight.

Laurie, fifteen, is struggling with a serious case of bulimia. One day she comes to my office in tears, explaining how upset she is at how her dad has been talking about his need to lose weight. Laurie and I agree that Joel should attend our next session to discuss this issue.

At the next session, Joel, a rotund gentleman farmer who is semiretired, explains that his doctor has told him that his health will improve if he loses some weight. Laurie responds that she can understand why losing weight seems like a good idea for her dad, and why it is not a good idea for her. Yet whenever Joel talks about his efforts to lose weight she can't help but feel that she should diet, too. Laurie explains tentatively, "It hurts me to hear you say you are too fat. It's like you're putting my own eating-disordered feelings into words."

"But I am too fat, honey," responds Joel. "I eat too much and that has made me too fat."

"Let's see if we can compromise here," I suggest. "Both you and Laurie need to eat good, well-balanced meals to deal with your eating problems. Can we agree not to talk about the need to lose weight when the family is together? It's not good for Laurie to hear or do that kind of talking." Both Laurie and Joel nod in agreement.

The next week, Laurie tells me how much things have improved. Her dad is eating better meals, and best of all, no "fat talk." Later, Joel confides in me privately that he struggles with binge eating. He tells me that eating meals patterned after Laurie's have helped him keep his bingeing under control. And yes, he does lose a few pounds.

## If You Have an Eating Disorder Yourself

If you are a parent with an eating disorder, helping your child either avoid an eating disorder or overcome an existing one presents a unique set of challenges.

Your own disorder puts your child at greater risk of getting an eating disorder than the average child. It appears from other research, however, that with good parenting, in spite of the parent's eating disorder, the child can remain unaffected.

### Why the Eating-Disordered Parent's Child Is at Greater Risk

There are a number of reasons why an eating-disordered person's child is at greater risk for an eating disorder themselves:

- When you model eating-disordered behaviors and attitudes, your child is more likely to come to the conclusion that these behaviors are normal, and have problems in the same areas.

- Eating-disordered parents may also overtly encourage their children to diet, or covertly promote such behaviors by only serving low-calorie foods, for example.
- Often, eating-disordered parents are uncertain about how to feed their children.
- Eating-disordered moms also tend to have more concerns about whether their child is growing properly or is the right weight and shape, which can lead to underfeeding, or in some cases overfeeding.
- Mothers with eating disorders are often overly involved in their children's eating and even their playtime activities.
- Because there is a genetic component to eating disorders, the child of an eating-disordered parent will remain at higher-than-average risk, despite their best efforts at protecting their child from eating problems.

Research indicates that parents' eating-disordered behaviors have more of an effect on older children and teens than on younger children. Even if you are the parents of younger children, you will be doing yourselves and your children a great service if you do what it takes to resolve your own eating issues.

Colette told me that in trying to keep her bulimia from her five-year-old daughter she sometimes left her child outside playing in the yard alone longer than she knew was right. Colette worries that soon her daughter will ask her why she spends so much time in the bathroom, or why she often doesn't join the family for meals. Other eating-disordered parents have told me that because they restrict the amount and kind of foods in the house, they are not able to offer their children the wide array of foods they know will foster a flexible, carefree approach to eating.

**What You Can Do to Keep Your Child Free of Your Eating Problems**
If you are an eating-disordered parent and are reading this chapter, you are probably wondering how you can possibly raise a child with healthy attitudes toward food, shape, and size. My experience with both anorexic and bulimic parents, however, is that when their child's health is at stake they are able to do what it takes to provide their child with the parenting the child needs to make progress, regardless of the seriousness of their own problems.

Single mom Pauline, in and out of treatment for her own unremitting eating disorder, was able to effectively help her own anorexic daughter gain weight, much to the surprise of all the professionals who were involved.

The best approach for you to take if you are a parent with an eating disorder is to be proactive about conveying positive messages about food and eating to your child, despite your own behavior. Here are some suggestions on how to do that:

- Try to muster the wherewithal to eat meals with your children; doing so will have immeasurably positive effects on their eating habits.
- Engage an experienced nutritionist to help you learn to feed your children in a healthy way.
- In cases when one or both parents have significant eating issues of their own, you may need to arrange for your child to see a nutritionist so that you can be less involved in providing food direction.

It goes without saying that the most precious gift eating-disordered parents can give their children is to seek their own recovery. Most adults will need professional support (psychotherapy and nutrition counseling) to recover from a serious eating disorder.

## In Summary

It should now be clear to you that your own body image and attitudes toward food, weight, and appearance have a direct and powerful effect on your child's own body image, food attitudes, and behaviors. You also now have a sense of how one child can be genetically more susceptible to an eating disorder than a child from another family. Our message is that though there is little you can do to change your child's genetic makeup, there is quite a bit you can do to model positive food attitudes and behaviors to your child. Your own dieting behavior, or critical or supportive comments you may make about your child's weight or appearance, for example, can send your child one of two messages: "I am unhappy with my body, and you should be with yours as well" or "It is not what you look like that matters to me, it is who you are as a person, and what you do." We hope that after reading this chapter, you will adopt (or continue employing) an approach that sends the latter message, not the former.

# 9

# Beyond the Family Circle:
# Friends, School, and Summer Camp

In this chapter, we will talk about the role of school, friends, and forces outside the family at both the onset and in the treatment of your child's eating disorder. Sometimes starving, bingeing, or purging behaviors are noticed first at school by teachers, coaches, counselors, or nurses, or by friends who may turn to these professionals for advice on what to do. We will discuss how you can best enlist these people in your effort to turn your child's disorder around quickly. Sometimes friends can create an environment that triggers the disorder. If this is the case with your child, we will discuss ways to address this problem, and give your child the tools she needs to alter her situation.

Class trips, summer camps, boarding school, and college present other types of challenges for parents who fear their child may be at risk for an eating disorder. It is important that you prepare your child, especially if she is at risk for an eating disorder, for the experience of living away from home for the first time in these settings, where her food behavior is often a preview of things to come. We will suggest ways for you to talk to your child before she embarks on such situations, and assess whether she is really ready to be away from home.

## Friends

### "Fat Talk" and Dangerous Friends
Research has shown that among girls, the simple fact that a child's immediate circle of friends regularly discusses dieting and weight can put them at risk for disordered eating. Called "fat talk," these discussions permeate a

social atmosphere where the shared understanding is that being thin is important, and being fat is bad. When this worldview serves as the basis for friendships it can exert a remarkably powerful hold over your child. While your child's weight- and body-conscious friends may have many positive qualities, for our purposes here, we will call them "dangerous friends."

The intense bonds a child can form with dangerous friends can foster highly contagious behaviors. Peers are such an important influence, in fact, that behaviors such as your child comparing her body with that of her friends, or teasing by her peers can have more influence on whether she develops disordered eating or an eating disorder than psychological or family factors.

The following are clues that your child may be making dangerous friends, or may be feeling social pressures that are putting her at risk for an eating disorder. You should be concerned if even one of the following is true for your child, and continue on to the next section, "What to Do about Dangerous Friends":

- Your child's best friend has an eating disorder, is dieting, fasting, has body-image concerns, or is preoccupied with being thin.
- Your child frequently compares her body to those of friends, other girls at school, popular girls, and fashion models. These behaviors have been shown to predict body-image dissatisfaction, which is often the first step in the progression to an eating disorder.
- Your child competes with friends in the area of weight, shape, and appearance. Doing so makes it more likely that she will experiment with dieting.
- Your child believes that thinness is a key requirement for membership in the popular group at school. Even children as young as nine have been shown to believe that they will be more likable by being thin. These girls are at higher risk for eating disorders and poor body image.
- Your daughter believes that she is unpopular, or feels insecure, socially incompetent, or unsupported by friends. Girls who hold any of these beliefs or feelings are at higher risk for developing an eating disorder than other girls.

## What to Do about Dangerous Friends

Dangerous friends are hazardous because they may be helping to set the stage for an eating disorder in your child. You need to be alert to those risks and be ready to counter them with positive messages. Children who are at greatest risk for an eating disorder are those who are under the influence of both friends and family with body-image concerns. If you have come to believe that your child's friendship circle shares a preoccupation with body image, then it is especially important that within the family, you do everything possible to counter those concerns and messages.

In addition to the tips in chapters 3 and 8 on what you can do to promote healthy eating attitudes and habits, the following are some suggestions on how to strengthen your child's defenses against dangerous friends:

• **Encourage supportive friendships.** Researchers believe that supportive friends can actually be protective against eating disorders. (For more information, see p. 145.)

• **Educate your child about the negative impact of "fat talk," and of critiquing their own and others' bodies.** Make sure your child knows that losing weight will not make her fundamentally more likable to others. If your child replies that in fact her group selects friends largely based on weight and appearance, you can inform her that people who make such judgments about others are not very good "friend material." Teens, especially, may appear to tune out advice like this from parents, but don't be disheartened; underneath their attitude of indifference, or sometimes even irritation or hostility, most children feel cared for when parents give advice, and actually hear what their parents are saying.

### Avoid Barring Your Child from Contact with Dangerous Friends

We suggest that you wage your campaign of positive messages within the family, because it is rarely effective to bar your child from associating with children you disapprove of. Attempting this will usually result in your child turning even more to those children, or becoming reticent about sharing what she is hearing from the "barred" friends. When it comes to issues with friends, you will probably be most effective as advisors rather than rule makers. One way to play this role is to try to help your child recognize how her friends are affecting her, and to help her strategize ways to render herself immune to whatever negative influences these friends might present. In the following case study, Phoebe's mother wisely gives Phoebe room to choose her own friends, but gently points out some negative behaviors she has observed in Phoebe's new friendship group and voices her concern that Phoebe might be tempted to adopt those behaviors.

Phoebe told her mother, Roslyn, that she was thrilled to find herself a member of her middle-school class's in-group after her stand-out soccer season. Several of the most popular girls in class, who were also on the team, had made it clear that Phoebe was now one of them. An invitation to the group's first "overnight" of the new year confirmed Phoebe's hopes, and she could hardly wait for the important day to arrive. Roslyn, however, was less than excited about Phoebe's social boost. She had noticed that all of the girls in this new group were very thin, and she suspected that several of them were flirting with eating-disordered behaviors. Still, she made a point of remaining neutral.

"Did you have fun?" Roslyn asked when Phoebe returned from her weekend with her new friends.

"It was so cool, Mom. I had the best time," Phoebe gushed. Later, catching Phoebe alone while she studied at the kitchen table after dinner, Roslyn asked the usual "mom questions," such as, "What time did you go to bed?" and "Which movies did you watch?" Then Roslyn tackled the questions she really wanted to ask. "How was the food?" she began.

"That was the weird part, Mom," Phoebe answered. "Though there was lots of food out to eat, nobody ate much."

"That does seem odd," Roslyn responded. "What do you think that was about?"

"I don't know, but I do know that these girls really like to talk about food and diets."

"Did you eat?" Roslyn asked.

"Yeah, but it was hard to find time to because everyone was so busy doing other things," Phoebe answered.

Roslyn cleared her throat. "I have to tell you that I'm a little worried about the influence these girls might have over you, Phoebe. We've talked lots about how girls your age can easily get into trouble with diets. I have the sense that these new friends of yours are at risk."

Trying her best to reassure her mom, Phoebe said, "I'll keep an eye out, Mom. I think it will be okay. You know me—I'd never give up my chocolate."

"Well, keep me posted, okay?" Roslyn replied. "If you're going to hang out with these girls often you'll need to figure out how to eat when you are with them."

"Will do," Phoebe answered as she got her books together and headed up to bed.

### Turn Your Child's Friends into Examples to Learn From

If you hear from your child that one of his friends seems to be developing an eating disorder, it is best to respond with sympathy and an explanation that these behaviors are often a way to cope with difficult problems. You should be available to listen to your child's concerns and thoughts about his friend's eating problem, and to take advantage of any "teachable moments," situations that lend themselves to palatable pontificating on your part. These moments may give you openings to do something as simple as encouraging your child to be concerned and sympathetic, or to point out that there are healthier ways to cope, such as talking out one's problems with a parent or a trusted friend, or even seeking counseling.

At dinner one night, Andy clearly wanted to talk about his close friend, Amber. "I can't believe she thinks she is too fat, Mom," Andy began. "You know, since she started talking like this I haven't seen her eat a thing at school," he added.

Tamara, Andy's mom, took a deep breath and said, "I'm really sorry to hear this about Amber. She's such a nice girl." Andy seemed interested in what Tamara was saying so she continued, "I wonder what's bothering her? It can't be healthy to miss lunch, and I wonder how well her mind is working if she isn't eating all day. Andy, does Amber seem concerned about what she might be doing to her health?"

Andy thought a moment and then said, "She just seems so depressed these days. She's not fun anymore."

"Have you talked to her about your concerns?" Tamara asked gently.

"No, do you think that would be a good idea?" Andy asked.

"Yes, if you feel comfortable about having that kind of conversation," said Tamara. "Sometimes just hearing that a friend is concerned is enough to turn something like this around. You could also talk to the guidance counselor you like, to see what she thinks."

"Let me think about it," responded Andy.

"Good idea, son," said Tamara, making a mental note to check in with Andy about this in several days.

Do not, however, assume your child is safe from eating difficulties just because he or she shows concern and insight into a friend's eating problems. Often those with problems of their own are the most likely to notice the problems of others. I have seen many parents who are perplexed at how their child, who is very concerned about a friend's behaviors, can still continue her own eating-disordered behaviors.

### Know Who Your Child's Friends Are

Sometimes simply keeping abreast of who your child's friends are and what they are telling her can help avert eating problems.

Amanda was well aware from many heart-to-heart talks with her daughter Brandi that several of Brandi's longtime girlfriends were headed toward eating problems. Brandi told her mom that these friends never ate lunch, but instead used lunch hour to pore over magazines such as *Seventeen* or *YM*. Brandi reported that just yesterday Talia, the ringleader of the group, pointing in horror at Brandi's usual Friday lunch of fish and chips, said to her, "You aren't seriously going to eat that, are you?" Brandi, who had recently recovered from her own eating disorder, was so angry and embarrassed that she was at a loss for words. She picked up her tray and stomped off, tempted, she told Amanda, to dump her food into the nearest trash can. She thought better of this move, because, as she told her mom, "That would mean they win!" Then Brandi uttered the magic words that mothers of adolescents long to hear: "Mom, what do you think I should do?"

Amanda responded tentatively, saying, "Well, you've been friends with these girls for a long time—"

"Yes," Brandi cut in, "but they have really changed since we started junior high. I know I changed, too, last year. When my eating problems began I acted a lot like they are acting now. But I'm better now, and I can't stand to be around them."

Amanda, again hesitating, answered, "Well, what are your options?"

"I would really like to spend time with my new lacrosse buddies," said Brandi. "They're always bugging me to join them for lunch. Maybe tomorrow I will."

"Sounds like a plan," Amanda agreed.

## Teasing

Just as the "fat talk" described earlier promotes a negative ideal of thinness among friends, so does teasing. Although most of us know better than to criticize or tease an adult about weight or size issues, it comes as a surprise to many to find out that children, too, are sensitive to teasing about these issues. Many children who are teased about their weight, even when the taunts are quite clearly exaggerated or untrue, believe that the insults are based in fact. Research has shown that the more a child is teased about his size or weight, the more dissatisfied he is with his body. Teasing, in fact, has a greater impact on body dissatisfaction than being heavy, and even bullying not related to weight can trigger an eating disorder.

Even relatively neutral comments about weight can lead to body dissatisfaction. Undue interest in a child's growth and size, for example, can easily be misunderstood by the sensitive child. BJ told me that she knew her aunt meant her no harm when she asked, as she did regularly, "BJ, what size are you wearing now? You've really grown since I last saw you." BJ confessed that she found herself thinking she needed to go on a diet whenever her aunt talked to her this way.

Sometimes even losing weight can cause problems with peers because it can evoke envy, which can then lead to rejection and teasing. This is a reminder to parents to teach their children that teasing about body weight and appearance is *never* acceptable, even if it is about weight loss, not weight gain. (For more on teasing, see p. 49.)

## Helpful Friends

We do not mean to imply that friends are always negative forces. Friends can play an important supportive role, and can actually help protect your child from an eating disorder.

Gabby's friends on the field hockey team have made it clear that they are girls who want to be strong; they eat what they like and think dieting is silly "girly" behavior. They become instrumental forces in Gabby's gradual recovery from an eating disorder.

Research indicates that in addition to being protective against eating disorders, support from friends increases the likelihood of a speedy recovery from eating disorders. When friends confront each other about their eating-disordered behavior in a kindly but direct manner, it can be a powerful inducement to turn away from those habits. This is especially true of purging behaviors, because purging, it seems, is the one eating-disordered behavior that can be turned around quickly. When friends confront friends about undereating or bingeing, it is harder to get such an immediate positive response.

It is usually obvious whether your children's friends are a supportive or a negative influence, especially if you take the time to engage your children in conversations about their relationships with their peers.

## School

### When Your Child's Disorder Surfaces at School

An eating disorder affects every aspect of a child's life, including his or her ability to do well in school and to be fully involved socially and athletically. A child who is undereating, for example, may have reduced energy and be less capable in sports and gym class.

In some cases, as we have noted, an eating disorder can go undetected because the child continues to perform extremely well in school and even on the playing field, despite significant eating problems. This happens most often with cases of anorexia, where the child's natural perfectionism is often directed toward both academic and/or athletic achievement *and* weight loss. For this reason, if you suspect an eating disorder, remember that continued high academic and/or athletic performance is no guarantee that your suspicions are unfounded.

### Enlisting Help from School Personnel

Sometimes starving, bingeing, or purging behaviors are noticed first at school by teachers, coaches, counselors, or the school nurse. Here, we will discuss a few of the many different ways that school personnel can help you when your child is battling an eating disorder.

- They may be the first to notice an eating problem.
- They may be able to intervene or bend rules at school to aid in your child's recovery.

- They may be able to help you find the professional resources you need.
- They may be able to play a protective, surrogate-parent role at school.
- They may help set limits and goals that help your child's recovery.

School administrators or coaches may set weight minimums that your child must meet before they can play sports or even stay in school. (For more information, see chapter 12, p. 224.)

Tatiana's story is a good example of how school personnel can help a child battling an eating disorder by bending rules or playing a surrogate-parent role. Tatiana is starting her freshman year of high school at the same time that she is trying to conquer her anorexia. She needs to have a mid-morning snack to increase her weight, but her high school's schedule does not allow it. All it takes is a note from the school nurse for Tatiana to be able to have a snack in study hall. Meanwhile, the school's guidance counselor, who has spoken to Tatiana's mother over the summer about Tatiana's effort to battle anorexia, offers to have lunch with Tatiana in her office. Since at this point in her recovery Tatiana is still too fearful about eating with other students, she jumps at the offer. Until Thanksgiving, Tatiana has lunch every day with the counselor in her office.

### School Programs or Activities That Can Trigger Eating Disorders

Just as your child's school and its personnel can be valuable allies in your fight against an eating disorder, so can the school sometimes play a role in the onset of the disorder.

An example is the local elementary school that decided to develop a heart-healthy curriculum after an enthusiastic health educator joined forces with an active PTA group. Both the educator and parents were excited about improving students' health by increasing exercise and reducing fat consumption. They instituted health classes that had children counting calories and fat grams and calculating the percentage of calories in the children's diet that were derived from fat. They also taught them how to eat in ways that would prevent heart disease and cancer, and encouraged regular exercise from jumping rope to jogging. Were it geared toward adults, there would be nothing unusual about this type of heart-healthy program. But keeping strict tabs on their own diet and exercise, even though it was an attempt to promote long-term health, was the last thing most elementary school children should be told to do.

Addie, a fifth-grader, told me that it certainly took the fun out of exercise. "Have you ever tried to jump rope for twenty minutes?" she asked, "Boring!" Valerie, a classmate of Addie's, blames her anorexia on learning to count fat grams when the program was in full swing, "It made me afraid of fat," she said. "I hadn't thought much about fat before the program started."

Because sometimes well-intentioned programs such as this can inadvertently trigger an eating disorder, it is wise to keep informed about and monitor all the programs and classes that your child is participating in.

## Summer Camp

If your child is recovering from an eating disorder or at risk for one, the prospect of summer camp can be anxiety-producing. How will she or he cope with the independence of camp life? Will eating or exercise problems reemerge or worsen? Here, we will outline some strategies for making your child's summer camp experience a success.

### Do Your Homework, Ask Questions

Often it is helpful when choosing a camp to inquire about the camp's procedures for dealing with children with eating problems. What you find out may be the decisive factor in choosing the best camp for your child. Although it is important to ask these questions, I notice that some parents are reluctant to mention their child's eating problem for fear that their child will be typecast as a "problem kid." I tell parents that if they are not comfortable with how the camp personnel respond to this information, it likely is not the best camp for their child.

### Make Staying in Camp Contingent upon Healthy Eating and Exercise

If your child has recently recovered from or is still in the throes of an eating disorder, you should make it clear to her that if she cannot maintain a safe weight at camp, or her health is jeopardized in any way, she will have to come home—no ifs, ands, or buts.

Just knowing that parents will take action if they lose weight, or if the camp staff becomes concerned about their ability to eat and exercise reasonably, is enough to keep some kids from doing so.

### Map a Plan before Your Child Goes to Camp; Stick to Your Promises

Before sending the child who has had observable food problems off to camp you will need to have a heart-to-heart talk with her, outline the ground rules for her camp experience, or map out a plan. You also need to promise yourselves that you will stick to your word, and not allow your child to remain in a situation where her eating or exercise behaviors could endanger her health or well-being. Not only would doing so be potentially injurious to her health, your credibility with your child as parents who can help her recover from an eating disorder may be irreparably damaged.

Emily, twelve, who was struggling with anorexia, had looked forward all year to attending a rigorous sports camp during the summer. But since September, Emily had been in treatment with me for anorexia. In May, I sat down with Emily and her parents and outlined a plan. Though Emily had made substantial progress (she had gained 10 pounds) and had impressed us all with her hard work, she still needed to gain about 5 pounds. And it was absolutely mandatory, according to her doctor, that she not lose an ounce.

With her parents' permission, I arranged to have the camp nurse weigh Emily weekly and call me with the results. Emily and I made a weekly phone date the evening of her weigh-in to discuss whether she was making progress and how she could modify her eating to cover her increased exercise. This plan worked well because we all understood that if Emily lost weight and if that weight was not restored within a week's time, she would be sent home. I had hoped she would gain weight at camp, but with the increased activity this did not happen. But Emily did not lose weight, either, which was most important. Once home she kept her food intake similar to her intake at camp and within a month had gained the last 5 pounds her doctor had ordered.

### Discuss Your Child's Situation with Camp Personnel before Camp Begins
In cases where you allow your child to go to camp but are concerned about her, you should let camp personnel know so they can intervene if necessary.

Paula's parents were worried that she would use the freedom of camp to revert to her overexercising patterns. They knew that if she jogged in addition to participating in all-camp activities, she was sure to lose weight. After some debate between themselves, Paula's parents decided to let the camp director know about their concerns. The director reassured Paula's parents that she would keep an eye on Paula and intervene if necessary, noting that it would be obvious to her and the camp counselors if Paula were exercising on her own. Paula's parents were especially relieved to hear the director tell them that they would be informed if things were not going well.

### Look at Summer Camp as a Test Run for Independent Living
When a child has made great strides recovering from an eating disorder, it is sometimes important to give her a chance to succeed or fail on her own. Summer camp can provide a ready-made opportunity for your child to demonstrate how far she has come in her recovery. This kind of experiment is best conducted in an environment you and your child know and feel comfortable with.

In the case of Liv, her parents decided she was ready for such an experiment. Most important, Liv herself was convinced she could handle it. Before she went to camp, Liv's parents set her down and reviewed their concerns with her. "Liv," her father gently began, "you know we've been worried about your eating. But we have been impressed at how you've done better the last several months."

"Going off to camp is a big deal if food is still a problem for you," Liv's mother Judith added. "Do you think you can handle it? You know that nothing less than three meals a day and substantial snacks will do."

Looking serious, seventh-grader Liv responded, "I think I can handle it. Don't forget, I've been going to this camp since fourth grade. I know I like the food and I know what to expect. Don't worry, you guys!"

Liv makes a good point. It is the fact that Liv has been to this camp several times without problems that finally tips the balance in favor of Liv attending camp.

### When Should You Limit or Prohibit Camp for Your Child?

If your child, unlike Liv, is still on very shaky ground—just beginning to battle her eating disorder, in the midst of a serious disorder, or recently relapsed back into a serious problem—you have legitimate concerns about her ability to manage food or exercise. In such cases, you may want to prohibit camp altogether. Limiting camp experiences to no more than one week in length until you are more confident makes sense in situations that are less serious. Consulting with your child's doctor can also help you decide on a reasonable and safe approach.

The bottom line on summer camps is that you should not send your child to an extended overnight camp unless your child demonstrates to you that she can do all of the following:

- Eat regularly and adequately.
- Maintain a healthy weight.
- Control disordered behaviors such as overexercising and purging.

## Going Away to College

Apart from summer camps or similar limited experiences, when a child goes away to college, it may be the first time he or she has lived away from home and on their own. This big change, compounded with new food choices, crazy schedules, rigorous academic demands, and new social challenges, makes it no surprise that the first several years of college are considered to be a time of high risk for the development of an eating disorder. Some eating-disordered college students struggle with the new freedom to eat or not to eat now that they are beyond Mom or Dad's watchful eyes. Other students have difficulty making food choices among the large array of delectable foods offered in campus cafeterias, or they founder when they find they do not have the same access to foods they are comfortable eating.

For all of these reasons, you should be particularly watchful as your child enters college. If your child has recently recovered from an eating disorder or is currently struggling with one, you need to first evaluate whether it is safe for her to go away to college at this juncture. If you decide it is, it is your responsibility to ensure that your child has the support and resources she needs at school or in the nearby community to protect her health.

**Should You Allow Your Eating-Disordered Child to Go Away to College?**
Although it may seem harsh, I believe you should not send your child away to college unless she demonstrates she has mastered normal eating and exercise, or the college has a well-respected treatment program in which your child can participate. Even in a situation where there is a good college-based program available, you should think carefully about the wisdom of sending a child with significant food problems off to college. Here are some facts and arguments to consider:

• **According to recent surveys, up to 20 percent to 30 percent of collegiate women are engaged in disordered-eating behaviors.** If your child has the bad fortune to find herself in a group of friends where eating problems are common, she may come to the conclusion that these behaviors are the status quo, and despair of being able to overcome her own problems in such an environment.

• **Because most college health services will treat your child as a responsible adult, you may feel cut out of the picture.** For example, most colleges will not allow you to make an appointment for your child, but will insist that your child make her own appointments. Most colleges will not inform you if your child misses an appointment or has lost weight or is having trouble with purging; you will only hear from them if your child is obviously taking a serious turn for the worst, or if her eating disorder is clearly interfering with her college studies.

• **With an active eating disorder, your child will not have the best college experience she could have.** Your child will get more out of college if she waits until her eating disorder is clearly under control.

Taking time to consider these facts and assessing your reaction to them can help you decide whether your child is ready to go off to college, and whether you are ready to let her go. You may find that you are not yet ready to turn over the responsibility of your child's recovery to her just yet. On a positive note, knowing that entering college is contingent upon making progress in her battle against her eating disorder can motivate your child to get her eating problems under control quickly.

**Shopping for the Right College**
Maureen's mother told me that whether or not a college had good eating-disorder resources figured heavily in whether or not they allowed Maureen to apply for admission. Given Maureen's significant eating-disorder history, her parents were not being overprotective, they were just being smart.

If your child has an eating disorder, you and your prospective college student should shop around for a college that has a program for treating eating disorders. Ideally, the college you choose will have an adequately staffed eating-disorder program right on campus, which will include experienced physicians (nurse practitioners and physician's assistants also can provide competent medical monitoring), therapists, nutrition counselors, and psychiatrists.

Some colleges provide all or some of these services free of charge to enrolled students. Others limit the number of visits students can make each semester. Still other colleges refer students who need these services off campus, which usually means that either you or your insurance carrier will foot the bill. Some colleges leave it up to the family to find community resources if their child needs that kind of support.

Issues to consider if the college of your choice does not provide the services your child needs include:

- Whether or not your insurance policy will provide adequate coverage.
- Whether or not getting to and from off-campus visits can be conveniently arranged.

If you expect your child will need continuing support at college, you may want to arrange either a visit with or a phone call to the college's health service or counseling center before your child selects a college to attend, or certainly before your child leaves for college. This preliminary call or visit will help you better understand the services that are available to your child.

**Making Contact with the On-Campus Treatment Team**
After your child has selected a college, if you are certain that he will need services, you should insist your child make an appointment to see a member of the college's eating-disorder team. You yourself may also want to visit with a member of the team to share your concerns and perspective. Once your child is working with a professional on or off campus, your main responsibility is to make sure he is making and keeping his medical, psychological, or nutritional appointments. Although as we have noted college staff and other professionals treating your child will treat him as a responsible adult, this does not mean you cannot or should not let the profession-

als who are involved with your child know of your concerns. Your perspective can help professionals provide insightful care.

### Make Staying in School Contingent on Maintaining Minimum Weights

Some college students do well with nothing more than regular phone check-ins with their parents or hometown nutritionist, therapist, or physician. Others do best making a connection with a professional either at college or in the surrounding community.

When students know that staying in college is contingent upon taking care of their bodies and overcoming some of their eating-disordered behaviors, they seem to be able to marshall their personal resources (though they may need substantial family and/or professional help as well) to overcome even a serious eating disorder. This approach works if parents hold firm to their decrees. In most cases, the student is able to stay in school and not have to take the leave of absence.

### Just Because She's in College Doesn't Mean She's All Grown Up

It is not unusual for first-year college students to gain 10 to 15 pounds or more, and in some cases grow in height as well. This phenomenon is so common that it has been labeled the "freshman 10" or the "freshman 15."

The substantial weight gains some first-year college students experience during fall semester can be explained several ways: College freshmen, often for the first time in their lives, are given the complete freedom to eat or not eat as they please, at a time when many have not yet learned to manage their own eating. Some freshmen gain weight because they are taking in additional calories in the form of alcohol and/or party foods, which are found in abundance at the many food-related social events associated with college life. For others, the freedom of being away from home may trigger a latent binge-eating problem. Sometimes the awareness that a student is gaining weight, for any of these reasons, is so demoralizing that she compounds her problem by consoling herself through food.

Another explanation is that the college years are a time during which many children finish growing. This is the time that many adolescents gain the pounds and even inches they need in order to reach their adult size and shape. While weight gain may seem to happen all at once, often because it is compounded by the dramatic change in eating habits we describe above, once eating patterns settle down (as they usually do later in that first college year) weight gain stops. College students usually fully develop by the end of their sophomore year, arriving at the weight and height that they will maintain as an adult.

If your child is alarmed to find that she has gained weight after entering college, you can remind her that while some of it may be due to the stress of adjusting to her new life, at least some of it is the normal weight gain of a still-growing young adult and should not be unduly feared.

If, despite your reassurances, your child is still concerned about undesired weight gain, you should keep the lines of communication open and let her know that you are available to talk about it if she chooses. As Holly's story illustrates, this is often a sensitive issue, around which parents sometimes fail to tread lightly.

Holly, a freshman, was excited to be taking her first trip home for Thanksgiving vacation. She told me later she would never forget her shock and embarrassment when the first words out of her father's mouth when he met her at the airport were, "My, you've put some meat on your bones." I came to know Holly well as we worked together to overcome the eating disorder that that thoughtless comment spawned.

Instead of this reaction, Holly's father would have done better to say nothing more than how glad he was to see her. This is a good example of the adage I recommend as a guide for parents and others when faced with a potentially sensitive weight increase in a loved one: "When in doubt say nothing." While no good ever seems to come from harping about weight gain, severe weight loss, on the other hand, carries with it serious medical risks and can be especially harmful to young people. As we have suggested in this chapter, these are situations that demand speaking up if they affect someone close to you.

If your child feels her weight gain is more than simply the freshman 10 or 15, but a sign of a deeper problem, she would be well-advised to make an appointment with an on- or off-campus nutritionist, as Holly did with me, for an assessment. Again, this is an area that you want to handle with sensitivity. You should not assume your child wants to talk about the weight she has gained or feels the need to do anything about it. Let your child take the lead on whether this is an issue that is up for discussion.

## In Summary

It is one thing to deal with a child's disorder at home, within the safe confines of the family circle, and quite another to send your child, eating problems and all, into the wider world of friends, school, summer camp, or college. We hope this chapter has given you a glimpse of both the risks inherent in those wider worlds and the many ways friends, teachers, coaches, and counselors in those worlds can provide support and guidance for a child struggling with an eating disorder.

Sending a child with eating problems away to school or to summer camp can be anxiety-producing. We have tried in this chapter to give you the confidence and direction you need to help your child make these transitions with ease, while never losing sight of the fact that eliminating the disorder must be your first priority. The more you know about the peer pressures she may be feeling, the quality of the supervision she will receive at summer camp, or the specialized resources available to your child at her school, the better equipped you will be to help her.

# PART THREE

# HEALTHY
# EATING GUIDE

We have described the various eating disorders and how to intervene and establish a collaborative rather than confrontational relationship with your child. In this section, we will outline the nutritional approach to solving eating disorders that has worked so well with the children I have treated over the past fifteen years.

Your goal as parents is to return to your child the confidence she has lost in her ability to eat in an organized fashion, and to know when she has had enough to eat. The method that we will outline for you in this section will restore your underweight child's normal weight and protect against binge eating and overeating by providing a blueprint for regular meals, snacks, and exercise.

Following the plan will take careful planning, patience, and perseverance. Yet it is not beyond the abilities of parents who care about their child and are committed to helping her get better. By now you realize that as parents you are the first and potentially most powerful allies your child can have in fighting her disorder. You also realize that it is of the utmost urgency to address the problem as soon as possible, with energy and vigor. Family interventions to change eating habits, in fact, are most effective with younger children. The younger the patient, the more important it is that the family be involved.

# 10

# Normalizing Eating
# with a Food Plan

The core of my nutritional philosophy is that in order to stop their destructive eating, anorexics, bulimics, and binge eaters must cease to diet and gain confidence in making food choices. By undereating, restrictive eating, and dieting, your child is setting herself up to binge eat. For an anorexic, it may take months to succumb to the temptation to binge, while for a bulimic the pendulum may swing from starving to bingeing on a daily basis. In either case, the goal is to normalize eating patterns while meeting the body's needs for both nutrients and sensory satisfaction. I tell my patients that recovery from an eating disorder, whether it is anorexia, bulimia, or binge-eating disorder, is predicated on accepting and practicing normal eating and exercise. When my patients tell me that they are afraid that if they stop dieting they will gain weight, I tell them, "People don't gain weight from normal eating, they gain weight from bingeing. And if you stop dieting, you will be less likely to binge."

My chief weapon in the battle to normalize eating is the Food Plan, which (depending on the disorder) is designed to reduce food-related anxiety and binge eating, restore a healthy weight, or bring about a slow reduction in weight. Eating-disorder sufferers often have lost the ability to recognize the signals for hunger and fullness. The Food Plan helps your child learn to recognize those signals by mimicking the patterns of appetite-based eating.

Nicole's grandmother likes to tell Nicole, "You're just like me, 'pleasantly plump.'" Her grandmother is right. Nicole, whose family on both her mother's and father's side are tall and big-boned, has always been chunky. Unhappy with her genetic heritage when it comes to size, Nicole begins to diet in the fourth grade, but without success. Within a year, she is purging, yet she still does not lose weight. By the time Nicole's mother brings her in to see me, she is fourteen years old. She begins each day vowing to diet, but by day's end, has binged and purged at least once. She weighs 200 pounds and is utterly demoralized.

When I first outline a Food Plan for her, Nicole responds as many of my patients do, saying, "This is way too much food. I know I will gain weight if I eat this much." I reassure her, replying, "No, this is minimal normal eating. A lot of people need more food than this. If you follow this plan you will take care of your nutrient needs, your body will be satisfied, and you will not have to binge. Bingeing is your body's way of getting the nutrients it needs when you undereat. You may need more food than this, but this is a start." I also explain that eating up to six times a day as the Food Plan directs will help raise her metabolism, which over time will help Nicole maintain a healthy weight.

As you read the following description of the Food Plan, keep in mind that you can tailor your child's plan to her own tastes and needs.

## The Basic Building Blocks of the Food Plan

The individual components of the Food Plan are simple. Your child should have three meals a day, two to three snacks a day, and normal portion sizes. I encourage my patients to make their own food choices within food groups and to choose one to two servings of "fun food," foods eaten for pure sensory pleasure, every day. Including fun food is a particularly effective strategy for overcoming an eating disorder because it protects against bingeing. There should be no more than a three- to four-hour interval between meals and snacks, and your child should know when the next meal or snack will be eaten. Your child's eating schedule must for the time being come first; other commitments must be scheduled around the Food Plan.

The importance of this last point, that fixing your child's eating disorder has to be your first priority, is one that Cara's mother does not grasp at first. In the year after winning her state's Junior Miss contest, Cara loses 30 pounds. Although she still has a very pretty face when I begin seeing her, it is hard to imagine her winning a beauty contest; her arms are spindly, her backbone protruding, and her breasts and buttocks are wizened. Where she once was able to convince a panel of judges that she possessed a sparkling intelligence to match her outward beauty, now she can barely carry on a coherent conversation.

Despite Cara's best efforts at sticking to the Food Plan I have drawn up for her, she loses more weight. As we explore possible solutions, it becomes clear that part of the problem is that she feels her mother, Helen, is more interested in feeding and caring for her new husband, Ted, than in her seriously anorexic daughter. Helen feels obligated to serve a nice, large meal at 8 P.M., when Ted arrives home from work. By then, Cara is no longer hungry and just picks at her dinner. In fact, appetite does diminish for many people if meals or snacks are more than three or four hours apart. We come up with the solution of Cara having a large after-school snack, which will leave her appropriately hungry for a late dinner.

But Cara also makes it clear to Helen what the real problem is, saying, "Mom, I feel you care more about Ted's eating than mine." Before Cara can make progress she needs to truly believe that fixing her eating problems is the family's primary goal.

Helen, though, is still not convinced this is the proper approach. She speaks to me privately, wondering if by coddling her daughter she will promote selfishness, or an unhealthy sense of entitlement on Cara's part. After all, she points out, Cara certainly, at age sixteen, is old enough and competent enough to fix her own dinner. I explain to Helen that Cara's eating disorder in essence has made her regress to the point where her needs and feelings are those of a much younger child.

To overcome an eating disorder, often families temporarily have to cater to their affected child's food needs in ways that the child, when she has recovered, will balk at. First, Helen makes a standing date with Cara to take her out for a restaurant meal once a week, just the two of them. After discussing it with Ted, Helen offers to have dinner ready for Cara at 5 P.M. I encourage Helen to eat with Cara if she can, but also to join Ted later for a snack while he eats dinner. It occurs to both Helen and Cara that Ted's dinnertime can coincide with Cara's evening snack, providing important family time. Since we began working together, Helen and Ted have come a long way in giving Cara the support she needs to make her recovery. Cara's story, though, is still a work in progress.

Sometimes, the kind of emotional and psychological regression I describe in Cara's case is even more severe. One seriously affected thirteen-year-old patient of mine for a time needed to be fed spoonful by spoonful by her mother before she began to eat on her own.

As you will see, your child's *pattern* of eating is more important at this stage than what is actually eaten. At Toronto General Hospital, this phase of recovery is called "eating with training wheels," and that is what your child is doing, learning to eat all over again as if for the first time. An exception to this rule is the child who is seriously underweight or losing weight and needs to be eating an increasing number of calories per day. (See chapter 11, p. 196, for more on adapting the Food Plan for the anorexic child.) Mastering these "training wheels" will pave the way for your child to gradually be able to eat freely, without the aid of the Food Plan. While your child is on the road to recovery, however, the Food Plan will help ensure that you are introducing adequate protein, calcium, calories, fat, vitamins and minerals into your child's diet. We also remind you that the Food Plan is based on minimum servings. Underweight anorexics, as well as highly active people, will need to eat more to meet their caloric needs.

This is what the Food Plan looks like:

### Breakfast
Calcium
Complex Carbohydrates
Fruit or Vegetable
Protein (optional)
Fat (optional)

### Snack

### Lunch
Calcium
Complex Carbohydrates
Fruit or Vegetable
Protein
Fat
Fun Food

### Snack

### Dinner
Calcium
Complex Carbohydrates
Fruit or Vegetable
Protein
Fat
Fun Food

### Snack

As you can see, the formula is simple and much like the way a healthy eater eats without thinking about it. (Most people, in fact, would do well to follow this or a similarly well-balanced food plan.) The variety comes in the foods that you choose to fulfill each of these requirements. Although I discourage my patients from counting calories, for those who insist on doing so, the plan, depending on food choices and portion sizes, ranges from 1,500 to 2,500 calories per day. Most girls and young women will need at least 2,000 calories per day and more if they are very active. Boys and men, on the other hand, usually need at least 2,500 calories.

The following is a list of foods that I suggest for each of the categories of the Food Plan, and a brief description of why each category is important to maintaining health.

## Calcium Suggestions

Milk, yogurt, cheese, frozen yogurt, ice cream, pudding, tofu, soy milk. (Not all soy products are fortified with calcium. Check the label to see that one serving contains 30 percent of the body's daily calcium requirement. This is equivalent to the calcium contained in a glass of milk.)

### Why Calcium Is Important

Most people know that calcium is essential for strong bones and teeth. Calcium is also found in the blood where it regulates nerve transmission, blood pressure, heartbeat, and muscle contractions. It is necessary for blood clotting and secretion of hormones and digestive enzymes. Because the role calcium plays in the blood is so vital, the bones act as a calcium reserve, providing adequate blood calcium even if one is not consuming enough dietary calcium. When this calcium reservoir is regularly tapped, bones become porous and weakened.

It is especially important that children through young adulthood consume adequate amounts of calcium, as the calcium we add to our bones up through our early twenties is what will sustain our bones for the rest of our lives. From our mid-twenties on, consuming enough calcium will ensure that we do not lose bone density, but will no longer improve our bone density. One of the saddest long-term consequences of anorexia is early and severe osteoporosis, which leaves young women with weakened bones and painful and impairing stress fractures. While consuming adequate calcium is only one factor (others are achieving an adequate body weight and resumption of menstrual periods) that protects bones, it is one strategy that can quickly be instituted.

### Adding Calcium to the Food Plan

Physicians suggest that children and teens with anorexia consume a total of 1,500 mg of calcium per day, slightly more than the 1,300 mg recommended for most children and teens.

The 300 mg of calcium in a cup of milk or yogurt is considered the standard for assessing other sources of calcium. For example, it takes 2 ounces of cheese to equal 1 cup of milk, or one serving. Swiss cheese, however, is much higher than most cheeses in calcium with a mere ounce (a generous slice) providing 300 mg. Most frozen yogurt and ice cream require a serving size about 1½ cups to 2 cups. One surprise is that cottage cheese is not a particularly good source of calcium. It requires 2 cups of cottage cheese to make a serving of calcium. Calcium-fortified soy products (tofu and soy milk) and calcium-fortified orange juice are reasonable alternatives to dairy products. Tofu provides substantial protein (18 grams per cup) as well.

The wide availability of reduced-fat dairy products (which are as good as full-fat dairy products in providing calcium and other nutrients) can be helpful in convincing your child to make improvements in this food group. Children are more likely than older teens to be open to using milk as a beverage at meals, which is an easy way to meet calcium needs. I discourage parents from engaging in battles over low- or nonfat dairy products versus full-fat products (see p. 59), since any of these meet your child's calcium, protein, and vitamin needs. The child that chooses lower-calorie dairy products will just have to get the calories she needs from eating additional foods. Some children are not averse to choosing higher-fat dairy products, which can help those with a small appetite gain weight.

Sari was one of a handful of my patients who was quite willing to switch to whole milk and Ben & Jerry's ice cream from 1% milk and frozen yogurt. Sari found that by doing this, she could restore her weight without having to substantially increase the size of her meals, an eating pattern she felt much more comfortable with.

Most eating-disordered patients' diets are woefully deficient in calcium, even though they may know that calcium is necessary for strong bones. The Food Plan calls for three servings, or 900 mg of calcium. Three servings of any of the high-calcium foods we have listed, plus the approximately 300 mg of incidental calcium found in grains, fruits, and vegetables, provides most children with adequate calcium. To achieve the recommended 1,500 mg of calcium per day for an anorexic, your child would have to have at least four calcium servings per day, or you will need to augment her diet with calcium supplements. I suggest that parents calculate how much calcium their child gets on average and have them make up the difference with a supplement. It is better to insist that your child take a supplement than to fight over her avoidance of dairy products. In tallying your child's calcium intake, you should include what she may be getting in a multiple vitamin. Most multiple vitamin supplements contain 300 mg of calcium (listed as 30% of the Daily Value).

Since it is hard for many children to remember to take vitamins or supplements regularly on their own, parents should get into the routine of giving them their daily supplements or reminding them to take them.

If your child already takes calcium supplements and feels this will take care of her bones, you can point out that in addition to calcium, dairy products contain protein and a host of other vitamins and minerals that are also important for healthy bones. In addition to providing 300 mg of calcium, a 1-cup single serving of a dairy product contains 8 grams of protein. This is not, however, enough to be considered a protein serving. In other words, your child can't have a cup of milk and think that she has fulfilled both her calcium and protein requirements in the Food Plan.

As we have noted (see p. 59), as long as a child is getting adequate calcium parents should not ban the use of diet sodas, since they are so widely consumed by normal eaters. Even though these drinks are of absolutely no nutritional value, as long as your child is not consuming voluminous amounts of them, thereby killing her appetite, you will be better off saving your energy for other, more important battles. If you do allow your child to drink soda, I suggest you encourage moderation in the same way that you might limit your child's television viewing time.

## Complex Carbohydrate Suggestions

Cereal, bagels, bread, muffins, crackers, pretzels, rice cakes, rice, potatoes, pasta, corn, grits.

### Why Complex Carbohydrates Are Important

Complex carbohydrates, or starches, are extremely important in maintaining health. Along with simple carbohydrates—the carbohydrates found in fruits, vegetables, dairy products, and foods that contain sugar—they are the ideal energy source for all the cells of the body. Complex and simple carbohydrates are the body's major source of glucose, the only energy that brain and central nervous system cells are designed to use.

Complex carbohydrates also provide the body with essential vitamins and minerals, particularly B-vitamins, magnesium, zinc, and even some iron. Whole-grain complex carbohydrates are good sources of fiber, which improves the health of the digestive tract, gives feelings of fullness, and helps prevent constipation. Some eating-disordered patients, hearing that high-fiber diets are lower in calories, may be tempted to overdo fiber. If your child has adopted such a diet, it is helpful to warn her that too much fiber (she may overdo high-fiber cereals for example) may cause rather than prevent constipation, inhibit the absorption of some minerals (especially calcium), and even cause dehydration. Anorexic children may in fact do best choosing lower-fiber carbohydrates to minimize feelings of fullness.

## Carbohydrates' Starring Role: Protecting Protein Stores and Preventing Harmful Fat Metabolism

Carbohydrates also play an important, "protein-sparing" role. When the body is not being fueled with enough carbohydrates, protein is broken down to provide the glucose the brain needs. Adequate carbohydrate intake protects protein from being used in this way, preserving the body's protein stores for muscle building and other equally important functions. (See "Why Protein Is Important," p. 168.)

One reason the body prefers not to burn protein for energy is that when protein is used for energy by-products are created which must be excreted through the kidneys. This can be hard on the kidneys and is one reason why the currently popular high-protein, low-carbohydrate diets are not recommended. Another is that too much dietary protein can cause loss of calcium from bone. In order to keep the brain nourished and protein stores protected, the body needs to be supplied with carbohydrates at least every four to six hours.

An adequate supply of carbohydrates also protects the body in another important way: it facilitates in the efficient burning of fat without allowing the build-up of potentially dangerous chemical by-products known as ketones. The creation of these compounds, which is called ketosis, can upset the normal chemical balance of the blood. Unchecked, ketosis can lead to dehydration, which, in turn, can damage the kidneys and cause the loss of essential nutrients in the urine. The loss of potassium, one of the essential nutrients, can lead to heart arrythmias. In extreme cases, ketosis can result in coma. The fact that low-carbohydrate diets can result in ketosis is one of the reasons most nutritionists advise against them.

Like many of the symptoms of anorexia, ketosis is an adaptation to famine conditions that allowed our ancestors to survive with a less than reliable food supply. In an anorexic, however, it signals an extreme stage of starvation that must be taken seriously.

## Famine Metabolism and Lack of Appetite

Even mild ketosis can interfere with appetite, another adaptation to famine. If your anorexic child says she isn't hungry when she hasn't eaten all day, she is likely relying on ketones for energy. The complete loss of appetite that accompanies ketosis can help turn anorexia into a chronic condition because undereating seems "easy."

If this happens to your child, it is wise to explain to her that her lack of appetite is a result of ketosis. Otherwise, she may erroneously conclude she does not need to eat. When my anorexic patients say they are never hungry, I tell them this means their body is moving into "famine metabolism." While the anorexic likes the idea that her body is burning fat for energy, I warn her of the dangers she faces when this happens. "At the same time your body is burning fat and producing the ketones that decrease appetite," I tell her, "in order to supply energy to the cells of the brain and the central nervous system, which cannot burn fat, it is also breaking down its own protein stores, including protein in muscle and organs." The loss of muscle tissue accounts for the spindly legs and arms that most anorexics develop. Of course, we can't see how the heart, lungs, and even the brain are affected by the loss of protein.

Finally, I add that another effect of famine metabolism is a general slowing of the body's metabolism as the body tries to get by on fewer and fewer calories. Most anorexics, except very young ones, are aware that a high metabolism is an asset to maintaining a thin body weight. The idea that they might be "damaging" their metabolism helps some anorexics eat better.

### Adding Complex Carbohydrates to the Food Plan

When selecting complex carbohydrates to fill out the Food Plan, you should encourage your child to choose full servings; for example, two slices of bread, one cup of pasta, one bagel, one English muffin, one cup of cereal or rice. Carbohydrate foods are good choices for snacks, especially if combined with a serving of fat or protein.

Eating-disordered children are likely to choose foods in this group over foods from the protein or fat group, as foods in this group (breakfast cereals and breads) are well known to be low in fat. Ironically, these foods are also likely to become favorite binge foods.

While higher-fat carbohydrate foods such as desserts, cookies, and chips are more commonly thought of as binge foods, many eating-disorder sufferers will stubbornly hold to their resolve to avoid fats and sugars even as they are bingeing. These "lower-fat, healthy" carbohydrate foods (breakfast cereal is a good example) are the only foods they may allow themselves to eat freely, because they are low in calories. Bingeing on these foods illustrates that too much of a good thing can be a problem. It appears that when we eat foods that are low in fat and/or protein we don't get the biological feedback signaling that we have had enough to eat. Patients tell me when they binge on low-fat carbohydrate foods they feel full, but not satisfied. Often, they end up eating an enormous amount of food, more than they might if they had eaten a serving of a high-fat dessert.

## Protein Suggestions

Meat, fish, poultry, cottage cheese, cheese, legumes (dried beans), eggs, nuts, seeds (sunflower, pumpkin, sesame seeds), peanut butter or other nut butters, or high-protein soy products such as tofu and tempeh and seitan (wheat-based meat substitute).

### Why Protein Is Important

It is hard to overstate the importance of the role of protein in recovery from an eating disorder. Protein is a vital nutrient needed to make enzymes, antibodies, hormones, muscles, tendons, ligaments, bones, teeth, hair, nails, and blood. Protein regulates fluid and electrolytes in the body, preserves the body's delicate acid-base balance, and is essential for blood clotting and for the transport of oxygen and nutrients throughout the body.

Protein foods also provide essential B-vitamins and minerals. Meat, fish, and poultry provide iron and zinc. Cheese and most tofu (check the label) provide calcium.

### Protein as Protection Against Overeating and Bingeing, and as Metabolic Enhancer

Researchers have shown in clinical trials what I have seen in my own practice: that eating-disordered patients who consume high-protein meals feel more satisfied and are less likely to overeat or binge later on high-fat and sweet foods or to binge at all. In addition, metabolic rate increases after a meal of protein. Relaying these facts to your child can help reassure a child who is resisting increasing their protein intake.

### Protein's Effect on Hair, Skin, Muscles, and Bone

Those who have experienced the ravages of weight loss can be told that increasing their protein intake will help their body begin to restore hair, skin, muscles, and produce the important hormones that protect bones. You should add, though, that unless eating more protein is accompanied by weight gain the body will not produce enough of the hormones (estrogen) that protect bones.

### The Importance of Protecting Protein

While we have stressed the importance of dietary protein in keeping the body healthy, protecting against bingeing, and enhancing metabolism, we also must point out the importance of protecting the body's protein. Unlike carbohydrates and fat, which can be stored in the body when not being used for the body's energy needs, protein in the body is always in use, so to speak. Proteins we eat are incorporated into everything from our skin to our bones and vital organs. It is a biological truism, however, that the body's need for energy "trumps" the maintenance of all these systems. Because cells die immediately without a constant source of energy, protein is taken from muscles, blood, and organs such as the liver and heart to provide calories to the child who chronically undereats.

**Why Eating Enough Protein May Be Difficult for Your Child**

Despite all these good reasons for eating protein, it is not always easy for the eating-disordered person. Many foods that are high in protein are also high in fat, which makes it a struggle for fat-phobic eating-disorder patients to find acceptable protein choices.

To counter the common fear of fat among eating-disorder sufferers, you can point out that in nature, protein and fat most often occur together, and suggest some low-fat, high-protein choices: legumes, such as kidney beans, garbanzo beans (chickpeas), dried split peas, lentils, and cannellini (Great Northern) beans, fish (water-packed tuna is a favorite of some fat-phobic children), turkey, chicken, and lean red meats. Cottage cheese is also available in reduced- and nonfat forms. Supermarkets stock wide varieties of already cooked legumes, ready to be eaten either heated or straight from the can. Two other meat substitutes are tempeh (a fermented soy product) and seitan (also known as "wheat meat," or wheat gluten). Staple foods in parts of Asia, both tempeh and seitan are served in many Chinese restaurants in this country and are available in the specialty food sections of bigger supermarkets. Some children are open to using protein powders or egg substitutes, although they will likely tire of using supplemental forms of protein, or eventually decide they want to socialize with friends over pizza or at a barbecue.

Although it is likely that your child's diet will be low in protein, you may find, as I do with many of my patients, that once they understand the benefits of increasing their protein intake, they are quite open to doing so, and even come to embrace protein in their diet. Most of my patients, in fact, report they "just feel better" once they begin to regularly consume additional dietary protein.

**Protein and the Vegetarian Child**

Many eating-disordered people follow a vegetarian diet, in part as a way of controlling food intake and weight. It is especially challenging for vegetarian eating-disordered children to get adequate protein since they do not eat lean meat such as chicken or fish. Most vegetarians who are not afraid of eating fat rely on cheese and soy products for protein. But eating these products may be beyond the ability of a vegetarian in the throes of an eating disorder. The low-fat proteins we mention earlier are often acceptable to the fat-phobic vegetarian: reduced-fat cottage cheese and cheese, low-fat tofu (available in some communities), and legumes. I tell vegetarian patients I am sorry that when protein choices must be limited to low-fat vegetarian foods it is such a short list, but the body cares more about getting adequate protein than about variety. I find that often after some time following the Food Plan, these children become more willing to expand their list of acceptable protein choices and eventually include even chicken and fish, which are naturally high in protein and low in fat.

By focusing on your child's need to consume adequate protein, you can avoid nonproductive discussions aimed at getting her to give up her vegetarian ways. Remember, it is more important at this point to get your child to eat protein, not to quibble about what kind of protein she will eat. It is worth reminding her that if she does not consume enough calories to provide for her energy needs, protein will be burned for energy and therefore will not be available to do the important things in the body that only protein can do.

While you may not convert your vegetarian child to eating meat, you should inform her that one essential B-vitamin, $B_{12}$, is only found in animal foods. Strict vegetarians, who do not eat any meats or dairy products, must be certain to take supplemental vitamin $B_{12}$ or risk long-term damage to nerves and muscles. Parents of vegetarians should be sure to check the $B_{12}$ content of the products their vegetarian children use. The recommended daily dose of $B_{12}$ for children is 1.8 micrograms (mcg) and for teenagers 2.4 mcg. Many soy products are fortified with $B_{12}$, and most general multiple vitamin and mineral supplements contain enough $B_{12}$ so that if taken daily, your child's needs will be met. Growing vegetarians are advised to take a general supplement to ensure they are providing their bodies with all the necessary nutrients, particularly iron, zinc, vitamin D, and $B_{12}$, as all of these nutrients are likely to be low in vegetarian diets. Vegetarians who avoid dairy products are also at risk for low calcium and protein.

**Adding Protein to the Food Plan**
Protein is optional at breakfast in the Food Plan but not for lunch and dinner. Some children may do better if it is added, others find that protein consumed at breakfast leaves them feeling overly full; still others find that they are too rushed in the morning to take the time to add protein to their meal.

Children who need to gain weight may benefit from protein at breakfast, but any food as long as it provides calories will do the trick. Children who are at risk for bingeing at breakfast or over the course of the morning should be encouraged to include a serving of protein at breakfast. Children who binge in the afternoon or evening should experiment with a serving of protein at either afternoon or evening snacks or both.

Aim to have your child consume one protein serving, or from 20 to 30 grams of protein per meal. This is the amount typical of a modest 3- to 4-ounce serving of meat, or 1 cup of legumes, tofu, tempeh, seitan, egg substitute, or cottage cheese. It takes either 3 eggs, 6 egg whites, or 4 tablespoons of peanut butter to equal one protein serving. (For more on how to recognize a normal serving size, see chapter 11, p. 182.)

Some of my patients have discovered that mixing and matching proteins works well for them. Samantha finds that protein really gives her a strong start in the morning, yet the three eggs' worth of protein that she needs is more than she can face in that form. With some experimentation Sam hits upon a breakfast that works for her: her mom scrambles two eggs for her while Sam spreads a tablespoon of peanut butter on an English muffin and pours a glass of juice. Sam has fun trying various nut butters and eventually becomes an ardent fan of cashew butter.

Proteins found in food vary in quality. Animal proteins (meats, fish, poultry, and dairy products) are the easiest to digest and of higher quality than plant proteins (dried beans, soy products, nuts, and seeds). High-quality proteins like those from animals contain the specific amino acids needed by the human body; plant foods are lacking one or more necessary amino acids. Yet plant proteins, if properly combined, can also provide the full complement of amino acids the body requires. Nutritionists refer to plant proteins that combine to create a more complete protein as "complementary proteins." Complementary combinations of protein include legumes and grains, or seeds or nuts paired with legumes or grains, or dairy products combined with plant proteins. Specific examples of efficacious pairings of proteins include chili beans and corn bread, a peanut butter sandwich, or a glass of milk with meals that contain vegetable protein.

Eating just a little bit of animal protein like fish or chicken, and of course beef, does the same thing, effectively complementing vegetarian proteins. For example, a few pieces of chicken in a stir-fry will improve the quality of the protein in vegetables and rice. Nutritionists believe that as long as complementary proteins are consumed over the course of a day and enough energy and total protein is consumed, vegetarian eaters do not need to worry about their protein intake.

Because they are making blood, bone, and muscle, growing children need relatively more protein than do adults. Low protein intake can lead to short stature; learning impairments; weakened, shrunken hearts; anemia; and muscle weakness. One of the most obvious signs of low protein intake is its effect on the skin. On low-protein diets, skin loses its elasticity and becomes dry.

As important as protein is, I do not recommend protein or amino acid supplements. At best, they are not necessary, and at worst, may even be dangerous. Protein drinks are often popular with people with eating disorders because they seem so "healthy." Their main health benefit, however, once the body's protein needs are met, is additional calories. When protein in excess of energy needs is consumed, that extra protein is stored as fat, in the same way the body stores excess dietary fat or carbohydrates.

Parents should watch that their child does not inadvertently take in too much protein. Several of my teenaged patients have had kidney problems resulting from overdoing high-protein drinks over a span of several months. Fortunately, in each of these cases as soon as they stopped the supplemental drinks, kidney function was restored. Although few cases of actual overdoses have been reported, single amino supplements are potentially even more dangerous than high-protein drinks if misused. These supplements have no known benefit and should be avoided because the body is designed to handle whole proteins, not single amino acids. An overdose of one amino acid may cause a toxicity or may inhibit the absorption of another amino acid. If the absorption of even one essential amino acid is inhibited, the body loses its ability to make the various proteins that the body needs to function properly. It is for this reason that combining proteins is so important, especially for the eating-disordered vegetarian. I mention amino acid supplements because I have seen parents encourage the use of supplements in an attempt to speed up restoration of their child's health. I do not encourage this approach, and remind parents that supplements, in fact, can cause an extra stress on the weakened body.

## Fruit and Vegetable Suggestions

Any fresh, cooked, dried, canned, or juiced fruits or vegetables.

### Why Fruits and Vegetables Are Important

Fruits and vegetables contribute key nutrients such as fiber, vitamin A, vitamin C, folate (also known as folic acid), potassium, and magnesium. Fiber helps prevent constipation and other intestinal problems, lowers cholesterol, may reduce risk of heart disease and cancer, and promotes feelings of fullness. Vitamin A is an important antioxidant that protects eyesight, promotes bone growth, and helps the body fight infections. Vitamin C is also an antioxidant which protects against infections. It also is essential for healthy bones, skin, teeth, and tendons and helps in the absorption of iron. Folate is essential for DNA synthesis and consequently is required for new cell synthesis. Potassium is crucial in maintaining heartbeat and fluid and electrolyte balance. Magnesium is key to the functioning of many of the body's enzymes, and for the release of energy from other nutrients. Fruits and vegetables also provide energy in the form of simple carbohydrates.

**Adding Fruits and Vegetables to the Food Plan**
The Food Plan suggests at least three servings of fruits and vegetables per day. Although many health experts think that getting closer to five servings is better for long-term health, I do not insist that those recovering from an eating disorder eat more than three servings (unless they are inclined to) since few normal eaters eat that well. Choosing to include a serving of fruit or vegetable at snack time is one way to increase the amount of fruit eaten; another way is to eat two servings at meals. Think of a typical serving size as any of the following: a piece of fruit, 1 cup of fruit or vegetables, 1 cup of fruit or vegetable juice, or ½ cup of dried fruit.

Parents often ask if cooked vegetables or frozen vegetables are as good as fresh. The answer is yes, as long as the vegetables are not overcooked and are frozen properly.

Though juice lacks the fiber of whole fruits, it can be a good choice, because fruit and vegetable juices contain virtually the same array of vitamins and minerals as do their fresh counterparts. I recommend that you minimize use of juices that contain less than 100% juice and are not tomato-, carrot-, or citrus-based. These usually contain little vitamin C and are not much more nutritious than soda. Ideally your child will include such juices as sparingly in their diets as they do soft drinks.

**Fruit and Vegetable "Heavy Hitters"**
When it comes to which fruits and vegetables to choose, nutritionists prefer that people select an ever-changing variety since different types tend to be rich in different nutrients. By alternating your choices, you maximize the odds that you will be getting all the nutrients you need. There are, however, certain fruits and vegetables that I call the "heavy hitters" of the plant kingdom, which contain an extremely rich variety of nutrients. I recommend introducing these to your child, and putting into heavy rotation those that your child likes. The heavy hitters include broccoli, carrots, cabbage, bok choy, spinach, collard and mustard greens, fresh tomatoes, sweet red or green peppers, citrus fruits and juices, papaya, mangos, apricots, kiwi, cantaloupe, strawberries, and bananas. A single serving of any of the following heavy hitters: winter squash, yams, potatoes and sweet potatoes, contains enough complex carbohydrates to count as a full serving of that group as well as a serving of the fruit and vegetable group.

Remember that pushing your child to eat fruits and vegetables he is reluctant even to try will likely result in an even stronger aversion to those foods. It is wiser to be content with the fruits and vegetables your child likes. As children mature so do their taste buds, so I advise patience in this area. In time most children become more adventuresome with fruits and vegetables.

If you are worried that your child is not eating enough variety from the fruit and vegetable group, you can provide a multiple vitamin and mineral supplement as "nutrition insurance." Knowing your picky eater is getting adequate vitamins and minerals will keep you from worrying excessively about the nutritional needs of your young child.

### Guarding against Overconsumption

Parents should be on the lookout for excessive consumption of fruits and vegetables, since your child likely knows they are high in vitamins and minerals and low in calories and fat (with the exception of olives and avocados). Anorexics in particular may try to overconsume fruits and vegetables in order to keep from gaining weight. Too many servings (more than five per day) of these foods can contribute to feelings of overfullness and to diarrhea or constipation.

Cindy, one of my young patients, had heard that apples could cause weight loss. By the time Cindy's mother made an appointment for Cindy to see me, she was eating ten big green apples per day and little else. She didn't make the connection between her almost constant stomach cramps and her apple consumption. Most nutritionists have a story of a patient who ate so many carrots or other dark green, yellow, or orange vegetables that their skin, especially the palms of their hands, took on a decidedly orange glow. Though this effect (due to high intake of carotene, a nontoxic form of vitamin A) is not thought to be dangerous, it does indicate an eating pattern that is out of balance. Of course, overconsuming apples (or any fruit or vegetable) and virtually nothing else, as Cindy was doing, could lead to nutrient deficiencies and serious gastrointestinal problems.

### Fruit and Vegetables and the Anorexic Child

If your child needs to gain weight, she should choose fruits over vegetables since most fruits have roughly twice the calories of equivalent servings of vegetables. Because fruit juices, like other fluids, are digested quickly, they are an efficient way to obtain the nutrients and calories offered by whole fruit without contributing to feelings of overfullness.

Unfortunately, many eating-disordered people are almost phobic about drinking any fluids that contain calories, preferring instead to drink diet sodas or water. As a parent, you may want to wait until your child is feeling more comfortable with her Food Plan before suggesting fruit juices. Fruit juices are surprisingly high in calories and helpful to the anorexic who needs to gain weight.

## Fat Suggestions

Peanut butter, cheese, some meats, egg yolks, nuts, fried/sautéed foods, butter, margarine, cream cheese, salad dressing, mayonnaise, sauces, muffins and other baked goods, bacon, chips, ice cream.

### Why Fat Is Important

Fat is as essential to health as every other nutrient we have discussed. Fat-phobic eating-disorder sufferers are surprised when I tell them that fat has an important role in regulating appetite. When we eat foods that include fat at meals and snacks, we feel satisfied and less likely to overeat. We also feel more satisfied between meals because fat is slower than other nutrients to digest.

While the body can store only a limited amount of carbohydrates, the body's other source of energy, it is able to store a large number of calories in a very compact manner in the form of fat. Having a ready source of stored energy allows us to miss an occasional meal without harm. Without stored fat, our ancestors would not have survived the irregularities of their food supplies. I tell my patients that we are here today thanks to the body fat of our forebears; because of those fat stores, entire populations were able to survive even severe famine.

Fat serves as a "shock absorber," preventing damage to organs, and helps maintain body temperature, keeping us from feeling too cold or too hot. Foods that contain fat also provide us with essential vitamins (A, D, E, and K) and essential fatty acids. In addition to all these important functions, fat helps the body absorb a number of essential nutrients.

### Dietary Fat vs. Body Fat: Are They the Same Thing?

Many people are confused about dietary fat and its relationship to body fat. It is important to clarify the issue here, because for an eating-disordered person, this typical misconception underlies the fear that they have about eating fat and can have dangerous consequences. I explain to my patients that dietary fat and body fat are biologically the same substance. Yet eating dietary fat will not necessarily increase body fat. The amount of body fat any of us has is determined primarily by genetics. To a lesser extent, how many calories we take in on average also affects the amount of body fat we have. If we regularly take in more calories than we need, our bodies are able to convert the extra calories to body fat *regardless of their source*. Calories come from protein, carbohydrates, fats, or alcohol.

My patients agree that the relationship between the dietary fat that they fear and their body fat is confusing. I sometimes say to them, only half in jest, that if the fat in food was called by another name, they would not be so afraid of it. One of my patients who had taken a course in nutrition suggested that in our sessions we refer to dietary fat as "lipids," the scientific name for fats. Separating lipids, which are important to maintaining health, from body fat, she felt, underscored in a powerful way another point that I like to make to patients: over the last fifty years, while the average American intake of dietary fat has decreased, the rate of obesity has increased.

### Starvation and Fat Metabolism

Now that we have clarified the difference between dietary fat and stored body fat, we can talk briefly about fat metabolism. When extreme food restriction becomes chronic, the body eventually is able to rely on stored body fat for energy. The disadvantage of burning fat for energy when food is restricted is that it results in the potentially dangerous process known as ketosis, which we mentioned earlier in this chapter. The body makes this metabolic switch to avoid life-threatening loss of body protein from muscle, blood, and organs.

### Adding Fat to the Food Plan

Although young adolescents or children are less likely than older youths to be fat-phobic, your child may have tried to cut fat drastically from his diet. If so, it is helpful to gently tell him that dietary fat is not harmful to health. Your child needs to hear, over and over again, that fat is an essential nutrient that must be consumed daily to promote growth and to preserve health by providing necessary fatty acids and fat-soluble vitamins. You can also remind him that he lives in a society that is overly focused on the health consequences of consuming too much fat. Like protein, including enough fat in his diet will help your child feel more satisfied and less likely to binge. I do not suggest children, or adults for that matter, count fat grams. If your child insists on doing so, however, you can inform him that he should have at least 65 grams per day (equivalent to 30 percent of a 2,000 calorie diet). Even diets with this much fat are considered to be low in fat by nutritionists. Most of my patients, when I tell them this, are surprised that the requirement is so high. You might also pass on to your child the nutrition science truism that too much or too little of a nutrient over time causes health problems. For example, extreme low-fat diets are associated with higher than normal blood fats (triglycerides), a reduction in "good" cholesterol (HDLs), and even an increase in total cholesterol.

Again, for those who count fat grams, a serving is about 10 grams of fat, or 1 tablespoon of salad dressing or cream cheese; or 2 teaspoons of mayonnaise, butter, or margarine (of course, reduced-fat products don't count). A "fat" serving of nuts is one-quarter of a cup. It takes 2 tablespoons of peanut butter or other nut butters, 2 eggs, 1 ounce or 1 slice of cheese to equal a serving of fat. Typical fun foods like cake, cookies, pie, and ice cream contain 10 to 20 grams of fat per serving and help provide additional fat necessary for adequate intake.

Since protein and fat often occur together in foods, I tell my patients who need to gain weight that they may as well be efficient and choose foods that provide both. Peanut butter, cheese, some meats (like sausages and hot dogs), egg yolks, nuts, and fried/sautéed high-protein foods are a bargain in that the eater can "get credit" for both a serving of protein and fat at the same time. Remember, though, that it takes twice the serving size to provide a serving of protein as it does fat. For example, 4 tablespoons of peanut butter equals one protein serving and two fat servings. You should make sure your child does not count two tablespoon of peanut butter as a full protein serving, even though it provides one fat serving.

Peanut butter, cheese, eggs, and nuts are more likely to be chosen by eating-disordered patients than high-fat meats or fried foods, probably because they are able to focus on the protein rather than the fat content of these foods, and also because they need little or no preparation to eat.

Another way to double up on food groups is to add a couple of teaspoons to a tablespoon of fat (butter, margarine, sour cream, cream cheese) to servings of complex carbohydrates such as bread, bagels, rice, or potatoes or add salad dressing to salads or mayonnaise to sandwiches. I have found that once patients accept that they need to eat fat, they may choose to experiment with fun foods as still another way to add fat to the diet.

## A Word of Warning about Servings

We would like to make it clear that the Food Plan template ensures *minimum* amounts necessary to ensure adequate nutrition, and should not be used to limit your child's eating. You should be sure that your child has *at least* one serving of each group at most meals. For example, a reasonable meal would be a cheese sandwich, a small salad dressed with oil and vinegar, and several cookies, even though each one of these items contains enough fat to "count" as a fat serving.

## Snack Suggestions

Anything from the calcium, complex carbohydrates, fruit or vegetable, protein, fat, or fun foods categories. One snack serving is equal to one to two servings from the calcium, complex carbohydrates, fruit or vegetable, protein, fat, or fun foods categories.

**Making Use of Snacks**

At first, you can suggest that your child use snacks to fill in any gaps; that is, to fulfill any food group requirements that she has left unfulfilled during the day's meals. If all those requirements have been met already, she can be encouraged to choose freely from any of the food groups, including the fun food group. Snacks are good times to practice mixing and matching foods. One traditional snack is cheese and crackers. For most people, one-half a serving of cheese and a half a serving of crackers hits the spot. (For some-one who needs to gain weight, whole servings or more of each would be a better choice.)

## Fun Food Suggestions

Any dessert, cookies, cake, ice cream, pudding, doughnuts, croissants, candy bars, chips, fries, non-diet sodas.

**Why Fun Foods Are Important**

Fun foods are desserts, snack foods, and "junk food" that usually contain simple carbohydrates and fats. I call them fun foods because they are eaten just for pleasure, not because they provide any particular nutrient besides fat. The benefit to normal as well as disordered eaters is that these fun foods impart a supreme sense of satisfaction, a satisfaction that can actually prevent bingeing.

**Adding Fun Food to the Food Plan**

Most foods in this group provide a generous serving of fat, so the hesitant eater can "get credit" for a serving of fat. However, normal eaters typically consume one to two servings of fun food a day, usually at the end of a meal or as a snack, in addition to the two to three servings of fats specified by the Food Plan. I consider this pattern ideal, but it may be more than a child recovering from an eating disorder can manage initially.

Eating-disordered people, even young ones, tend to avoid fun foods, however, because these foods have the reputation of being unhealthy. Most find that consuming these foods creates anxiety and guilt, and for some, fun foods can seem to trigger overeating episodes. Eating-disorder sufferers often avoid these foods except during a binge, or when a purge is planned. It is your challenge as parents to try to reframe fun foods as helpful moderators of appetite rather than as triggers to a binge.

I encourage my patients to voice the fears and feelings that these fun foods give rise to. I explain that if fun foods were, in and of themselves, unhealthy to eat they would not be allowed into our food supply. Another point worth making is that the healthfulness of one's diet is best assessed by looking at its total nutrient composition, not by assessing the nutritional quality of each food. Since fun foods effectively prevent overeating and bingeing, they are important components of a healthy diet. If nutrient needs are met by well-chosen foods at meals, there is nothing wrong with eating several moderate servings of desserts or snack foods over the course of a day.

You can also point out to your child that after fulfilling nutrient needs everyone has unfulfilled caloric needs. Unless met, those needs lead to weight loss or binge eating, depending on the eating disorder the child is struggling with. I explain it to my patients this way: "Your Food Plan does a good job of meeting your protein and other nutrient needs, but it is low in calories. To remedy this you could eat either more dinner, three apples, or a bowl of ice cream—your choice." Put this way, many patients see the appeal of choosing a fun food. If they choose ice cream instead of cookies or a brownie, I point out, they are also getting a nice dose of calcium as well.

I like a serving of fun food consumed at the end of a meal because it puts a natural boundary around the meal. It is helpful to point out to a bulimic or binge-eating child that once dessert is eaten most normal eaters stop eating. Not surprisingly, in a controlled experiment of binge eaters, one study found that after meals containing protein, subjects could stop further eating by consuming "sweet-tasting, palatable food." Research has also shown that you can have a powerful curbing effect on appetite by following a relatively high-protein meal with a dessert. However, desserts eaten out of the context of a high-protein meal can lead to binges for those with eating disorders.

In hospital and residential eating-disorder treatment centers, patients are required to consume some type of dessert with meals to help patients learn to tolerate the anxiety and other negative feelings these foods provoke. The idea is to encourage the casual but regular inclusion of desserts into your child's diet, not to approach fun foods as special treats to be consumed infrequently. The latter approach can make desserts even more desirable and more likely to trigger a binge when eaten. Consuming fun foods twice a day effectively destigmatizes them and makes them less desirable.

## In Summary

The basic Food Plan that we have outlined for you in this chapter forms the crux of this book and of our nutritional approach to solving eating disorders. By explaining in detail the function and importance of each component of the plan, we hope you now have a more complete understanding of what normal, healthy eating looks like.

Because the Food Plan is simple, logical, and easily memorized, children and adults alike can adopt their own version of the Food Plan whether they are trying to solve a serious eating disorder, trying to outgrow some dangerous disordered eating habits, or simply want to eat better and feel healthier. If it is sensitively introduced, the Food Plan can be helpful to just about anyone. Our families use the Food Plan template for planning meals and making bag lunches or packing for car trips. We find it helpful when making choices at restaurants, and for just about any situation that requires some preplanning.

Much of the value of the Food Plan, however, lies in how it is adapted to fit individual situations and people. In the following chapter we will detail how you can tailor the Food Plan to your child's own needs.

# 11

# Getting the Most out of the Food Plan

As we demonstrated in chapter 10, the Food Plan is nothing more than a detailed blueprint for daily meals and snacks. For the eating-disordered child who fears losing control over her eating, or fears gaining weight (even though that is precisely what she may need to do), the Food Plan provides your child with the assurance of knowing exactly what and when she will be eating. Following the plan will, over time, both normalize your child's eating, and ensure that as this process is taking place, she is getting enough nutrients from the five major food groups (protein foods, complex carbohydrates, fruits and vegetables, high-calcium foods, and fats).

This chapter is devoted to tips on how to make the Food Plan work for your child, offering more detail on how to best implement the plan, parenting approaches that work best with it, and specific ways you can adapt the plan to the anorexic, bulimic, or binge-eating child.

## Tips on How to Make the Food Plan Work

### Adding What Is Missing

When drafting your child's first Food Plan, I advise that you use one of two approaches. You can sit down with your child and, using the template in chapter 10, p. 162, help her design her own version of the Food Plan. Or you can take your child's current diet, and using the plan as a guide, work on gradually adding the components that are lacking. The second technique is one that professional nutritionists often use, comparing the child's eating pattern with the Food Plan template, and asking, "What is missing from your diet? What do you need to add to fulfill the Food Plan?" Many eating-disordered patients like this approach because it feels therapeutic and collaborative. I find that it is one that can be easily adopted by parents working with their child. Most children, especially older teens, respond best if they are put in the "driver's seat," with parents remaining primarily in an advisory role when it comes to food choices. Be prepared to make suggestions if your child requests them, but let her take the lead in how she will begin to improve her nutrition.

### The Rule of Threes

I like to give my patients catchphrases or slogans to keep them focused on their goals and make the Food Plan easier to internalize. One is the Rule of Threes, which reminds them that the cardinal rule of the Food Plan for most people is that they should have three meals and three snacks a day, with no more than three hours between each meal or snack.

### The One-Cup Rule

Teaching your child the One-Cup Rule reminds her that if she is in doubt about how large a serving size she should eat, she can use a one-cup measure as her rough guide. This rule is based on the idea that one cup is approximately what most people consider a normal serving. It works for most liquids and solids, with the exception of very rich foods. Most people, for example, would surmise that one cup of shelled nuts is too much to eat at one sitting, as would be one cup of something rich like butter or chocolate chips. For nuts in the shell, however, one cup is about right.

While the One-Cup Rule is meant to be used more as a mental guide, a way of sizing up food on the plate by looking at it, some eating-disordered children at first cannot feel confident about serving sizes unless they physically measure their food. Parents should not prohibit measuring, but should assume that it is a temporary behavior, and will end as your child gains confidence in her ability to know when she has had enough.

### Normal Serving Sizes Are Normally Served

Even after explaining the One-Cup Rule, children with eating disorders will probably still need some guidance about serving sizes. You can start by explaining that the Food Plan is based on normal serving sizes, or portion sizes that people generally eat. Consuming less than normal serving sizes offers no advantage to a child who is recovering from an eating disorder. Instead, less than satisfying meals and snacks are likely to trigger bingeing, purging, or continued weight loss.

But what is a "normal serving size"? In the United States, where restaurant portions are notoriously overlarge compared to other countries and cultures, this is not always easy to determine.

Here are a few guidelines: a single scoop of ice cream at your local ice-cream shop is a normal serving size, as is a hamburger. School lunch programs comply with standards nutritionists have set delineating normal serving sizes, so visualizing a school lunch tray can help you and your child recognize what a normal serving is. An apple or a banana, no matter the size, is a serving of fruit. A simple rule of thumb for meats, fish, and poultry is that a modest serving is the size of a deck of cards or an outstretched palm or balled fist. This means that your child should eat at least this amount to fulfill a single protein serving. The eating habits of parents and siblings, provided they have no eating problems, can also help the child struggling with an eating disorder determine appropriate serving sizes.

While most school and college food services serve what nutritionists would call "normal" servings, many restaurants and delis do not. The recent trend in "supersizing" makes eating out a challenge for the child trying to eat normally. Because of this, those recovering from an eating disorder may want to wait until they feel they can confidently estimate normal serving sizes before eating out.

If you do decide to eat at a restaurant, be prepared to help your child, if necessary, negotiate the perils of an overlarge meal. If you know from experience that your child is likely to feel extremely guilty about overeating, and tempted to cut back the next day or purge, try suggesting that your child eat no more than one-half of a portion. Or, when your child seems overwhelmed by a New York–style deli sandwich that looks like it could serve a family of four, try suggesting, "Would you like me to cut that sandwich into a serving size for you?"

Remember, though, that for most children, no real harm is done if they consume all of a larger-than-normal portion at a restaurant. Most of us eat slightly more at restaurants than we do at home. This is not a health problem unless most meals are oversized, as the body is able to average out varying caloric intakes.

When eating at home using packaged foods, on the other hand, you will need to serve larger serving sizes than what the manufacturer recommends. Since serving sizes listed on packaged food labels are usually half of a normal serving size, you should double the portion size specified on those package labels.

Remember, if in doubt about a normal serving size, one cup is a close approximation. By initially serving your child one-cup servings, you can help her internalize the concept of "normal serving sizes." Over time, she will absorb this lesson and eventually be able to come to the dinner table feeling confident in knowing how much she should eat. She will not be overly fixated on serving sizes because she will know that any approximation of a "normal serving size" is just that, an approximation. Eating slightly more or less than a normal serving size at any given meal will not be cause for alarm, because she will feel confidence in her ability to maintain a healthy weight, despite these normal fluctuations in meal and snack sizes.

I cannot overemphasize the benefits that will accrue to your child when you are confident about portion sizes. Confidence breeds confidence. If you master and internalize the concept of normal serving sizes, so will your child.

## Eat When Hungry, Stop When Satisfied

Although this sounds simple, anyone with an eating disorder can tell you that it is not. Having an eating disorder renders most sufferers, at least initially, unable to accurately assess their own level of hunger and satisfaction. Being able to read and respond to natural internal hunger and satisfaction cues is in fact one sign of having recovered from an eating disorder. One of the first goals I work on with my patients is encouraging them to pay attention to the first, often faint, signals of hunger or fullness from their body. This is one of the early and important benefits of following the Food Plan, since adhering to it will effectively "recalibrate" your child's perceptions of hunger and satisfaction. Encourage your child to pay close attention to the signals her body is sending her at various times in the day as she follows the Food Plan. What is her body telling her right before it is time for a meal or snack? How does her body feel right after she has finished that meal or snack? Gradually, she will begin to trust her body when it signals to her when and how much to eat.

I find that for most patients, it is easier to recognize and accurately interpret signs of hunger than those of fullness. I tell them, "If you are hungry the odds are high that your body needs food, even if you have fulfilled the Food Plan." Fullness, though, is a much harder sensation for the eating-disorder sufferer to accurately discern. Often anorexics, especially, will feel full before they are able to fulfill their Food Plan. I suggest that they follow it anyway, noting that over time, following the Food Plan will calibrate their "fullness sensation" so it, too, can be a helpful guide to how much to eat and when to stop eating.

I call this approach to food "eating in tune." The child who is eating in tune may occasionally leave a bite, or ask for a smidgen more of something. You should be suspicious, however, if your child's eating strays substantially from the Food Plan. Until an underweight child attains a healthy weight, you should insist that she follow the Food Plan.

**Calibrating Hunger and Fullness for the Child**
**Who Needs to Gain Weight**
For the child who needs to gain weight, your rule of thumb when it comes to hunger and fullness should be that your child can eat more than the Food Plan specifies when hungry, but when full, should eat *at least* what the plan specifies. If your underweight child is losing weight following the Food Plan, regardless of her reports of fullness and lack of hunger, her plan must immediately be altered to include more food and calories.

**Calibrating Hunger and Fullness for the**
**Normal Weight or Overweight Child**
If weight is not an issue for your child, and he is too full to eat all that the Food Plan specifies for a meal, try moving a serving or two from the meal to the next snack.

If your normal weight or overweight child is gaining weight following the Food Plan, it is probably because he is still binge eating. In the spirit of problem solving, you should help your child figure out why this is so. Often binge behavior continues because either the child is not fully following the Food Plan or his Food Plan is inadequate in some way. Continued problems with binge eating usually indicate the child's plan is too low in calories, too low in protein or fat, does not include enough fun food, or there is too great a span between planned meals and snacks.

**Structure Now Means Freedom Later**
The paradox of the Food Plan is that though it seems extremely scripted and rigid, following it will actually over time give your child the tools she needs to eat in a carefree, natural way, trusting her own ability to eat when she is hungry and to stop eating when she is full.

Some children find immediate relief in the Food Plan and the guidance it provides. Others, like Claudia, whose doctor told her she needed to gain 15 pounds, found the idea of following a Food Plan demeaning. She insisted that at sixteen years old she knew exactly what she needed to do to gain weight, "I know how to eat, I'm not a baby! I certainly don't need a Food Plan to tell me what to eat," she told me indignantly. I suggested that she see what she could do in a week's time to gain the weight her doctor instructed her to. A week later Claudia had lost, not gained weight.

Although she was not happy about it, she began working with me to develop a Food Plan for herself. Most children in Claudia's situation need specific meals and snacks planned. I brought Claudia's mother, Miranda, to the session so that the three of us could put our heads together to come up with an individualized Food Plan. One advantage of following the Food

Plan, I reminded Claudia, is that if she does not gain weight, it is the plan's fault. Claudia brightened at this thought, and became more enthusiastic about the plan. The truth was that she was overwhelmed with guilt when she lost weight and knew her parents were almost sick with worry. The idea of shifting the burden of beginning to eat from her shoulders to the Food Plan was immensely appealing to her.

Within half an hour, Claudia, Miranda, and I came up with four different versions of the Food Plan using foods Claudia likes for the three meals and snacks Claudia needed to be eating. By mixing and matching, Claudia realized she would not be bored. I promised her, as I do all my patients, that Food Plans are to be continually revised so that the foods Claudia wants to eat are included.

Excited by the possibilities of the Food Plan, Claudia followed her plan scrupulously the next week and came to her next appointment feeling proud of her accomplishment. When a weight check revealed that she had lost, not gained weight, she was devastated. How could all of her hard, painful work have resulted in failure? Most parents, when they see such results, are either incredulous, since they have seen how much their child has eaten that week, or are angry, assuming their child has somehow "cheated" during the week. In Claudia's case, her parents were baffled and disappointed.

First I explained that they needed to understand the extraordinary mental effort and physical discomfort involved when an anorexic child like Claudia begins to follow the Food Plan. Then I comforted Claudia and her parents by explaining that what she had just experienced is absolutely the norm. When an anorexic begins to improve her diet, her metabolism can jump sky-high so that as she eats more, she loses more weight. I concluded by reassuring them once again that the Food Plan will work if they give it a chance and if Claudia continues to add food to her plan until she is consistently gaining weight.

"All we have to do now," I told them, "is figure out what you need to add this week. We will keep adding to your plan until you are gaining at least one pound per week." Claudia stuck to her Food Plan, and as time passed, found that she was able to gain the weight she needed and eat in a more carefree, unscripted manner.

### No Food Is Forbidden
Your child will also find it liberating to hear that, contrary to common belief, no food, in and of itself, is fattening, forbidden, or addictive. In fact, any food can be incorporated into the Food Plan, although I usually advise adding "scary" or potentially binge-triggering foods after the Food Plan is firmly in place.

Deirdre's story is a good example of how to slowly incorporate forbidden foods into the plan. Deirdre is a chronic binger. Like many children who have fearful aversions to certain foods, she, upon first adopting the Food Plan, chooses a "safe" fun food—in her case, fat-free pudding. She feels safe with the pudding because it is fat-free and is available in single-serving sizes. After using the pudding for several weeks, Deirdre grows confident in the Food Plan's ability to maintain her weight. Then I pose an experiment, suggesting that at lunch Deirdre substitute a prepackaged brownie for the pudding. We pick lunchtime for this experiment because at school there is no opportunity to binge.

The experiment is a success. Deirdre describes how thrilled she is with the power she now feels she has over brownies. She really *can* eat just one. A week later, though, she binges after school. Like many eating-disordered patients, she is quick to place the blame on the fun food component of her Food Plan, in her case, the brownie she had after lunch.

"Wait a minute," I say. "It is much more likely that your binge was caused by skimping on your Food Plan." Sure enough, that day at lunch, Deirdre had let her worries about her weight interfere with the plan and had skipped eating her sandwich. I remind her that one or two brownies per day, or their equivalent, will not cause weight gain, but bingeing will. With renewed commitment to the Food Plan, Deirdre was soon eating her lunchtime fun food with confidence.

I tell my patients that as long as they avoid certain foods they will continue to find them scary. They need to work at learning to eat scary foods just as a person who is afraid of heights works at his phobia—one rung of the ladder at a time. When the bingeing or rapid weight gain they anticipated does not materialize, they are able to reassure themselves that these forbidden foods do not in and of themselves have the power to trigger binges. No food, in fact, does. Yet because no good results from terrifying a child who has a serious eating disorder, exposure to feared foods should not occur until the child feels comfortable following her Food Plan.

### Less Than Perfect Eating Is Perfectly Okay

Keep in mind that the Food Plan is a general guide. If on most days your child's eating approximates that of the Food Plan you have adopted, you can be confident that her nutrient needs are being met. I encourage parents not to become overly fixated on following the Food Plan precisely. Remember, your child does not need to eat perfectly to be perfectly healthy.

The Food Plan is based on what scientists believe each of us should eat to meet our nutrient needs, a sort of statistical average diet. Just as a non-eating-disordered person may eat unevenly from day to day but over the course of a week or a month eat a balanced diet, so can you allow a certain amount of leeway as your child follows the Food Plan.

Having said this, I must add that you have cause for concern if your child is losing weight or bingeing. Since it is a nutritional truism that undereating eventually results in either weight loss or bingeing, it is likely that the Food Plan is not adequate and should be revised, that either serving sizes are too small, or that too many low-calorie foods are being chosen.

**Individualize Your Child's Food Plan**

Another appealing aspect of the Food Plan is that it can be tailored to fit your child's natural eating patterns. Protein and fat servings are optional at breakfast, because many children do well with a lighter breakfast, knowing that they will get their protein and fat later in the day. The morning snack is also a flexible component. I have noticed, for example, that college students who have a late breakfast and an early lunch may not be hungry enough for a morning snack.

Some children prefer to eat four or five small meals a day rather than the standard three. This works well for children who are very hungry when they come home from school and particularly in families where dinner is served late. Providing a snack that includes all the components of a meal (most importantly, protein and fat) helps prevent the overeating that can happen at this time of day if children eat more typical snack foods, such as pretzels or chips. Fruit, certainly a healthy snack, by itself is not satisfying enough to stave off the hunger that can trigger a binge. Many of my patients find that crackers and cheese or peanut butter eaten with a piece of fruit is very satisfying. Another popular snack is yogurt and granola and a piece of fruit. For those who want something hot, macaroni and cheese works well. The Food Plan can be adjusted to fit this pattern simply by diminishing serving sizes at dinner to restore its overall balance. Most children do this naturally; if they eat a bigger after-school snack, dinner is smaller.

What you should avoid is the situation where your child fills up on less-than-nutritious snacks in the afternoon and then picks at dinner because he is not hungry. A small dinner is acceptable if your child's after-school snack is well balanced and contains enough protein to constitute a protein serving. By the end of the day your child should have fulfilled all the food groups indicated in the Food Plan; whether these essential servings are consumed as snacks or meals is not important.

Anorexic children whose primary goal is weight gain may have to add additional food groups to snacks, or increase the size of servings in both meals and snacks. It is not unusual, however, for the anorexic child to take advantage of her parents' willingness to individualize her Food Plan and perhaps almost unconsciously begin to make lower-calorie food choices or to skimp on snacks. It is worth repeating that if your child is losing weight, it means she is not eating enough and that more servings or higher-calorie food choices must be added to her Food Plan. In this situation, exercise patterns should also be reassessed. (See chapter 12 for more information.)

## Make Incremental Improvements Your Goal

Both you and your child should be aware that very few people can pull off a wholesale adoption of the Food Plan from the outset. Your goal should be incremental improvements in diet, using the Food Plan as your template. By continually encouraging your child to add to her diet and cheering her on with each success, the task of going from barely eating at all, in some cases, to a three-meal, three-snacks-a day regimen is not nearly so daunting. As your child progresses in her recovery, she will eventually be able to choose a well-balanced diet using a variety of foods.

## Provide Confident Food Advice

As we stress throughout this book, it is immeasurably reassuring to an eating-disordered child when parents are confident that they know just what their child needs to eat to get better.

I often tell parents to exude confidence when determining portion sizes at meals. You can tell your child that the portions that you usually serve at mealtimes are normal portions, and that you guarantee that eating these normal portions distributed across three meals and three snacks will not cause weight gain. To gain weight, you might add, most people have to eat substantially more than the Food Plan template.

You may come to a point, however, where your child is not satisfied with your answers, or seems concerned about nutrition information you are unfamiliar with. This may mean it is time to bring in the services of a nutrition professional. (See p. 206, and chapter 14, p. 262, for more information.)

## Treat the Food Plan Like a Homework Assignment

Alice's parents found that approaching the Food Plan like a school homework assignment was effective. As with homework, they expected Alice to "just do it," no excuses allowed. And like homework, their job as parents was to make sure she had the time, the place, and the tools (in this case the food) necessary to complete her assignments. They also needed to be prepared to offer their help and support if their daughter was struggling with her assignments. There are many ways that a family can approach the Food Plan as "homework assignments." In my experience, most families find a way that works for them. Some parents, like Alice's, find it helpful to look at the strategies they use to get their children to do their homework or household chores. Alice was allowed to watch a half hour of television on school nights (*Seinfeld* reruns were her favorite) if she got her homework done first. Why not, her parents thought, use the same strategy to help Alice finish dinner and dessert? Alice had to complete her homework and her Food Plan before the television was turned on. Alice came up with an even better idea: "How about if I finish my dinner before *Seinfeld*, but eat my dessert during the show?" Her parents agreed to give the amended plan a try, and they and Alice were delighted when it worked. As Alice's story illustrates, letting your child make suggestions about Food Plan homework assignments can work well, as long as you feel that the assignment represents a substantial enough step on her road to recovery.

There is no question that these homework assignments are more easily accomplished if your child is enthusiastic and motivated to adopt the Food Plan. The truth is, however, that many children are not, at least initially. Although it is more of a challenge for parents when your child is less than eager, I recommend experimenting with this "homework assignment" approach to get your child started on a Food Plan anyway. If instituted properly, the Food Plan will eventually win your child over with its logic, and help put her on the road to recovery.

## Sample Food Plan: Belinda's Story

The following case history illustrates how the Food Plan can be used to achieve gradual weight gain.

For the first time in her life, Belinda begins struggling with food issues the summer before her first year of high school. The technique I use with her, as with all of my patients, is to give her a copy of the Food Plan template. We painstakingly go through the plan, starting with breakfast and filling each food group in with foods Belinda either likes or feels comfortable eating.

I start the process by saying, "What do you want to eat for your carbs at breakfast?" Belinda suggests cereal, to which I respond, "Perfect. Remember that a serving size is a cup of cereal. Can you think of another carbohydrate you like, in case you get tired of cereal?" To this, Belinda responds, "Well, I like bagels." "Another good choice," I say. "Putting cream cheese or butter on the bagel would give you a fat serving. How about that?" "Noooo, I am certainly not ready for that," Belinda says. "That's okay for now," I tell her.

Belinda's parents are instructed to prepare meals that meet the Food Plan guidelines. Using one of Belinda's favorite dinner meals, grilled chicken, I show Belinda and Mimi how a dinner based on the Food Plan might look. I point out that most families just naturally prepare meals that meet the Food Plan guidelines, and I make it clear to Mimi that I expect meals (especially dinner) to vary day to day. I also explain that in the beginning, at least, Belinda will be more successful following the plan if the Food Plan groups are fulfilled using foods Belinda is comfortable with. Belinda, like a lot of girls I work with, has recently given up eating beef. Mimi agrees to fix two tofu hot dogs, another of Belinda's favorites, when she is serving beef to the rest of the family.

Next, I note approvingly that the Food Plan that Belinda, Mimi, and I have created calls for frequent meals, an eating pattern that eases the feelings of fullness that anorexics often feel when first adopting a Food Plan.

I point out that Belinda's current Food Plan does not call for eating desserts, and we discuss the efficacy of one or two desserts a day as protection from both anorexic relapses or from bingeing. Belinda, like most anorexics, is quite worried about the possibility of bingeing, even though she has not engaged in this behavior before.

We work on coming up with some dessert options, and I encourage Belinda to add whatever foods she feels comfortable with. Often, I will ask my patients, "What do you want to add, or what do you think you can add?" I also make sure to provide abundant positive feedback and encouragement at any suggestions that add substantial calories.

## Parenting Approaches That Work with the Food Plan

The following tips outline the attitudes and approaches that will work best for you as you help your child adopt a Food Plan.

### Be Patient

At first your child will probably be unable to agree to add enough food to actually increase their weight. Yet as long as she has shown a willingness to change something, remain supportive and positive. Often with my patients, I happily agree to changes knowing full well that their next weigh-in is unlikely to show any weight gain. When the next visit arrives, I say in a matter-of-fact manner, "It looks like your body is telling us that you need to add more food. What are your ideas?" Being patient does not mean that you should not expect weight gain. It means you should matter-of-factly keep adding to the Food Plan until your child is gaining weight.

Often children with eating disorders will draw a blank when it comes to what foods to add. If this happens with your child, you should refer back to the original Food Plan template to "see what is missing." Pointing out that your child is missing protein, fats, or carbohydrates often will help the reluctant child generate her own ideas of foods that she can eat. Or, you can simply prod her to choose a food from our list of suggestions in chapter 10.

## Be Firm, Don't Collude With Your Child

Sometimes it is hard for parents not to collude with their child when first adopting a Food Plan, serving her frugal portions of the few low-calorie foods she will eat. To gain the minimum one pound a week doctors like to see, however, your child will have to accept bigger servings and richer foods. As you become used to using the Food Plan, you will become better at assessing when increases are called for to help your child achieve this rate of weight gain, and how much food to add.

Alexis's parents unintentionally colluded in a different way. Alexis's weight loss began during a serious, two-week bout with the flu. First she lost her appetite and then a very sore throat made eating uncomfortable. She lost 12 pounds, a trend that continued when her parents bought their dream house in another part of town and Alexis had to endure a stressful midyear change of school.

Like many anorexics, Alexis felt compelled to be involved in food preparation and shopping. It was a way for her to have contact with food without actually eating. She was her mother's best kitchen helper, sometimes cooking the family's entire dinner without taking a single bite herself. Her family colluded by continuing to allow Alexis to prepare food, and also letting her refuse to eat it. Hearing about Alexis's behavior reminded me of my bout with teenage anorexia, when I would prepare fancy hams, artfully decorated with cloves and pineapple. I, too, never took even a single bite of those dishes I painstakingly prepared.

My role with Alexis was to help her parents regain control of the family's food preparation and get her own eating back on track. Alexis was allowed to help with cooking, but only with dishes that she was willing to eat.

To Alexis, eating was no fun, it was "a drag." Although I expressed sympathy for these feelings, I reviewed the Food Plan with her, and explained that it outlined the minimum amount she had to eat to maintain her health. Alexis decided that she would simply tell herself she had to eat. On her second visit, she agreed that it would help if her mom packed her a lunch that matched the Food Plan. On her third visit, I suggested she add another snack so that she had a total of three snacks per day. Alexis suggested she have a milk shake before bed. This, I told her, was a great idea. Gradually, as her own eating normalized, her need to cook for others without partaking herself diminished.

## Don't Become the "Eating-Disorder Police"

Just as we have warned you about the dangers of colluding with your child, or caving in to her strong-willed desires to eat little or nothing at all, so must we warn you against going to the opposite extreme and becoming the "eating-disorder police."

Lavonne's parents were rightfully alarmed by her weight loss. Their worry caused them to be excessively watchful of her every bite. They found themselves pressuring her to eat just one more bite, and often, to eat far more than was necessary. The Food Plan helped Lavonne and her parents relax a little, and feel confident that they knew fairly precisely what and how much she needed to eat.

**Rewards and Penalties: Should You Use Them?**
I advise parents never to use rewards and penalties to promote weight loss in bulimic or binge-eating children, since these methods send the message that your love and approval are predicated on how your child looks.

Rewarding weight gain, on the other hand, does not seem to be fraught with such difficulties. Research has shown that rewarding weight gain results in increases in both caloric intake and weight.

Before you institute an elaborate system of rewards, however, a few caveats about their use are in order:

• **Reward actual weight gain, not improved eating behavior.** Why? Because increased eating, even significant leaps, does not always lead to weight gain. If you reward improved food behaviors you may find your-selves in the nonproductive situation of giving your child lots of rewards while he or she continues to lose weight.

The deviousness that often goes hand-in-hand with anorexia, even among essentially good children, can also make rewarding food behaviors, not weight gain, backfire. My patient Nicholas told me that he had become expert in hiding food in his napkin at dinner. Had his parents rewarded him for eating a good dinner, he would have felt that he was pulling one over on them, and would have likely spent his time thinking of other ways to deceive them at meals.

• **Don't be overly hasty in rewarding weight gain.** This is important because weight changes in anorexic children can be volatile. Marti and Frank agreed that their daughter Melissa would be able to pick out a new CD if she gained 2 pounds. Just as they hoped, Melissa immediately improved her eating, gained the 2 pounds, and happily went shopping for the latest Britney Spears CD. A week later, the 2 pounds had vanished and Melissa had even lost a few more. Frank insisted Melissa hand over the CD until her weight was back up, which, as you can imagine, did not go over well with Melissa. The Johnson family ended up in even more of a pickle when they rewarded their daughter's weight gain with the puppy she had always wanted. Of course, when she lost the weight, they couldn't take the puppy back.

It is better, experts think, to reward weight gains in increments of 5 pounds or so, and after the increase has been maintained for a week or more.

• **Save substantial gifts for substantial gains.** I have seen parents use pets, special vacations (one mom promised her daughter a winter cruise), permission to take a special art course, or signing up for a summer sailing camp as rewards for weight gain. If you choose to give such rewards, I suggest that you make sure your child first puts in a substantial amount of time and effort and makes truly significant progress. Not only will you feel that your reward is justified if you do this, but children are less likely to have relapses if they have made substantial progress.

• **When possible, try to offer activities rather than possessions as rewards.** As our examples of the CD or the puppy used as rewards show, parents can get into binds when they promise objects or possessions rather than access to a cherished activity.

If your reward is an activity, however, and your child loses weight, permission to participate in the activity can easily be withdrawn. Garrett was told by his doctor that he needed to regain over 20 pounds. His parents found that he made regular progress if they allowed him to go driving with one of them (he had just received his learner's permit) on the weekends immediately following the weeks in which he gained at least one pound.

• **If you do reward with objects, keep them small.** An exception to the rule of avoiding possessions as rewards is small objects. Stickers are a good example of a reward small enough that they seem to avoid many of the complications we describe above. I have seen parents effectively use stickers to "acknowledge" days when their child has successfully followed the Food Plan.

• **Avoid offering rewards for finishing meals or snacks.** Parents are often tempted to reward their children for finishing meals and snacks. Experts advise against this as they have seen too many patients eat their meals and snacks yet lose weight because they were also surreptitiously over-exercising or purging, or still not eating enough to match their metabolic needs.

• **Honor your promises.** If you do decide to reward weight gain, it is essential that you not waver on delivering the promised rewards when a goal is achieved. Conversely, your child must not receive the reward if she fails to gain the requisite amount of weight.

## Protect Your Own Eating Habits

Sometimes parents can become so involved and invested in getting their child to eat that they find that their own eating patterns are affected. In the case of my patient Charlotte, her anorexia was so advanced when I first began to see her that her mother, Marilyn, had to take over almost all meal and snack preparation before Charlotte could make progress. Charlotte was so "hungry" for her mother's company and attention that she even demanded that Marilyn eat meals and snacks with her. Marilyn began to worry that she herself was gaining weight. I made it clear that Charlotte's food needs were unique to Charlotte, and although she needed Marilyn's involvement, there was no benefit in Marilyn ignoring her own body's signals and overeating just to get Charlotte to eat. A number of mothers and several fathers have told me that they have gained weight trying to help their child eat more.

When some patients have realized that they inadvertently caused a parent to gain weight, they have felt extremely guilty and tried to use their guilt to justify reducing their food intake. Other girls, particularly those who are in the early phases of treatment, may demand that their mothers eat what they have to eat and suffer as they do by gaining weight against their wills. You should be on guard against this phenomenon, and support your child's Food Plan without making your own eating an issue.

One approach is for you to make it clear that your own eating patterns are not up for discussion. While you should keep your own efforts to lose weight private, those efforts should not affect your effort help your child recover from her eating disorder. Remember to keep the focus on your child's eating, not on your own.

## Rely on Weight Monitoring to Calm Weight-Related Anxieties

Regular weight checks are a necessity for the underweight anorexic child and can be very helpful for the bulimic child or binge-eating child who worries that improvements in eating will translate to weight gain.

The regular weight checks that a doctor or nutritionist usually conducts can give your child an important sense of confidence. I do not usually encourage parents to monitor their child's weight at home because only rarely have I seen parents handle this successfully. You and/or your eating-disordered child may lack confidence in the accuracy and reliability of your home scale, or you may have difficulty interpreting changes in your child's weight. Knowing that there is a scale in the home, your child is apt to want to weigh herself repeatedly as well.

Julie, one of my severely anorexic patients, would weigh herself every hour that she had access to a scale, even if it meant setting her alarm so that she could weigh herself throughout the night. Her parents tried hiding the scale, but Julie would search until she found it. Eventually, they threw the scale out. Not only is this out-of-control obsessive behavior, but the child's fear of weight gain can be aggravated by frequent weigh-ins.

After hearing my reasons for eschewing weigh-ins at home, some parents may still want to experiment with them. If this happens, I respond, "I can't argue with success. If weigh-ins at home go well and lead to progress, then go ahead with my blessing." (For more on weight monitoring by a professional, see chapter 14, p. 262, and Appendix B.)

### Your Goal Is to Aid in Recovery, Then Return Control of Eating to Your Child

Remember not to lose sight of the fact that the purpose of the Food Plan is to address the immediate problem of helping your child learn to regulate his own eating. Once your child is consistently managing his food responsibly we encourage you to gradually return control to him. We also remind you that just because you are closely involved in your child's eating, this is not license to be overinvolved in other areas of his life.

## Adapting the Food Plan for the Anorexic Child

### Adding Calories to the Anorexic's Food Plan

For anorexics, the idea is to augment the Food Plan continually until your child is gaining weight. When weight gain stops, you need to add more food to the plan, until your child has achieved a healthy weight.

The abject fear most anorexic children have about gaining weight too quickly or gaining too much weight makes it prudent for parents to incorporate additional calories gradually. Your child's body weight will be your guide as to how slowly or how quickly you can, or need, to do this. If your underweight child is losing weight, you must insist she increase the pace of her caloric additions. If her weight is stable then one or two weeks in which little to no weight is gained can usually be tolerated without jeopardizing your child's health. If she does not begin to gain weight after that, however, or continues to lose weight, you should consult a professional.

Because rapid, unchecked weight gain will be your child's biggest worry, it can be helpful to tell her that such an occurrence is highly unlikely, mainly because it is very hard for an underweight person to gain weight. Because the starving body resists gaining weight, it takes well above and beyond a normal intake of food for most anorexics to begin to restore weight. Another reason out-of-control weight gain almost never happens with anorexics is that if a child has been undereating for any length of time, she is likely to feel quite full even after modest food intake, and will at first find it hard to eat the large quantities necessary for even modest weight gain.

From a medical point of view, gaining weight quickly rarely causes problems. The exceptions are the rare cases in which a severely anorexic child who is being tube-fed is at risk for complications from refeeding (see chapter 6, p. 94, for more information).

Although, as we have said, we do not encourage calorie counting, when your goal is weight gain, it is helpful to keep in mind that each addition to the Food Plan should total at least 300 calories. Most anorexics can tolerate additions of about 300 to 500 calories per day. Since most protein and fun food servings are about 300 calories, adding a serving of either is an easy way to add on to the plan. A single serving of the other food groups (calcium, carbohydrates, fruit, and fat) are about 100 calories, so more of these would have to be added. Vegetables are so low in calories that most nutritionists do not allow vegetables to be counted toward any additions aimed at weight gain.

When Kirsten needed to add to her Food Plan, I asked her what she wanted to add. Her first suggestion was a protein bar. Since I knew that was about 200 calories, I applauded her choice and then asked what she could add from the calcium, carbohydrate, fruit, or fat groups. "How about a yogurt?" she suggested. "An excellent choice," I responded. Kirsten and her mother figured out that she could add the protein bar to her afternoon snack and the yogurt to her breakfast meal. The next week, despite her good additions to the plan, Kirsten's weight was down again. Knowing that her lunch did not include a fun food, I suggested she add a dessert to lunch. Kirsten liked the idea of finishing lunch with a bowl of ice cream and a cup of tea.

As Kirsten's story illustrates, with a little basic math, most parents can figure out how to add the calories their child needs using the foods their child is most interested in.

### When Your Child Has Achieved a Healthy Weight

When your anorexic child has achieved her weight goal, you should (as I usually do with my patients who have achieved this breakthrough) advise her to continue following the Food Plan until it is clear that her weight is stable and she is no longer in danger of losing weight. At this point, she can begin eliminating some of the servings that are above and beyond the Food Plan Template. I advise my patients to pay close attention to their sensations of hunger and fullness, aiming to avoid both going hungry and feeling overly full. Any reductions in the Food Plan must be made very, very slowly, and only after it is clear that your child is maintaining her weight. This may not occur for a number of months after your child has regained all of her lost weight. While your child's weight is in flux, her weight should be checked periodically. Reductions in the plan can continue as long as she is able to maintain a normal weight.

It is important that you make sure, however, that your child does not cut down to below what the Food Plan template calls for. Eating below the Food Plan template may lead to less-than-adequate nutrient intake and/or a relapse. After your child has maintained a normal weight for a while, she will likely find that her body weight has become less responsive to under-eating. This is normally how the body protects itself against weight loss. For the recovering child, however, it can be read as a license to undereat: "See, Mom, my weight is okay, so I must be eating enough." If you allow this to continue unchecked, your child may conclude that if she eats any more she will gain weight. Again, you should insist your child eat at least the number of servings outlined in the Food Plan template.

As your child recovers from her eating disorder, her goal (as well as yours) should be to internalize the Food Plan, becoming less preoccupied with following it to the letter, but retaining the spirit of the plan as a guide to good eating for the whole family.

## Hypermetabolism of Anorexia: When Metabolism Shifts from Very Slow to Very Fast

Anorexia in its most severe stages causes the body to adapt to starvation by slowing its metabolism down to a snail's pace. But when the anorexic begins to eat again, she triggers a process of bodily repair and restoration that can cause her metabolism to shoot through the roof. This phenomenon is known as "hypermetabolism of anorexia," and is one that parents who are dealing with an underweight child should be aware of. If your child has reached this stage, she may need to consume up to twice the calories that would normally be expected of a healthy child or, in fact, of a recovering bulimic or binge-eating child.

For the child, this is a unique predicament that can be difficult to adjust to. Although your child may initially lose weight quickly, she soon finds that even though she is eating almost nothing, very little further weight loss results. She concludes that her caloric needs are in fact modest. This is an example of the "famine metabolism" at work that we mentioned in chapter 10, p. 166. Loss of body weight and muscle mass, and the increased caloric efficiency of her body as it responds to starvation has caused her metabolic rate to drop to a very low level, and her weight loss to slow or even stop. To lose more weight, the anorexic may have to restrict even further.

When food intake is improved, the body begins to repair itself and to restore weight, a process that requires a tremendous number of calories. This refeeding leads to an increase in metabolic rate, likely caused by the caloric costs of growing lean body tissue and restoring depleted fat stores, as well as the increases in protein synthesis, heart rate, and body tempera-ture that go along with improved nutrition.

When hypermetabolism of anorexia occurs, the anorexic's Food Plan must be regularly increased until the anorexic approaches normal weight levels. After weight has been restored, most anorexics are able to maintain a normal weight on normal food intake. Some, however, will need to eat more than normal for a year or longer to maintain normal weight.

Some anorexics may gain a little weight when calories are initially increased even if their total intake remains far below normal. Parents should not be misled into thinking this means their child can survive on below-normal calorie and nutrient intakes. This little blip upward in weight is usually temporary and unless the child truly improves her food intake, she will begin to lose weight again or won't gain another ounce.

The high calories needed for most anorexics to gain weight is so far above what they can eat comfortably that most cannot create an effective Food Plan on their own.

When we started working together to overcome her anorexia, my patient Traci agreed to having a "regular" dinner (meaning a dinner typical in amounts and food choices for her family) that matched the basic Food Plan template. When Traci's weekly weigh-in showed that she had lost weight, I instructed Traci and her mother, Joan, to make sure Traci added something (either another serving or increase the size of servings) to her base plan of three meals and snacks. This routine was to be continued until Traci began gaining weight, at which point her Food Plan could plateau.

At its peak, Traci's expanded Food Plan included several generous servings over the basic Food Plan template, with additions made to the calcium, fat, and fun food groups. She typically began the day with a big bowl of cereal and milk and a generous-size glass of juice. Several hours later she ate a large muffin and drank a glass of milk. A typical lunch was a sandwich made with a whole can of tuna and mayonnaise, two cups of milk, a small bag of chips, and three good-sized cookies. Traci's afternoon snack was a bowl of granola and yogurt (a cup of each) and a piece of fruit. At dinner, one favorite entrée was an ample serving of salmon served with a baked potato and steamed carrots (both with pats of butter) and topped off with a dessert. Before bed, she ate two cups of ice cream.

Traci's story illustrates just how large the recovering anorexic's food intake may need to be in order for her to begin to gain weight. Within a month Traci had gained 3 pounds and had memorized the Food Plan. As is typical, during the first several weeks, Traci complained of uncomfortable fullness, but by the end of the month she felt appropriately hungry before meals and comfortable afterward.

Anorexics such as Traci who need to gain weight often find it more palatable to add additional servings of fun food rather than to add yet another entrée or supplementary servings of other foods. The difficulty of meeting their extraordinarily high caloric needs means that they should not be discouraged from eating more than the recommended two servings per day of fun foods as long as nutrient needs are met by adequate servings of the other food groups.

**Don't Take Your Child's Anger Personally**

It is perfectly normal for your anorexic child to go through a period of anger, defiance, and outright rebellion when she first begins to eat more and gain weight. This period of poorly controlled emotional outbursts can be hard to take when you are used to the model behavior of the classic anorexic. I advise parents not to take this behavior personally; it is to be expected as your child faces the frightening prospect of letting go of her eating-disordered behavior.

In Carla's case, not only did she argue about serving sizes, she became exceedingly cranky at mealtimes, speaking to her parents in ways she never had before. Even her behavior outside of meals was far from pleasant. One way to look at this development is that the anorexia arrests development so that when the child begins to eat and gain weight she is thrust headlong into the turmoil of puberty. Most parents, as Carla's did, find a balance between allowing more expression of negative feelings yet limiting how disruptive the child is allowed to be. Carla's parents found that sending her to her room for a 15-minute cooling-off period was effective when she went on one of her yelling tirades.

## Adapting the Food Plan for the Bulimic Child

**Explaining the Food Plan to Your Child: Why Purging Doesn't Work**

When fourteen-year-old figure skater Amelia first came to see me, she was engaging in self-induced vomiting as a means of controlling the weight that her binge eating made a constant worry. We first had to address Amelia's fear of weight gain, since it was interfering with her efforts to stop purging and improve the size and quality of her meals. At first Amelia was incredulous when I explained to her the limited effect vomiting has on calories. Studies show that regardless of the size of the binge, the body holds on to about 1,200 calories. Researchers have also shown that over time, most bulimics gain weight. This is because purging leads to larger and larger binges, and does not rid the body of nearly as many calories as bulimics believe it does.

I told Amelia that she would have no hope of controlling her binges and her weight unless she was following a reasonable and satisfying Food Plan. Intrigued, she agreed to try the Food Plan, with the understanding that until the Food Plan was fully in place she should expect to continue to have some trouble with bingeing.

When you sit down to discuss the Food Plan with your child, it is helpful to be aware of the following facts:

- Bulimics who stop purging usually simultaneously stop bingeing.
- Purging with laxatives causes a decrease in caloric absorption by approximately 10 percent only.
- Purging by self-inducing vomiting eliminates some calories, but as I told Amelia, about 1,200 calories are retained.
- Purging with diuretics provides no decrease in caloric absorption at all; any change in weight associated with diuretics results from the loss of body water.
- Most patients do not gain weight as the result of recovering from an eating disorder unless they are underweight.
- Long-term bulimics and binge eaters who have gained above their normal weight as the result of their eating disorder most likely will lose some weight with normalized eating patterns.
- If your child's weight has not changed in spite of the bulimia or binge eating, she is most likely to remain at or near her current weight as she recovers.

One approach that is almost always essential if parents are going to be successful in helping their bulimic or binge-eating child is to let her know that her bingeing and/or purging make "perfect sense," but they have tragically backfired. In other words, bingeing is a natural reaction to undereating; while purging, in this day and age, is not an uncommon response to overeating. Though you may be appalled when you learn the details of your child's bingeing and purging behaviors, it is best to let your child know that more than anything else, you are worried about her, especially about the possibility of her eating behaviors becoming chronic. The life of either a bulimic or binge eater is not what you want for your child.

**Encourage Experimentation with the Food Plan**
If your child is suffering from bulimia or binge-eating disorder, you should be aware that he is disheartened about his ability to control his body weight. I have found that often these patients are quite receptive to experimenting with a Food Plan that will help them maintain a healthy weight. A collaborative ("Let's figure this out together"), supportive ("I know how worried you are about your weight"), confident ("The Food Plan will take care of your weight over time") approach reduces the child's anxiety and allows experimentation with a Food Plan.

**Modify the Food Plan and Your Involvement with It to Support Progress**
I cannot overemphasize the fact that in order to be effective, the Food Plan, as well as your involvement as parents, must respond to both progress and lapses. For bulimics, the Food Plan must be continually modified until your child is no longer bingeing or purging, and his weight is stable. Usually, this means a gradual shift from his eating-disordered pattern of eating toward the Food Plan template. When bingeing and purging, as well as the restrictive eating that triggers bingeing and purging, has stopped, you can gradually reduce your involvement in your child's "food business." The Food Plan that is protecting him from bingeing and purging then becomes his long-term Food Plan. A child who is at this stage will be able to adhere to the Food Plan with little thought; the Food Plan will have become almost second nature to him.

Conversely, when you notice signs that he is regressing (meaning bingeing and purging has increased), you should assume that either he is not following the Food Plan or that the Food Plan has become somehow inadequate and needs to be modified. Most likely you need to add more food to your child's plan, or make sure that his food choices are not being restricted in a way that is triggering bingeing.

**Add the Foods Your Child Is Bingeing On**
One effective technique is to add the foods that your child is bingeing on to her Food Plan. I assume if a child is bingeing on sweets her Food Plan is deficient in sweets. If this is the case with your child, perhaps another serving of fun food needs to be added. These foods, even if they are high in calories or fat, if eaten in normal amounts, will not cause a health or weight problem.

Although she was trying to solve her bulimia with a Food Plan, Brianna confessed to me that she was still bingeing after school on chips, cookies, and candy. Brianna's mother, Tammy, tried dealing with the problem by hiding these binge foods in the house. (She was reluctant to simply throw them away because she did not want to deprive Brianna's younger brother of these foods.) But Brianna, who was often alone in the house in the afternoons, knowing these foods were hidden somewhere, would scurry around the house until she found them. It felt almost like a game. Try as she might, Tammy was never able to keep these foods hidden from Brianna for more than a day or two. Brianna was frustrated because her pants were getting tighter and a weigh-in at my office confirmed she had gained five pounds over the past month.

I suggested Tammy add a single serving of chips, cookies, or candy to the half sandwich and juice or milk she fixed for Brianna's afternoon snack. It was Brianna who suggested that Tammy buy a "lockbox" in which to keep the supply of snack food. "Mom," Brianna said, "I want to stop playing this game with the treats. I know I will be more satisfied having a serving of them with my snack, but I want to make sure I leave the rest of them alone." Though the lockbox was an extreme solution, it worked for Brianna and her family because it was Brianna's own idea and one that she truly believed would work.

### Encourage Proper Snacks

Bingeing can also indicate that your child is just grazing or nibbling on snacks rather than eating a properly prepared, generous snack that either she has fixed or has been fixed for her. A proper snack has boundaries, meaning that its completion signals that it is time to stop eating. Rather than crackers eaten out of the box while watching TV, a proper snack would be crackers eaten at the kitchen table and served on a plate with a glass of milk or juice and possibly some sliced cheese or fruit.

Regina's story illustrates this common mistake. Because she wanted to lose weight, Regina did not plan to have an evening snack. But when she got hungry while doing her homework, she grabbed a big bag of pretzels or chips from the pantry and ate until she was uncomfortable. She ended up bingeing almost every evening. The solution for Regina was to take a study break at nine o'clock, the time she reported that she first generally noticed her interest in eating. I instructed her to at 9 P.M. take a plate and two to three normal serving sizes of foods she felt like eating, letting her appetite be the guide to what she chose. "It doesn't matter," I told her, "what you eat because you are adequately meeting your nutritional needs by following the Food Plan throughout the day." If she felt like pretzels she was to measure out one serving size and be sure to add another serving of a food she would like to eat with pretzels. Usually Regina chose a piece of fruit. Some nights she felt more like a serving of fun food, and wondered if that was okay, since she usually had dessert at dinner. "No problem," I told her, "as long as it is one normal-size serving."

### The Food Plan and the Older Bulimic

Bulimics in their mid- to late teens are more apt to respond to their parents' attempt to institute a Food Plan by rebelling. Because of this, you may find more success by focusing on ways that your child can be more responsible for the consequences of her eating disorder. Try having her replace food she binges on, or clean up the kitchen and bathroom after binge/purge episodes. (For more information, see chapter 4, p. 67.) Bulimics in this age range may need the assistance of a professional nutritionist to help them develop a Food Plan, as food issues are often so emotionally charged that they and their parents end up fighting about food, which is never productive.

## Adapting the Food Plan for the Overweight, Binge-Eating Child

### Explain That the Food Plan "Legalizes Eating"

One of the great benefits of the Food Plan for children who are battling binge eating or overeating is that it makes eating, which in their minds has become a taboo activity, permissible again. Explaining this to your child can turn a reluctant child into a willing participant in the Food Plan. Instead of feeling that everything they eat is too much and will cause weight gain, as they usually do, binge eaters are relieved to find that the Food Plan legalizes eating. When they no longer need to expend all their efforts on self-control or reducing their eating, they paradoxically find they are more in control, and are less likely to overeat or binge eat. Most children whose eating disorder has caused unnecessary weight gain, in fact, find the Food Plan refreshing as well as an easy way to maintain a healthy weight.

### Ban All Dieting and Weight-Loss Programs

You should also make it clear that restricting caloric intake and other active efforts to lose weight will slow your child's recovery from bulimia or binge eating. Until bingeing and purging are under control, even healthy weight loss approaches are counterproductive. (See chapter 2, p. 25, for more on dieting as risky behavior.)

When I first began treating my patient Nigel, he expected me to immediately put him on a restrictive diet to treat his binge-eating disorder. He was surprised and pleased to find that getting well called for nothing of the sort.

Nigel's problem was that his increasing weight had begun to interfere with his ability to be an effective member of his sailboat crew, the sport he loved more than anything else in the world. He complained that he felt slow and awkward and no longer able to climb the mast. At only seventeen, Nigel had experienced anorexia and bulimia over the last two years and, most recently, several months of binge eating that had led to a weight gain of over 50 pounds.

Nigel was so dissatisfied with his body size that he made food choices and binged in ways that were almost abusive. "I hate my body so it doesn't matter how I eat," he admitted thinking as he ate until he felt sick most evenings.

On his first visit Nigel, who was about ready to graduate from high school, described not eating all day and then spending the evening eating potato chips and ice cream while he studied or watched TV. He later told me how shocked he was that I didn't suggest he give up the chips and ice cream but instead helped him plan a reasonable breakfast, lunch, and dinner according to the Food Plan. At our second visit, I suggested he purchase chips in single-serving bags so he would know when he had eaten more than a serving. He even found little cups of ice cream that he remembered eating as a child at birthday parties. These helped him judge what a normal serving was, as did going out with his dad for an ice-cream cone on the weekends. By his third visit, Nigel said he was able to eat all three meals and hold his evening snack to two small bags of chips and one or two servings of ice cream. Nigel also reported that his pants were noticeably looser. On his fourth visit, he reported that a recent weigh-in at his doctor's office confirmed that he had lost five pounds. Nigel continued to lose weight and found that as long as he ate well during the day he usually had only enough appetite for one serving of fun food in the evenings.

Nigel's parents were thrilled that he seemed to be getting his eating under control, but needed to be cautioned that they should not aggravate his binge-eating habit by insisting or encouraging him to make low-calorie food choices or strive to lose weight.

### Stop Criticizing, Give the Food Plan a Chance to Work

It can be extremely difficult for parents of an overweight, binge-eating child to be patient enough for the Food Plan to begin first to normalize their child's eating patterns, and then to reduce the child's weight through healthy, normal eating. Sometimes, in fact, it is the parental pressure to diet and lose weight, and the criticism implicit in that pressure, that keeps the child from making progress.

Taylor had gained nearly 100 pounds during several years of binge eating. Although she was doing her best to follow the Food Plan we had worked out for her, and was making good progress at normalizing her eating patterns, she had not yet begun to lose weight. Taylor's mother, Janet, knew better than anyone how unhappy and insecure the extra weight made her daughter feel. Those feelings came to a head one day when the two of them were walking along a busy city street. A homeless man shouted out to Taylor, "There goes a really fat girl." As the tears welled up in Taylor's eyes, Janet felt as though the insult may as well have been aimed at her, so painful was it to watch her daughter's reaction.

Yet although she could sympathize with Taylor's pain, Janet was baffled by Taylor's inability to lose weight, despite months of working with a Food Plan. Janet said to me, "I just don't understand why Taylor can't adopt a low-calorie version of her Food Plan so she can begin losing weight. That's obviously what she needs."

What I saw during my sessions with Taylor was that she was being held back by the very fact that she knew her parents had trouble with her weight.

Just knowing that her parents assumed she was still bingeing and still disapproved of her food choices (since they had obviously not led her to shed pounds so far) pushed Taylor to overeat at times.

Often, I hear parents of binge-eating patients ask why their child simply can't eat less than their current Food Plan stipulates. I told Janet what I tell all of these parents: "Your child's weight will take care of itself over time if she follows a version of the Food Plan that is comfortable for her. In fact," I added, "dieting will put Taylor at increased risk for serious binge eating." Then I gently tried to address the issue of Janet and her husband's attitude toward Taylor, which I pointed out had more of an effect on their daughter than they realized.

"Any pressure from you to lose weight will continue to put Taylor at risk for overeating and binge eating," I told them. "No child comes with a blueprint that informs us of their best weight. But we can rightfully assume that normal, natural eating free of the pressures of parental expectations, will lead to the maintenance of a weight that is normal and natural." I reminded Janet that except for when she was on severely restrictive diets, Taylor has always been on the chubby side. It was those rigorous diets, of course, that set the stage for Taylor's bouts of binge eating, and her significant weight gain. I agreed with Janet that although Taylor's natural weight was probably substantially less than her current weight, it might be higher than what Janet or Taylor thinks is ideal. I added that all of us, Janet, Taylor, and I as Taylor's nutritionist, needed a big dose of patience as we focused on supporting Taylor's increasingly normal approach to eating. It was no big deal in the long run, I reminded Janet, if Taylor occasionally overate or even made poor choices; both are normal behaviors for teenagers.

Realizing that Taylor's eating and weight pushed so many buttons with them, Janet, Taylor, and I all agreed I was the best one to help Taylor with her food choices. Janet's job, as Taylor's mother, was to love and support her and forget about food issues unless Taylor asked for her assistance.

## When Is Professional Help Called For?

There are various circumstances under which you may find that you are unable to work with your child around a Food Plan. In such cases, you should consider enlisting the help of a professional nutritionist. (For a more detailed discussion about when professional assistance is called for, see chapter 14.) They are briefly summarized below.

• **When you feel you need help negotiating your child's Food Plan.** There are times when families find themselves at an impasse with the Food Plan, and their child's progress has stalled. In such cases, your child may respond better to the plan if it is administered by an outsider, who can keep you involved and show you how you can be most helpful.

• **When your interventions result in escalating control battles.**

• **Any time you have difficulty being consistent about setting limits for food behaviors, or enforcing limits that you have set.**

• **When you begin to feel like the eating-disorder police and worry you are being too harsh in your reactions to your child's behavior.** One benefit of having a professional involved in overseeing the development of a Food Plan is that it protects you from becoming angry and frustrated with your child when progress is slow. For instance, if your child follows the plan and instead of gaining weight, loses weight, you might be tempted to say, "I told you that you need to eat more!" or something similarly chiding and negative. A professional is more likely to be able to respond matter-of-factly, "It looks like we need to make another adjustment in your Food Plan." Your child is also less likely to turn on you if she has difficulty following the plan, but will instead look to her nutritionist for further guidance.

• **When your child needs additional assurance that her weight will not be allowed to spiral out of control when she adopts the Food Plan.** Enlisting the service of a professional nutritionist in such cases helps show your child that you are sympathetic to her concerns about body weight and will do what it takes to help her manage her food intake.

## In Summary

After reading this chapter, you should have a better sense of how adaptable the Food Plan is to widely varying circumstances. The highly specific nature of the Food Plan, which outlines exactly what kind of foods are to be eaten, how much is to be eaten, and at what times, gives the anorexic permission to eat again by providing the assurance that she will not overeat. The plan gives the bulimic and binge eater permission to eat by setting firm boundaries on how much and when she can eat.

You should also have a much better sense of the nuances of the Food Plan, how to best adapt it to your child's specific needs, and how to alter the plan as your child gradually regains his health. You will know the Food Plan has succeeded when it becomes superfluous, when your child has internalized its structure, rationale, and logic to the point where he can eat "in tune" without even thinking about it. This is what we call "normal eating," and it should be the goal of every eating-disordered child.

# 12

# Normalizing Exercise

Fifteen-year-old David, the son of a hardworking journalist father and a scientist mom, is a dedicated three-season athlete. In the fall he captains his high school's junior varsity soccer team. In the winter months, he skis with the school cross-country ski team, and in the spring, he runs track. Since January, however, David's exercise routine has become increasingly compulsive.

After a break from exercising over the holidays, David concludes that he is a little overweight and out of shape and begins going to the gym with friends. While his friends soon lose interest, David continues to exercise daily, using his study halls at school if necessary to get his workout in. By March he feels compelled to complete a two-hour weight lifting and Stairmaster workout every single day, in addition to training with the track team.

David becomes increasingly interested, even obsessive, about what foods he eats. When David first comes to see me, his mother, Connie, tells me, "I knew something was wrong when my all-American boy began reading food labels and cookbooks." David will not allow himself more than 1,500 to 2,000 calories a day when his body actually needs closer to 3,000 calories. David's parents bring him to see his pediatrician, who finds dangerously high levels of nitrogen in David's blood. This abnormal finding is probably the result of David's extremely high protein intake, the pediatrician informs David and his parents. Just in case, however, David is checked for kidney disease, which the family is relieved to find is not his problem. David has devised a diet for himself similar to the high-protein diets described in the sports magazines he reads. Every day he drinks several high-protein shakes made from a mix he purchased at the local health food store. In addition to the shakes, David limits himself to chicken, turkey, nonfat yogurt, and small servings of plain bagels or rice, vegetables, and fruit. He has three small meals a day and absolutely no snacks, no matter how hungry he is. He stays away from soda, chips, and desserts and eats more vegetables if he is hungry. David tells me it is easier to cut out all high-fat foods than to eat them in small amounts.

By April, David says he is burned out mentally and physically. He notices that he has much less endurance, and his times are getting slower instead of improving as the track season progresses. He seems always to be suffering from pulled muscles. Yet David's obsession with restrictive food intake and excessive exercise increases. He thinks constantly about what he is going to eat next or when he will schedule his next exercise session. By mid-May, he hates going to track because he has no energy, and he finds no enjoyment in activities he once found fun, such as golf or computer games. "I don't even have the energy to laugh anymore," David says, tears welling up in his eyes.

Often the compulsion to overexercise goes hand in hand with an eating disorder, and in some cases can even play a role in its onset. When this happens, the emotional and physical consequences—rapid and severe weight loss, stress fractures, or cardiac complications—can be devastating. In this chapter, we will explain how, just as you have worked on normalizing your child's eating pattern with a Food Plan, so can you help normalize his exercise habits. Exercise is another variable in our global approach to solving an eating problem. This means that whether your child exercises too much or too little, you and your child can experiment with different exercise approaches and see what works best.

In this chapter, we will first help you recognize what excessive exercise looks like. If you determine that your child has been overexercising, we will show you how you can come up with a rational plan of exercise that will keep your child fit and happy, and also ensure that she attains or stays at a healthy weight for her body size and type. For the eating-disordered child who is averse to exercise we will offer strategies for developing an approach to physical fitness that will leave your child feeling positive and enthusiastic.

## How Much Is Excessive? Early Warning Signals

You should be alert if you suspect your child is involved in excessive exercise because often such behavior is the first step down the path to a serious eating disorder. If you suspect that your child is overexercising, but are not sure, the following checklists will help you analyze your child's behavior and determine whether or not you need to take action. The first checklist contains moderately risky behavior, and the second contains higher-risk behaviors.

If your child exhibits two of these moderately risky behaviors, you should be watchful that her exercising does not escalate. If your child exhibits three or more of these behaviors, you have a problem that needs to be addressed.

## Moderately Risky Exercise Behaviors

❑ Does not give herself a regular "rest day."
❑ Engages in exercise that is planned, goal-oriented, strictly adhered to.
❑ Only exercises alone.
❑ Exercises more than one hour a day.
❑ Exercises more than coach recommends.
❑ Exercises rather than spending time on typical social, educational, or work activities.
❑ Exercises seemingly without enjoying it, where the primary motivation is calorie burning and weight loss.
❑ Purposefully increases exercise to counter increased food intake (for example, adds another 30 minutes to Stairmaster routine after eating a dessert).

## High-Risk Exercise Behaviors

If your child exhibits even one of the behaviors on this checklist, you should consider intervening.

❑ Exercises more than two hours a day.
❑ Weight loss coinciding with an increase in exercise, especially if your child is underweight, and especially if the weight loss exceeds 5 pounds.
❑ Insists on exercising in dangerous situations such as running alone at night, or when injured or sick.
❑ Seems obsessed with exercise and unable to control the need for it.
❑ Purposefully increases caloric expenditure during daily activities (for example, jogging from one class to another wearing a heavy backpack or preferring to stand rather than sit).
❑ Is highly anxious if unable to exercise.

To give you a little perspective, it is helpful to know that current exercise recommendations from the American College of Sports Medicine for maintaining health and fitness is to accumulate one to five hours of exercise per week. While this averages out to 20 to 60 minutes of exercise per day, three to five days a week, those minutes do not have to be consecutive, or even on the same day, but can be banked during the course of a week. Your child's ten-minute walk to and from the bus stop, for example, counts toward her cumulative weekly exercise tally. Any sustained movement at the intensity of a brisk walk is considered acceptable exercise, which means that even everyday activities such as raking leaves, vacuuming, or sweeping can be counted as part of weekly exercise.

In our exercise-obsessed society it is easy to overlook the fact that moderate exercise is all that is needed to maintain health. By informing you of these exercise recommendations, we do not mean to imply that you should keep track of your child's exercise by adding up the minutes she devotes to exercise. Nor should you insist that a child who exercises less than these recommended guidelines be forced to exercise more. Instead, we hope this information gives you the means to assess, in a general way, whether your child's level of exercise is appropriate.

## Anorexia and Exercise

Excessive exercise is a common practice of anorexics, often in the form of solitary aerobic activities such as distance running or using a Stairmaster at a gym. Researcher Alayne Yates calls dieting and exercise "sister activities," noting that a serious investment in one is likely to be accompanied by a preoccupation with the other. For the underweight child who already has an eating problem, even mild exercise can prevent her from gaining the weight she needs to restore health and can put her at risk for short- and long-term medical complications.

Because anorexics can sometimes feel surprisingly energetic despite the fact that they are starving themselves, they may not realize that they are overexercising. They may rationalize their behavior by asserting that they want to stay healthy and fit, or stay competitive in their chosen field of sport. Anorexics will also often overdo everyday activities, such as walking up a flight of stairs or walking the dog, performing the activity repeatedly to maximize caloric expenditure. Where one trip up a flight of stairs will do, they will take multiple trips up and down for no other reason than to burn off calories.

Extremely low-weight anorexics may exhibit tic-like physical movements such as rocking, toe-tapping, or pacing, or they will insist on standing when they could be sitting. These behaviors, over which the anorexic has little or no control, are believed to be caused by starvation. When anorexia progresses even further and body weight falls to an even lower level, this type of excessive activity tends to decrease, again an adaptation to a new, even more extreme level of starvation. In spite of a formerly addictive relationship with exercise, the anorexic now may even find it hard to walk up a flight of stairs. As she pulls out of this extreme phase of starvation with nutritional rehabilitation, her desire to exercise returns. Sometimes this happens with a vengeance, which can lead to another cycle of excessive exercise.

**Anorexia and Exercise Limits**

Angela, whose family had recently moved from Argentina so that her father could take a medical fellowship, suffered from a classic case of anorexia. Culturally, Angela was equally at risk in Argentina and the United States. Although eating disorders are relatively rare elsewhere in South America, Argentina has rates that rival those of America and Europe.

After we began to work together, Angela made dramatic improvements in her food intake, adding higher-calorie foods like nuts, granola, sports bars, dried fruit, and cream cheese and bagels to her daily Food Plan. She even began eating red meat again, which pleased her meat-eating parents. Yet her weight did not improve. She continued to take kickboxing classes two to three times per week, walk her dog after school, and go on long bike rides on the weekends with her best friend. We continued to pare down her exercise, but with no effect on her weight. It was only after she stopped all forms of exercise that her weight began to increase. Some anorexics can eat enough to fuel a fair amount of exercise. Most, however, like Angela, cannot.

As Angela's story illustrates, exercise limits are often necessary because excessive exercise makes it hard for anorexics to gain weight. Even low-intensity exercise, such as walking, expends calories that the anorexic can ill afford. In addition to burning calories, exercise also increases overall caloric requirements by raising metabolic rate. Weight and endurance training are particularly harmful for extremely low-weight anorexics because these activities increase overall caloric needs.

Exercise limits are also important because often the anorexic's heart and bones have weakened to the point where even moderate physical exercise can be dangerous. Because anorexia can significantly weaken bones in as little as six months, it is wise to consider limiting exercise fairly early on.

Exercise limits for the underweight anorexic who is not making hoped-for weight gains is often a key component of treatment. Exercise limits can be a powerful motivator for some patients who will do almost anything, including gaining weight, to continue participating in their chosen sport. You should be careful not to set weight goals so high, though, that your child feels they are unattainable and rebels against the entire plan. Consulting with your child's doctor about a safe weight for exercise can help you set a reasonable goal. As with other types of limits and goals we have described, it is important for you as parents to stick to your word. If your child attains her weight goal, you must allow her to resume at least some exercising, or risk losing all credibility and authority.

Usually weight goals are set in a stepped, or tiered fashion. As your child attains increasingly higher weights, she or he is allowed to do increasingly more exercise. In situations when weight gain has stalled, however, a more absolute, all-or-nothing approach is sometimes necessary.

Marissa managed to gain the 10 pounds she needed to before her pediatrician would allow her to play volleyball, and to maintain it in order to stay on the team. But after volleyball season ended, Marissa found it hard to continue gaining weight. She was taken aback when her pediatrician told her that she had to gain another 5 pounds before she would be allowed to participate in the spring track season. The doctor explained that since Marissa's period still had not returned it was clear she needed to gain more weight before she was truly on the road to recovery.

Restoring your child's normal weight is key to ensuring a full recovery. Children who gain some weight, but remain underweight are at high risk for a relapse or for developing a chronic eating disorder.

Some anorexics may point to the fact that they have increased their food intake as reason to allow increased exercise. But unless they are eating enough to attain their weight-gain goals, I recommend continued exercise limitations. Because the caloric needs of the recovering anorexic are often so great, it is the rare anorexic who is able to sustain a reasonable rate of weight-gain while engaging in regular exercise.

In the most severe cases, where a child cannot comply with exercise limitations and the excessive exercise is causing health problems, hospitalization or residential treatment may be your only alternative. (See chapter 14, p. 265, for more on inpatient or residential treatment.)

Sometimes an anorexic's tendency toward excessive exercise will actually predate the eating disorder. In such cases, it is likely that the overexercising is a problem in and of itself, separate from the child's eating problems. Simply treating the eating disorder may not be enough; specific efforts to address the overexercising are called for. (See p. 215 for more information.)

## Bulimia and Exercise

Thirteen-year-old Monica recounted how, in the throes of her bulimia, she would force herself to run after bingeing even if such vigorous exercise would cause painful stomach cramps. Exercise performed in this manner is considered a form of purging. Several months later Monica began to self-induce vomiting, which became her principle method of purging. It is not unusual for bulimic patients to go through different phases of the disorder, each with a different form of purging.

Although overexercising tends to be less of a problem with bulimics, when they do engage in excessive exercise, it is usually part of an effort to compensate for a binge. Doctors rarely set exercise limits for patients who are of normal weight, since they tend to regulate only those behaviors that have a direct impact on their patients' health. This can be frustrating for parents who recognize that their child is overexercising.

I encourage parents to work out a reasonable plan for their child's exercise regardless of whether or not her weight is a problem. I do not, however, advise parents to set exercise limits for their normal-weight children if it is likely she will fight the limit tooth and nail or become secretive about her exercise activities. Parents should always choose their battles wisely.

For bulimics like Monica who use exercise as a form of purging, as you work on helping them reduce exercise, you will also have to help them manage their bingeing. Limiting exercise can increase a bulimic's anxiety about bingeing. This anxiety can lead to increased self-induced vomiting, or to restrictive eating. As you institute exercise limitations, it is imperative that you also be ready to help your child develop a Food Plan (see chapters 10 and 11), which will help prevent your child from replacing exercise with more extreme eating-disordered behaviors.

## Binge-Eating Disorder and Exercise

Binge eaters often do not exercise, usually because they associate exercise with restrictive dieting and other methods of weight control. They think, "What is the point of exercising when my eating is so out of control? Any calories I work off will just come right back, doubled, tripled, even quadrupled, the next time I binge."

Binge eaters also tend to believe that adhering to a pattern of healthy exercise is harder than it actually is, and do not think they are able to meet those ideal standards. Gigi was typical of many binge eaters I see. She believed that the only exercise that would be meaningful would be that equivalent to a three-mile run. Anything less, she told me, "won't count."

Sometimes, the binge eater is so demoralized about his eating behavior and body weight that he has given up hope of incorporating exercise into his life. I have found that patients such as these rarely respond well to the message of "exercise more, it will help you lose weight." They have already heard this enough from family, friends, and society in general, and it has not worked yet for them. Instead, it is more effective to be empathetic and support whatever their current approach to exercise is.

Some patients are so focused on their perceived "failure" to exercise that they believe that is the reason their weight has increased. I encourage patients to keep their food issues and their exercise issues separate, and gently try to redirect their attention to correcting their binge-eating behaviors. "Eating patterns have a more potent effect on your weight than exercise," I tell them. "Regular exercise will improve your health, so we will want to incorporate that in the future. For the time being, we need to focus on your eating patterns." You are ready to exercise, I add, when you can engage in it for fun, relaxation, or health rather than for weight loss.

## How Parents Can Help Normalize Exercise

**Inform Your Child of the Dangers of Overexercise**
As concerned parents, it can be helpful to broach the subject of excessive exercise by informing your child of some of the dangers associated with it. If your anorexic daughter has stopped getting periods, her bones, without the requisite levels of protective estrogen in her body, are especially at risk for stress fractures.

You can then explain to your child that gaining weight is the only way to make her bones stronger. If her overexercising is keeping her from gaining weight, then she must either eat more or cut back on exercise. For most anorexics, the latter choice is less frightening than the former.

**Assess Your Child's Willingness to Collaborate**
Much of how I approach exercise with my patients depends on the severity of their eating disorder, the degree of weakness and malnutrition that we are dealing with, and the patient's willingness to collaborate in devising an Exercise Plan.

Some eating-disordered youths will welcome guidance in the form of a detailed weekly plan of exercise, and are even relieved when someone steps in to regulate or rein in their excessive exercise. When I suggest that they "take a break from exercise," they realize they have been secretly hoping for permission to do just that, after weeks or months of torturing themselves by demanding higher and higher levels of athletic performance.

## When Are Exercise Restrictions Warranted?

My rule of thumb is to consider exercise restrictions for patients whose weight is low enough to be considered anorexic and/or their exercise is excessive.

If your very thin child is engaging in regular exercise, consulting with your pediatrician to determine if your child's exercise level is putting her at risk is a wise idea.

In cases of severe weight loss, your doctor will likely bar your child from all exercise until significant weight is restored. After your child begins gaining weight, increasing amounts of exercise can be allowed. In less severe cases of weight loss you can allow moderate exercise as long as your child gains weight at a reasonable rate.

## Drafting an Exercise Plan

The following are our guidelines for drafting an Exercise Plan.

• **Work with your child's pediatrician or other medical professional.** It is important to work with your child's pediatrician or another medical professional because for seriously ill children grave consequences can result from mismanagement of exercise. In addition to the bone fractures and cardiac complications we have already discussed, obsessive exercise can also endanger a child because the exercise itself puts him or her in dangerous situations. The obsessive exerciser may exercise in unsafe situations such as running alone in dangerous neighborhoods. Exercising in the dark or in inclement or extremely cold or hot weather can also be dangerous.

Most doctors will ban or severely limit exercise until the anorexic patient has gained substantial weight. Underweight patients who cannot comply with their doctor's "exercise orders" are likely to be hospitalized.

While you may wish that your child's doctor would devise a comprehensive plan that covers all contingencies related to exercise, most doctors, as we have noted, do not involve themselves in setting exercise limits unless their patient is very underweight or is experiencing medical complications. Instead, they leave exercise limitations up to parents or, if you are seeing other members of a treatment team, to a nutritionist or therapist. These professionals can provide guidance as you work to normalize your child's exercise habits.

• **Know your child's exercise excesses, abilities, and limits, and tailor your plan accordingly.** As you are collaborating with your child to come up with a reasonable Exercise Plan, keep in mind what your child's excesses are and try to target those excesses with your plan. Fiona was concerned about her daughter Michelle's increasingly addictive approach to exercise. She and Michelle decided together that the first goal of Michelle's Exercise Plan would be to institute one rest day a week, to disrupt the cycle of escalating exercise. At first Michelle felt "deprived" on days she was not allowed to run. But she found her run the morning after her first rest day exhilarating; she hadn't had such a good run in months. Later, Michelle told

Fiona that she hadn't seen the value in rest days until she truly made them "restful" days.

Knowing your child's abilities and limits as an athlete will also help in drafting an Exercise Plan. For a competitive athlete who normally exercises more than the average child, it is reasonable to tell them "No more exercise than what your coach recommends." If your child is not a competitive athlete, you may find that setting a limit of two 10-minute walks on weekdays is appropriate.

For some children, parents might allow no more activity than getting themselves to and from school and 30 minutes of window shopping at the mall two days a week. Other children may prefer 15 minutes of swimming or biking every other day. Plans should always be contingent on your child's physical condition and whether or not he or she has attained weight-gain goals.

• **Involve your child in drafting the Exercise Plan.** Parents should make sure to involve their child in discussions about exercise. One mistake Tricia and Don made in coming up with an Exercise Plan for Megan, their anorexic daughter, was that by not consulting with her, they ended up limiting her exercise at a level "higher" than she deep down hoped for. As a result of this misstep, Megan concluded that her parents thought she was lazy and overweight, typical of the distorted fears of an anorexic.

• **Exercise Plans should be experimental and adjusted downward.** My rule of thumb is that if your anorexic child is not gaining weight at the rate of at least one pound a week, you should adjust her Exercise Plan downward.

Leila was sent home from boarding school because of her noticeable and worrisome weight loss. Her parents were not concerned about her overexercising because all Leila did was walk. But Leila didn't just take short walks, she walked for hours every day. When Leila's weight did not budge after a week on a Food Plan we devised, I suggested she limit her walking to no more than one hour a day. When that failed to bring the needed change in weight, she agreed to reduce her walking again, to 30 minutes a day, and then to every other day. Not until her only exercise was playing with her dog for 15 minutes a day did she manage to begin gaining weight. Leila's case illustrates how tying exercise limitations to weight gain in a collaborative manner reduces rebellion on the part of the child. Two weeks after we launched her Exercise Plan, Leila was suggesting different ways she could reduce her exercise.

It is important to note that if Leila had been *losing* weight instead of simply failing to gain weight, the gradual reduction in exercise that we describe in her case would have had to have been accelerated to protect her health.

As these case histories demonstrate, the key to drafting a successful Exercise Plan is to pick the right approach for your child and to be ready to alter it if it becomes clear that it is not working. An approach that is right for one child may not be appropriate for another.

• **Stick to your word.** I cannot emphasize enough that if you as a concerned parent decide to make your child's athletic participation contingent on achieving a certain weight level, you must follow through on your promises to restrict exercise. If you don't you will have lost the credibility that is essential to helping turn around your child's eating disorder. If you conclude that barring your child from a cherished activity is beyond your capabilities, you may want to consult a medical professional who can "lay down the law" for them.

• **Regardless of your child's weight, excessive exercise should be curtailed.** Even when a child does not have a weight problem, and is not exercising in order to lose weight, I still caution parents to be watchful. Excessive exercise in and of itself can predispose your child toward other eating-disordered behaviors.

• **Anticipate stumbling blocks, explore solutions.** It is helpful while you and your child are drafting an Exercise Plan to visualize its implementation. You might ask, "What would make this goal difficult to achieve?" or "What problems would you have following through on this goal?" Once you identify a potential stumbling block, work with your child to come up with a creative solution to help you overcome the obstacle.

Spencer's story is an illustration of how you and your child can do this. Spencer and his parents jointly decided that he would have to wait to join the intramural basketball team until his weight improved. Spencer, anticipating that he would find himself wanting to jump rope or jog after school, asked his parents to help him plan alternative activities after school. Since Spencer clearly missed the structure basketball gave to his day almost as much as he did the opportunity to exercise, Spencer's father, Keith, encouraged Spencer to consider other, less active organized activities. Before long, Spencer was an avid shutterbug and an active member of the photography club.

Whether your approach is experimental or directive, you must be absolutely confident that your child can safely undertake the regimen you plan. If you are uncertain about whether or not his physical condition can withstand the plan you are contemplating, consult your pediatrician.

## When Is It Okay for Your Child to Resume Exercise?

Determining when your child can resume exercising should be based on her medical status, rate of progress, and body weight. One indicator is the return of her monthly periods, which indicates that she has arrived at the minimal weight needed to protect bone health. Many doctors, however, allow moderate exercise before resumption of monthly periods as long as the child continues to gain weight. Consulting with a doctor who is experienced in such matters can be helpful at this juncture.

Although you may feel that your child should not exercise at all until she regains her normal weight, I have found that prohibiting exercise completely until then usually does not work. Your child, who is likely already rebelling against your efforts to help her, is not liable to comply with such a restriction, and the effort will only serve to further strain your relationship. If there is any question about whether your child is well enough to exercise, check with your doctor. Instead of engaging in a battle of wills in this area, I recommend that if her health is not medically compromised, the exercise she engages in is not excessive, and she is meeting weight gain goals, that you allow it. This does not mean, however, that she cannot benefit from discussing the risks of overexercise.

At the risk of sounding like a broken record, we will say this one more time: It is crucial that exercise not interfere with continued weight gain when a child is underweight.

## When Your Child Flouts Exercise Restrictions

I have worked with numerous patients who have confessed they continued to exercise in spite of restrictions on exercise. Jenny told me she did calisthenics in her basement. Mary confessed she went running when her parents were out of the house. Sometimes the child cannot keep from engaging in the uncontrollable hyperactive behaviors that we described earlier in this chapter. Because such flouting of exercise restrictions is not uncommon, I advise parents to do their best to enforce exercise restrictions when their child's health is endangered. At the beginning of treatment, or if your child is "hooked" on exercise, it is often necessary to make sure your child is not left unsupervised. Occasionally I see parents who are at their wit's end trying to enforce exercise restrictions. I ask them how they enforce curfews or limit after-school plans, and then encourage them to apply the techniques that have worked in those areas to exercise limitations. If you feel that you have been unsuccessful in all your efforts to modify your child's behavior, consider consulting with a seasoned professional who can help you develop an effective approach.

My patient Carolyn confessed to me that she got away with doing hundreds of sit-ups in her bedroom while she was under an "exercise restriction." Carolyn's parents eventually caught her in the act. They did not ban the sit-ups completely, but instead, in the spirit of compromise, and after first checking with their doctor about the safety of this plan, insisted she keep them to under fifty per day. As Carolyn continued to gain weight, her interest in exercise declined. By the time Carolyn had gained 20 pounds and was out of danger, according to her doctors, her exercise habits were more typical of other teenagers.

Erin's obsessive need to constantly be moving finally led her mother, Marta, to the realization that she would need to take a leave of absence from her job as a nurse in order to help Erin gain weight. Because of her tendency to think of every possible means to burn calories, Erin, whose weight was dangerously low, required almost constant supervision. On one occasion, Marta was at first pleased that Erin wanted to clean out the family's storage closets. When she realized that Erin was just looking for surreptitious ways to burn calories and prevent necessary weight gain, she had to step in and forbid Erin to clean the closets. To distract Erin from her obsessive focus on exercise and fill her time while she recovered, Marta regularly took Erin to the library and to their local bookstore, places where Erin felt comfortable just sitting and reading.

If your child's weight is as dangerously low as Erin's, you may want to think about rearranging your home or apartment so that walking and stairclimbing are minimized. While you may have to severely curtail your underweight child's activity for a while, do not go so far as to enforce bed rest, which could lead to even further and quicker bone loss. If continued trouble limiting your child's activity makes it impossible for her to regain the weight she needs, she may need the type of supervision that only a residential or hospital program can provide.

## Organized Athletics and Eating Disorders

Sports provides positive experiences for children and teens, and often improves their feelings about body and self. Children can experience newfound discipline, a work ethic, and teamwork. They learn to value their body for what it is able to do rather than just how it looks. Yet involvement in sports can also lead to lower self-esteem if the child does not measure up to his or her or the coach's expectations. Competitive sports can also promote a self-imposed, unrealistic drive for perfection, and as a result, a high level of stress.

All of these factors increase the risk of developing an eating disorder. Athletes who excel and kids with eating disorders also share another trait: a tendency to be compliant. If the coach says jump, they ask, "How high?" So it is no surprise that a number of studies have found that eating disorders are more prevalent among athletes than among kids who are not involved in sports.

Some children are convinced that their well-being and self-esteem are dependent on the high level of regular exercise and the intense competition of organized athletics. This idea is enforced by our culture, which places a high premium on fitness, exercise, and competition. Parents, teachers, coaches, peers, and teammates all reinforce this view, which makes it important to counter those pressures with support and information about why, in their case, it is actually protective of their health to cut back on exercise. Following are guidelines for parents of competitive athletes.

### Monitor Coaches and Other Adults Involved in Your Child's Sport

Although I have found that most athletic coaches today are sensitive to the risks for eating disorders inherent in organized sports, this is not true of all coaches. Comments by a coach about weight or shape, or assertions that weight loss will improve performance can trigger overexercise.

Allison was lucky enough to have a parent who was vigilant enough to halt negative coaching behavior before it got the best of her daughter. Allison, a naturally chubby child, blossomed into a curvaceous young woman who loved to figure skate. Carol, Allison's mother, had heard from some of the other skating moms that Allison's skating coach, a national champion in her heyday, had a habit of pulling skaters aside to suggest they watch their diets and try to lose a few pounds. Not wanting to put her daughter at risk for an eating disorder, Carol made it clear her daughter was not to hear a word about weight and dieting from the coach.

The unfortunate truth is that some coaches are so focused on winning, or creating star athletes that they may lose sight of the child's best interest. In some cases, coaches are excessive exercisers themselves and set the wrong example for their charges with their own behavior.

It is always a sensitive issue to suggest that coaches change their approach. You may want to check with other parents to see if they have similar concerns. Several parents may make more of an impression on a coach than isolated comments from one concerned parent. It may be necessary to share your concerns with the coach's supervisor if there is one. Sometimes, if there is no recourse and the coach refuses to amend his or her approach, it may be necessary to prohibit your child from participating. This should be done as a last resort. If your child argues that they want to participate in spite of the coach, you can allow for a trial period in which the child must prove that they can participate without regressing into their eating disorder.

## Be Especially Vigilant If Your Child Is Involved in a "Thinness-Demand Sport"

Sports such as gymnastics, figure skating, ballet, dance, diving, and distance running are among those eating-disorder experts call "thinness-demand sports." This means that the sport places emphasis on or favors a specific body type, usually thinness or small stature. Other sports that can foster a preoccupation with weight and size are those with weight classes or weight requirements, such as wrestling or crew. You should be exceedingly watchful if your child is involved in one of these sports.

Abigail is a serious ballet student who was recently accepted to an Ivy League college. She dances three to four hours per day and sometimes six to eight hours on weekends if her troupe is performing. She constantly worries about the fact that at 5'5" and 125 pounds, she is heavier than ideal for dancing. Abigail is referred to me by her primary care provider because she has reduced her food, fat, and protein intake, lost 15 pounds in six months, and is now suffering from irregular periods, heart palpitations, and dizziness. While happy with her weight loss, Abigail is worried about her health and about the bingeing she finds herself doing more and more often.

Abigail is, I explain to her, in one of the highest-risk categories for an eating disorder: girl athletes involved in a thinness-demand sport (ballet ranks at the top of these). She must deal with the appearance demands of her sport in addition to the cultural pressures all girls face to look thin and be attractive. Of course, boys who are involved in a thinness-demand sport are also at high risk. In sports like distance running, for example, coaches may believe that performance is improved by reducing body fat and lowering body weight.

Although Abigail's food restrictions are the cause of most of her physical symptoms, the real work she has to do is to accept her natural dimensions, and not try to make her body size and shape conform to the ideal of the reed-thin ballerina. She finds that when she accepts the fact that her body was fine at 125 pounds, she is able to gradually improve her food intake and return to her normal weight. As is common, Abigail is rewarded by a dramatic improvement in how she feels as she restores her weight. Though tempted to add rope jumping to her ballet training to moderate weight gain, Abigail resists, remembering that she has promised her parents and doctor that she will not overexercise.

Abigail realizes that her natural dimensions have not kept her from excelling in her local dance company, but they could keep her from becoming a successful professional dancer. She has already begun making choices, including going to college, that are leading her away from the dance world.

We do not suggest that parents discourage their children from involvement in sports. You should, however, be watchful if your child falls in love with a sport that does not favor her natural body type and be ready to sensitively help your child understand the realities of her sport.

## When to Bar Your Child from Participating on an Athletic Team

If your child's weight is dangerously low, restricting her from organized or school-sponsored athletic programs until her weight has improved may be necessary to protect her health. If your child is in this situation, you should be working closely with your child's doctor. Even in cases that are not quite so severe as to endanger health, restricting participation in sports, or even discussing the possibility of such a measure, can provide powerful motivation to begin gaining weight. Barring a low-weight child from participating in organized sports is easier to do than regulating access to recreational activities since children need their parents and often their physician's approval to participate. It also protects your at-risk child from medical problems that heavy exercise might aggravate.

The question, of course, is "At what point should I consider forbidding my child from participating on his or her athletic team?" You should consider such measures if:

- Your child's weight is so low that she is at medical risk.
- Your child is continuing to lose weight despite your best efforts to help.
- Your child's approach to exercise is so compulsive he is overexercising, especially exercising more than one hour per day and/or refusing to include "rest" days.

(For other signs of overexercise, see our "Early Warning Signals" checklists, p. 210.)

## Broaching the Subject of Athletic Limits with Your Child

Sometimes, even though parents know without a doubt that their child must be barred from participating in athletics until becoming healthy again, it can be hard to figure out how to broach the subject and to convince their child that this is so. If you are in this situation, you might start by explaining to your child that her eventual goal should be to resume a regular pattern of exercise and participate once again in her chosen sport. But while she is malnourished and underweight, exercise is not only not conducive, it is counterproductive to regaining health. (For more on difficult conversations, see chapter 7.)

Another effective strategy, as we have mentioned, is to bring in a professional who can clearly state your concerns as parents in medical or health terms and who can support limits on exercise.

Though it may seem harsh, "outnumbering" a young teen or child with professionals who support your plan is often effective. Professionals add clout and credibility.

### Talk to Your Child's Athletic Coach and Pediatrician

If you suspect that your child is engaging in excessive exercise and feel that your child's coach can be more of an ally than adversary to you, it may be helpful to talk to the coach as well as your pediatrician. They can help you devise a reasonable Exercise Plan or a scaled-back schedule of team sports until your child's weight has improved. Hearing both a coach *and* doctor explain the rationale behind the Exercise Plan can have quite an impact on a child. Although meeting with both coach and doctor together would be ideal, it is not easy to arrange such a meeting between two busy professionals. Meeting with each separately will also work. If your situation urgently calls for a joint meeting, it is usually the doctor or another professional who will arrange the discussion.

If you do have a frank conversation with your child's coach, be sure your child is informed, or even better, included in the discussion. Children, especially teenagers, can feel betrayed if they find out after the fact about conversations that were held about them by people who are central figures in their lives.

### How to Bar Your Child from Organized Athletics

If you determine that measures have to be taken to reduce your child's participating in an organized sport, you should first make it clear to your child that restrictions on sports participation are necessary because she is not restoring weight at a safe rate. Next, you should seek ways to institute a gradual reduction in exercise, as your child will probably respond best to this type of cutback. In cases where you have the support of your child's coach, this may be possible. In some cases, however, your child's coach may take an "all or nothing, either you are on the team or you are not" approach. One common solution is that the child is allowed to practice on a reduced schedule, but not allowed to play in games or take part in competitions until she has gained a significant amount of weight. School-employed coaches may be more accommodating since they are required not to discriminate against an athlete who has legitimate health reasons for participating at a reduced level.

If your child is adamant about continuing with her sport, you can respond, "All right, as long as you are gaining a pound a week and your doctor says it is okay." If two weeks later your child loses a pound instead of gaining a pound, you can say, "Until your weight is clearly increasing, no exercise outside of your team practices." Team practices are easier to monitor and regulate than other types of exercise, because all it takes is a call to the coach saying, "Due to medical reasons and until further notice, my child will only be able to participate in practices three times a week," or whatever the limit you and your medical professional have decided on.

There is no doubt that patients of mine who have been barred from their favorite activities because of their low weight are the ones who recover the quickest. The extra incentive of wanting desperately to return to a loved sport seems to give these patients an important edge in overcoming their eating disorder.

## Exercise Guidelines for Anorexics

Although we have recommended experimental and gradual restrictions on exercise for many types of eating disorders, we must stress that in severe cases of anorexia, all forms of exercise may need to be halted immediately to safeguard your child's health.

If you find yourselves in this more extreme situation where you are dealing with a child who is an excessive exerciser and has lost a tremendous amount of weight, my advice is to consult immediately with a trusted medical professional. If a patient is very low weight, below the fifth percentile in weight for her age (see Appendix B for more information on assessing body weight), her doctor will most likely restrict her from any physical activity beyond day-to-day tasks until the child shows that she can responsibly handle more exercise. At that point, permission may be given for a gradually increasing amount of exercise.

At seventeen, Eleanor is a tall girl like her mother, almost 5'8", and bigger and taller than her peers. When Eleanor's parents notice that she is jogging several hours at a time, has dropped a dangerous amount of weight, and seems to be continuing her weight loss with no end in sight, they become alarmed. Their daughter, they realize, has developed a severe case of anorexia.

Eleanor's weight at her first visit with me is 115 pounds, far too low for someone of her height. Her skin is pale, and her hair is dry and thin. She is clearly nervous, hyperactively tapping her toes and wringing her hands through the entire visit. When she visits her physician, he bars her from all exercise until she gains 10 pounds.

At first Eleanor is angry about the restriction. But she complies because she really does not have the energy she formerly had to devote to exercise. In a month's time she has gained back 5 pounds and is begging for permission to exercise. But her doctor holds firm: Eleanor needs to gain at least 10 pounds before any exercise is allowed. Like most of my patients, Eleanor buckles down and gains the weight because "she has to." Over a two-month period she gains the 10 pounds her doctor insisted on. Eleanor tells me that at first it was horrible not exercising. She reports nightmares in which she gains 50 pounds in a week's time. Of course, this frightening dream does not come true, and Eleanor's weight gain is actually quite slow.

Having gained the prescribed 10 pounds, Eleanor is allowed by her doctor to do what she wants for exercise as long as she continues to gain weight. Eleanor's parents are surprised that the doctor gives her such general guidelines. After talking with me, they realize that the doctor's guidelines are based purely on health issues, and that they can restrict her exercise further if it is in Eleanor's best interest, and particularly if they feel she will be compliant.

The next week Eleanor, her parents, and I all sit down together to talk about an Exercise Plan. It is important we hear from Eleanor first so I ask, "Now that you have earned permission to exercise, what do you think is a reasonable amount?" Eleanor replies, "Well, I used to run five miles a day, but I think that is too much. I was thinking of trying two miles." I then invite her parents to add their thoughts. "Eleanor," her mom says, "we would really like you to incorporate a couple of rest days. We understand now how important that is." Eleanor is taken aback by this suggestion, but upon reflection realizes that if she wants to participate in the after-school activities she is interested in, she will have to forgo exercise two days a week anyway. She agrees to two rest days a week. Eleanor realizes during her exercise moratorium how limited her life has become because of her obsessive exercise. In the next two months, she adds an after-school choral group and a pottery class.

If you are dealing with a sick eating-disordered child, one of your biggest challenges is to be at once firm about limits and restrictions, and yet hopeful that she will soon recover. I advise talking in the most serious of tones about the gravity of your child's disease, yet almost in the same breath, offering hope that with your help she can quickly turn the eating disorder around. You need to make your child feel that almost before she knows it, she will be free to engage in the activities she enjoys.

## Exercise Guidelines for Bulimics and Binge Eaters

Although excessive exercise is more likely to be a feature of anorexia than of bulimia or binge-eating disorder, children with bulimia or binge eating can also have trouble with exercise. When bulimics overexercise, it is often to compensate for binges. Attempts to restrict exercise often trigger fears of weight gain, and the bulimic is prone to begin restricting food intake as well.

In order to prevent this from happening, your bulimic child needs to hear over and over again that excessive exercise is not what will help her lose weight (if that is really what she needs to do); it is eliminating bingeing that will really make the difference. You can point out that it is possible to actually gain weight while exercising at a high level if binge eating is a regular habit. On the other hand, by eliminating bingeing, it is possible to maintain weight or even lose weight with no regular exercise. Though popular magazines emphasize the amount of calories burned during exercise, in reality the number of calories expended by increased exercise is minor compared to the number of calories the typical bulimic might consume in a binge. For example, a three-mile jog will burn up about 300 calories, the same amount of calories in a good-sized bagel. Although the size of binges vary quite widely, binges in the 5,000-calorie range are not unusual.

If your child, like many, does not understand the concept of calories, it is helpful to frame your message this way: "By not eating enough, you are setting yourself up to binge. Reducing exercise is not what is making you binge, not eating enough is." Bulimics need to hear repeatedly that it is food restriction that "drives" binge behaviors and that it is binge behaviors that lead to weight problems. It can be helpful for the bulimic to hear you say, "Yes, though it does seem logical that you should eat less if you are cutting back on exercise, this is the last thing someone recovering from bulimia should do. High levels of exercise can actually increase the likelihood that you'll binge, because you're not getting the nourishment your body needs to meet the extra demands of your exercising."

Introducing a Food Plan at the same time you are setting limits on exercise can help prevent continued bingeing and/or purging. (See chapters 10 and 11 for more information.)

Because bulimic children fear that they will gain weight if they cut back on exercise, periodic weight checks can be used to reassure the child in this situation that in fact their weight is stable. Irene helped her sixteen-year-old bulimic daughter overcome her fear of weight gain by arranging for Chelsea's weight to be checked at the doctor's office every two weeks. Reassured that her weight would be closely monitored, Chelsea agreed to experiment by cutting the length of her exercise sessions for the next two weeks, from 90 minutes on her exercise bike to 45 minutes. When Chelsea saw for herself that her weight remained stable, she offered to try one rest day a week for the next several weeks. Two months later Chelsea had pared down her exercise even further, to 20 to 30 minutes of biking per session and two to three "rest days" a week.

When you arrange an "exercise experiment" such as Chelsea's with your child, you should be watchful that your child does not sabotage the experiment by overeating on the days she does not exercise. Usually when this happens, it is not an intentional effort by the child to make the experiment backfire, although that does happen on occasion. You can explain to your child that it is not fair to evaluate the Exercise Plan if eating is out of control, and that testing the effect of less exercise on body weight will have to wait until her eating is stable.

## Exercise Guidelines for the Physically Inactive Child

If your child is not physically active, or is less physically active than most, you face a different kind of challenge. It is important to be careful not to overdo admonishments about exercise, since this can lead to increased resistance to exercise on the part of your child.

The fact is that some kids are naturally less interested in exercise than others. Children who are fortunate enough to have found a sport or an active hobby they enjoy have a ready-made form of exercise. Saying "go outside and play" to those who do not have such a sport is helpful for some kids, but for many it simply promotes more resistance. Most kids, and adults, too, enjoy exercise more if it has some purpose, such as playing with siblings, or with Rover, or taking Rover for a walk, doing errands, yard work, housework, or shopping at the local mall. Try to arrange family outings and events around some mild exercise such as taking a scenic hike, swimming, or canoeing. Remember that any physical activity, whether it is window shopping, sweeping the floor, or vacuuming, constitutes exercise. You should avoid insisting that your child play sports she does not enjoy, or jog if this is something she is not interested in. The last thing you want is to forever turn your child off to the pleasures and health benefits of regular exercise. Policing an Exercise Plan will add additional strain to your relationship with your child. Most parents eventually find it fruitless to engage in a battle of wills in this area.

Twelve-year-old Grace gradually became chubby as she approached adolescence. She was more of a bookworm than an athlete, and her parents had always been happy that Grace liked reading so much, but they were also pleased to see that Grace clearly enjoyed her twice-weekly karate lessons. Concerned about Grace's weight, her parents made an appointment to see me. Their first question was, should they insist that Grace get more exercise? Before answering their question, I wanted to know more about Grace and her eating behaviors. I asked them whether they had observed any binge-eating behaviors in Grace. Both parents were adamant that, no, Grace was not a binge eater or a bulimic. Though she liked her regular snacks and did not feel dinner was complete without a serving of dessert, she ate quite healthily. I told Grace's parents that I suspected that Grace's body was getting ready to go through puberty and a height growth spurt, which would likely even things out. It was also possible that Grace's natural body size was stockier than either of her parents. Although we have noted that it is likely that a child will inherit the body type of one or both of their parents, this is not always the case. Children inherit a set of genes from both parents, both recessive and dominant. Occasionally, it does happen that thin parents have a heavier child. If the child's eating behavior does not explain their size, then genetics—the expression of recessive genes in this case—is the most likely explanation.

The best thing to do, I told Grace's parents, was to support her continued reasonable eating and her interest in karate. The karate, along with the exercise Grace got walking her dog and playing with her friends, provided her with plenty of exercise. These are good practices, I reminded them, that will help Grace stay healthy no matter what her size.

## In Summary

While there are no hard and fast rules about what constitutes too much exercise, we remind you of the following guidelines: for children involved in coached sports, exercise that is more than the child's coach expects is likely to be excessive. Exercise sessions that last more than one hour, multiple exercise sessions per day, or exercise on a daily basis without any rest days are other signs to watch out for, as is exercise that is associated with weight loss and/or loss of menstrual periods. If your child is underweight, your child's doctor should be consulted before devising an exercise plan. Even modest exercise may be too much and can defeat your efforts to help your child return to a healthier weight. You should also be watchful of children who exercise in an effort to lose weight, counteract binges, or explicitly to burn calories.

You should tread carefully if you are concerned about your child's inactivity. It is better to plan family outings and encourage your child's interest in active pursuits than to badger your child about the need for regular exercise.

# 13

# Relapse Training

For bulimics and binge eaters, the biggest fear surrounding the adoption of a Food Plan is that they will lose control, lapse back into their destructive habits, and never be able to stop eating. Most anorexics' fears revolve around uncontrollable weight gain. As recovery progresses they may also begin to fear they will relapse into restrictive eating. Because these fears are so prevalent and strong, I make a point to include relapse training in my patients' treatment plan.

Your child, too, needs to be prepared for relapses of binge eating, vomiting, or restricting during periods of stress. As we have told you before, few eating-disorder sufferers are able to stop cold turkey. Instead of setting your child up for disappointment when she does relapse, it is wise to encourage her to be realistic and tell her that ups and downs are a normal part of recovery. What she needs, and what we will try to give you in this chapter, is a framework for managing the occasional relapse. It is of the utmost importance that whatever you do, you do not ignore relapses.

We will start by destigmatizing relapse, showing you how perfectly normal a part of recovery from an eating disorder it is. Then we will show you how to look closely at the factors that played a part in the relapse. Was your child trying to compensate for overeating by skipping the next meal, or undereating? Is your child getting enough protein? How you, and consequently your child, react to the relapse often means the difference between whether you succeed or fail in your effort to conquer the eating disorder.

Relapses point to possible weaknesses in current approaches and give you and your child a chance to practice problem solving, to formulate an improved approach that will prevent more serious relapses in the future. To help you do this, we will outline various relapse prevention strategies. I find that most people, once they are on the road to recovery, can learn to recognize the signs of an impending relapse and, by employing the relapse prevention strategies we outline here, halt the starve-binge cycle on their own.

## Relapse Training Strategies

### Destigmatizing Relapse

By the time you reach this chapter, we hope that your child has adopted a version of the Food Plan, is gradually learning to recognize feelings of hunger and fullness, is eating in a more organized fashion, and is meeting her nutrient needs. At this point, it is wise to discuss the likely possibility of relapse, and to begin the process of destigmatizing it in your and your child's minds.

It may help to discuss with your child some of the case histories that we detail in this chapter, and note how common relapses are when fighting a truly powerful force such as an eating disorder. Success or failure, you might tell your child, is not measured by one binge-eating or restrictive-eating incident, or one slip back into purging behavior, but over weeks, months, and even years.

If you were to chart your child's eating-disordered behavior, is there a clearly discernable trend of improvement since you adopted the Food Plan, despite the presence of a few setbacks here and there? If so, that is all that matters. You can tell your child that the fact that she has slipped up a few times along the way is not only okay, it is normal. Even normal eaters, after all, occasionally overeat or undereat, and yet they manage to revert to "eating in tune" once again. Slipups, in fact, can be valuable because they highlight areas of weakness or strategies that need to be revised. They provide us "teachable moments." You can also tell your child that she is most likely to suffer a relapse during the first six months after the adoption of a Food Plan.

Children need lots of assurance that you, their parents, are not angry when they have a relapse, but are concerned. It is important that struggles with eating-disordered behaviors are not interpreted or treated as disobedience. Parents should remember that eating disorders are essentially a mental disorder, in some ways much like depression or anxiety. Just as you would not tell a clinically depressed child to just "snap out of it," you would not want to tell an eating-disordered person to "just stop it." Making sure that you do not treat a relapse as disobedience means that you should never punish a child for his eating-disordered behavior, or for a relapse into those behaviors. Instead, I suggest that you take a positive approach, and reward your child when he successfully follows the Food Plan.

Rewards that have worked well with my patients include letting a bulimic child rent a video of her choice on the weekend following a binge- and purge-free week, and letting an anorexic child pick out a new pen or some other small item when her weight goes up at least 2 pounds. (See p. 65 and p. 193 for more on how to use rewards.)

### Analyze the Relapses: What Are Your Child's High-Risk Situations?

Next, tell your child that you and she are going to play detective and analyze each of her relapses. I encourage my patients to work backward and recall every detail that led up to the relapse and may have played a part in triggering it. Patients are instructed to use "lapses" to learn what behaviors or thoughts put them at risk for returning to eating-disordered behaviors. Was it skipping exercise and then worrying about subsequent weight gain? Was it opting not to have dessert with lunch and then feeling deprived all afternoon? How long did the relapse last? What eventually made it stop? Relapses usually fall into a few broad categories, which are described in the following sections.

*Restricting Food Intake*

Relapses are often triggered when the child deviates from the Food Plan and restricts her food intake. She may feel that she ate too much the day before and is trying to compensate. Usually it is reducing foods in the protein, fat, or fun food categories that trigger a relapse. More often than not, relapses into binge-eating episodes indicate the child is nutritionally deprived in some way.

My patient Jane, who is recovering from bulimia, suffers the prototypical relapse when she weighs herself one morning and discovers that after one month on the Food Plan she has gained a pound. Jane is so disturbed at the number she sees on her scale that, ignoring her Food Plan that day, she skips lunch. By dinnertime, she is ravenous, but once again picturing the number on her scale, she summons up all her willpower, forgoes the protein-heavy, rich entrée component of dinner, fills up on salad and says "no thank you" to dessert. Not surprisingly, Jane binges later that evening.

Although it is clear that checking her weight caused the restricting (for more on the advisability of monitoring one's own weight, see chapter 11, p. 195), which in turn caused the binge later that day, I focus on Jane's eating, or lack of it. I try to help her see how she could have prevented the binge by eating enough to feel satisfied rather than starved later in the day. I also inform her that fluctuations in weight up to 5 pounds are normal, even in people who are maintaining a stable weight.

*Facing Dangerous Foods*

Another common relapse trigger is being confronted by a food that your child finds particularly dangerous. Often bulimics and binge eaters believe that they must avoid coming into contact with certain foods at all costs. Although initially avoiding trigger foods may help your demoralized child make some progress, as long as some foods are forbidden the child remains at risk for a relapse. After all, no one can guarantee that your child's taboo food will never be encountered. I remind patients that no food, in and of itself, has addictive properties. If they have trouble with a particular food, it is not the food that is causing the problem, but that their eating disorder is still active. It is for these reasons that we included the "No Food Is Forbidden" guideline in chapter 11, p. 186.

Jessica fervently believed that she was addicted to chocolate and that if she took even one bite she would be compelled to binge. She had many "war stories" to prove her point, including the one about single-handedly finishing off a half-pound bag of M&Ms in one sitting. I reassured her that I could imagine her successfully avoiding chocolate for the rest of her life, and noted that certainly, no one *needs* to eat chocolate to provide essential nutrients. I also told her that chocolate is the one flavor that is universally loved by people across the world. Realizing that if she had the choice, she would rather be able to learn to eat chocolate than to never taste it again, Jessica and I mapped out a plan that would eventually overcome her fear of chocolate.

First and foremost, Jessica needed to be interpreting the Food Plan generously and conscientiously, eating two fun foods per day. Once Jessica was following the Food Plan effortlessly, she was ready to incorporate chocolate as a fun food into her daily diet. She decided that the small packs of M&Ms, which she knew to be less than 300 calories, would be her first planned foray into the world of chocolate. Jessica excitedly told me how after lunch she set aside a few minutes to enjoy her M&Ms. Because she had eaten well, she found that she really didn't want any more than the modest amount in the small bag.

*Abandoning the Food Plan Prematurely*

Sometimes, lapses result from the child's impatience with the Food Plan. She may tire of the fact that following the Food Plan requires a steady focus on food, and tell herself, "I am getting better, I don't need to think about food all the time any more. In fact, I think the Food Plan is fueling my obsession with food and weight. I would be better off without it." She jettisons the plan, only to find that she quickly falls back into the disorder.

Revisiting your child's Food Plan can be helpful at such junctures. You may need to revise the plan to keep it effective in protecting your child from relapsing. It may be that the child's schedule or food preferences have changed so that she has had difficulty following her original Food Plan. I have found that patients who have a written plan are better able to weather the occasional lapse. Try experimenting with writing out a Food Plan for your child, specifying acceptable foods for different meals and snacks.

Some children only need written plans detailing foods to be eating during "risky" times, such as afternoon and evening snacks. Other children do best by referring only to a generalized written version of the Food Plan, a plan no more specific than the Food Plan template. This allows for plenty of variety but still reminds them which nutrients each meal and snack must include. Janna knew that her lunch should provide protein, carbohydrate, fat, fruit, and a serving of calcium and fun food. After several weeks of looking at this formula, which she had written out for herself, she could, almost without thinking, pack her school lunch according to the general template. Her favorite was a turkey sandwich made with mayonnaise and cheese. The sandwich was a nutritional bargain because it provided protein, carbohydrates, fat, and calcium. With a can of juice or a piece of fruit and a dessert, her lunch fulfilled the Food Plan perfectly.

### Dangerous Moods

Relapses can also be triggered by certain moods: anger, loneliness, depression, frustration. While it is impossible to shield your child from these normal human emotions, it is helpful for her to learn to identify them and learn that the onset of one of those moods puts her at risk for relapse.

Many people with eating disorders have fallen into the habit of eating (or not eating) in response to unpleasant moods or feelings. It can be helpful to explore with your child whether disordered food behaviors actually improve his negative moods. Often the response is, "Yes, I feel better at least for a while." But patients who binge tell me that the guilt and regret they experience in the aftermath of the binge really is not worth the temporary improvement in mood. In the end, they still have to deal with their original unpleasant feelings.

Sometimes a relapse can actually be an early warning sign of incipient depression, anxiety, or other form of emotional distress. In such cases, engaging in some self-reflection and seeking help from a psychotherapist can help resolve both the emerging emotional problem and the resurgent eating-disordered behavior that it is causing.

Many people with eating disorders also struggle with depression. Treating the depression with medication and counseling allows the patient to direct her energy toward overcoming her eating disorder. (See chapter 14, p. 263, for more on the use of medications to treat eating disorders.)

In some cases, depression may predate the eating disorder. Margo's parents, Jim and Karen, had suspected that depression had played a role in the onset of Margo's eating disorder. Margo had quite successfully weathered the dual storm of her parents' divorce and her own anorexia. But when Margo suffered her first serious relapse into the eating disorder, they all realized that between the arduous process of helping Margo recover from her disorder and renegotiating their relationship as divorced parents that Margo's depression, which may have played a role in the onset of her eating disorder, had slipped through the cracks.

When Karen first suggested that Margo see a counselor, Margo was less than thrilled. To her surprise, however, the weekly counseling sessions over the course of several months led to a noticeable improvement in her eating. When the counselor recommended that Margo try a course of antidepressants, Margo found, as many do, that in addition to improving her mood, the medication helped her feel freer to add more foods to her daily diet because she was less afraid of overeating.

*Dangerous Places*
Sometimes it is not a scary food or mood that sets off a relapse, but a place or setting that your child may associate with bingeing or purging. Binge and purge habits form easily. Sylvie got in the habit of bingeing and purging while watching television on Saturday afternoons. Once Sylvie's parents understood the problems she had on weekends, they were able to help her find activities that precluded bingeing, such as taking a bike ride or going shopping with a friend.

For some children, a large part of the appeal of an eating disorder is the opportunity to "get away" with their destructive eating without being detected. Their "dangerous place" is anywhere they are alone with food. For children who are attracted to the surreptitious aspect of disordered eating, the solution is to make sure that you are always present during meals and snacks. When Garrett, an anorexic, was left alone to eat, he found himself feeding at least part of every meal or snack to the family dog. To him it was a game; he enjoyed seeing how little he could eat without his parents knowing about it. Lena felt "obligated" to binge and purge when her parents went out for dinner and a movie because she knew she had guaranteed uninterrupted time. You can be of particular help in such cases by being with your child for an hour or so after every meal and snack. (Few bulimics can still purge an hour after eating.) In Garrett's case, his parents made sure that one of them could be present for his meals. At first, it was difficult for Lena's parents to give up their weekly movie date. They felt that Lena was certainly old enough to be left on her own, and that their constant supervision was not age-appropriate. But when I encouraged them to view Lena's eating disorder as a disease, and their close attention like a crucial course of antibiotics, the decision to spend those evenings with their daughter was easy. They decided to substitute their weekly evening out with a weekly lunch date, and Lena finally began to make progress in her recovery.

Parents of teenagers who baby-sit should discuss whether baby-sitting is aggravating their eating disorder. Often the unsupervised time alone, the sense of privacy provided by another family's home, and access to new and different foods can be a setup for a binge.

It is difficult to overemphasize the importance of close parental involvement during meals and snacks when your child is battling a serious eating disorder. But as any parent knows, attempts at close parental supervision are likely to annoy, if not outrage, a child if they are not handled sensitively.

My severely anorexic patient Eliza confessed to me that what she feared most when left alone was the possibility that she might overeat. Yet in a moment of clarity, Eliza confessed to me that when she ate alone the exact opposite happened: she overreacted to her fear of overeating by skimping on serving sizes or skipping them altogether. Although Eliza had not purged yet, she was contemplating it. She knew that both purging and undereating were impossible if her parents were present.

I encouraged Mona and David, Eliza's parents, to think of Eliza's Food Plan as medicine that it was their responsibility to administer. They needed to be careful, however, not to be overbearing, which can happen when parents are too rigid in their approach. Over time, Mona and David learned to be sure that one of them was with Eliza whenever she ate, and continued this practice until she was well on the road to recovery. They found that a low-key, undemanding, and inconspicuous approach worked best with Eliza. Anything more obtrusive would be intolerable to her, and she would tell them so, in no uncertain terms. Yet Eliza told me privately that although it sometimes annoyed her that her parents were always around when she was eating, another part of her felt safe in the knowledge that her parents took her eating problems seriously.

*Stress*

If your child gets too busy, too excited, too anxious, or too tired—in other words, overstressed—she can be at risk for a relapse. Stress can make it harder for your child to concentrate on keeping her food and exercise behaviors on an even keel. When you know that it is a time of unusual busyness, excitement, or anxiety—for example the holiday season, when meal schedules may be altered and when more snack foods are served—it is important to be extra-solicitous around preparing foods and scheduling meals. If circumstances are conspiring to create a level of stress that inter-feres with your child's recovery, you and your child should sit down and pri-oritize the extras in both your lives. Remember that the first item on your list of important things to accomplish should be your child's recovery.

When the Martins' daughter, Leslie, relapsed, the family decided that they all needed to jettison some activities. Leslie, in particular, had to con-sider paring down her many school-related activities. Her parents had heard excuse after excuse for why Leslie was losing weight again, all of them legit-imate; she simply didn't have time to eat lunch or snacks and also keep up with all her activities. Without making a big deal out of it, Barry, Leslie's father, who had a relatively flexible job, rearranged his schedule. He wanted to be able to fix Leslie her afternoon snack, and sit and talk with her while she ate it. Leslie, for her part, dropped one after-school meeting so she could be home for snack time. Barry and Leslie found that a bonus to this arrangement was that their relationship deepened just through spend-ing those few minutes together most afternoons before Leslie took off for sports practice.

*Dangerous Mind-Sets: Threats to Body Image*
Brittany, a young teenager who has struggled with anorexia and now bulimia, told me she was shocked to find when she was looking back over her diary's entries for the past few years that since eighth grade she signed every diary entry with a postscript: "P.S., I'm fat."

"Gee, I must have been telling myself I'm fat for a very long time," she told me. "It's no wonder I have an eating disorder now." I asked Brittany where she thought the "I'm fat" came from. "I started my period that year and I think I probably gained some weight, too," Brittany remembered. "I know that made me feel more self-conscious about my body. But what I remember most, and I have never told anyone this, is that a boy I liked at school started to tease me about being fat. The teasing didn't last very long, because I think he figured out it really hurt my feelings. I know I started my first diet then."

As Brittany's story illustrates, sometimes it is a threat to the child's body image that can set off a relapse of an eating disorder. Usually, as your child normalizes her eating and her body weight, she starts to feel more in con-trol, more confident, and more hopeful, and her body image problems begin to improve substantially. Occasionally, however, despite improved body image, you will still see signs of low self-esteem, anxiety, or depression. Children who continue to struggle with these other issues should be evalu-ated by a psychotherapist. They may need specific treatment and medica-tions to overcome these problems.

Sometimes your child will have genuinely made strides in improving her body image, but her newfound sense of self-esteem may be fragile, and easily affected by anything from a random negative comment to an argument with a friend. It is striking that for many teens the antidote to any negative experience is a return to eating-disordered behaviors. "Going on a diet" becomes the solution to every problem. Children who have increased their self-esteem by becoming successful at dieting and weight loss will need to learn to appreciate other skills and traits that they possess as they recover.

As she worked hard to recover from her eating disorder, Elyssa had to work equally hard to find a new basis for her self-esteem. Before, her main source of pride, and the object of all her friends' admiration had been her 10-pound weight loss over the summer before she entered high school. Now, Elyssa had to find other ways to think about who she was besides a successful dieter. With some effort, she was able to identify that she was kind to her younger siblings, she worked hard at school, she had a good sense of humor, and a keen fashion sense.

Just as with relapses triggered by other stressors, relapses caused by unresolved body-image problems or attacks on a newly formed sense of self-esteem can actually be helpful in pointing out where you and your child still need to do some work. Lingering body-image problems will interfere with your child's ability to make progress in her eating behavior, and until they are addressed and resolved, will continue to increase the likelihood of relapse. We refer you to chapter 8 to help you explore the possibility that your child's persistent body-image problems reflect a learned response from you. Body-image problems that remain in spite of normalized eating should not be ignored and are best addressed by a psychotherapist.

### Unintentional Changes in Weight or Eating

Some relapses are triggered by changes in weight or eating behavior that are outside the control of the recovering child. Ellen's experience is an example of this type of relapse. After eating a special dinner out, Ellen and her family all experience the horrible gastrointestinal complications of food poisoning. No one in Ellen's family eats anything solid for two days. By day three, everyone is back to normal eating except Ellen. Secretly thrilled by her newly flat stomach and by the fact that she doesn't feel very hungry, she plans to continue her liquid diet as long as she can. Ellen's mother, Marianne, realizes that Ellen may be tempted by these circumstances, and is at risk for serious relapse.

Marianne makes it a point to discuss her concerns in private and not at a mealtime because she knows that such discussions are almost always best held when food is not present. Simply laying out her concerns in a logical manner helps Marianne illustrate the folly of Ellen's plans. Marianne begins by saying she does not know if Ellen is tempted to continue to undereat, but she can understand how easy it would be to do just that. Then Marianne reminds Ellen how hard Ellen and, in fact, her whole family, has worked to overcome the eating disorder and asks if she can do anything to help.

Notice that Marianne refrains from accusing Ellen of deliberately under-eating, a tactic that usually works to keep this type of conversation from escalating into a full-blown argument.

Other situations that put recovering children at risk are having an oper-ation, traveling, going to camp, new or difficult personal relationships, and major life transitions. All of these are situations that, to varying degrees, temporarily take control of eating away from your child.

### Changes in Exercise Routine

Any change in routine, including your child's exercise routine, can increase risk of relapse. Rebekah's relapse occurred during her family's "dream vacation" to a resort in the Bahamas over winter vacation. All meals were included in their hotel stay, and the food was delicious. There were so many planned activities that Rebekah found she couldn't get in her usual daily run. Certain that with the richer food and no exercise (Rebekah still had trouble thinking of anything less than a brisk run as exercise) she had gained weight, Rebekah planned to go on a low-fat diet as soon as she returned home. Sensing Rebekah's increasing anxiety about her weight, her parents arranged for a check-in visit with me as soon as they returned home the next week. First, I wanted to know how Rebekah had eaten, and asked her to recall, with some specificity, what she had eaten during her vacation. While Rebekah had indeed eaten a wide array of excellent, rich foods, she had stuck to her basic Food Plan.

Much to Rebekah's surprise, a weight-check showed that her anxiety about missing her usual exercise was unfounded; she had not gained a pound. Before the trip, she had resisted the notion that any sustained body movement counts as exercise. Although she swam, snorkeled, explored the resort, and walked on the beach, she told herself that those activities "didn't count" and would not keep her from gaining weight. But after checking her weight upon her return, Rebekah finally accepted the fact that heavy exer-cise was not essential for weight maintenance, and so was able to expand her definition of exercise.

Over time, Rebekah's enjoyment of outdoor activities increased as she came to realize that while exercise was good for her health, it was only a minor factor in maintaining her weight. The primary benefit to her was that these activities were simply fun.

## Recognizing a Relapse: What Are the Early Warning Signs?

As you can see, a variety of situations are likely to lead to a relapse. The challenge for you and your child is to identify those that she is most susceptible to and to learn to recognize their early warning signals. It is always surprising to me how often parents miss the obvious because they really don't want to believe their child is in trouble again. They put on blinders, rationalize that their child "has the flu" when she purges, or assert that she missed a period because she is under stress.

Likely early warning signals of relapse include:

- An increase in thoughts about weight, shape, and size
- "Feeling fat"
- Actual and significant changes in body weight
- Increased interest in dieting or exercise
- A rekindling of the desire to overeat or purge
- Regular episodes of binge eating, dieting, or purging
- Loss of menstrual periods

Encourage your child to be attuned to what her mind and body are telling her: Are the thoughts and feelings she is experiencing an early sign of emotional distress, an indicator that food-related behaviors need attention, or both?

## Coping with the Unexpected: Developing Relapse Prevention Strategies

Now that you are familiar with the various situations that commonly trigger a relapse, and are attuned to the early warning signals that precede those episodes, it is time to begin to develop some preventive strategies.

When I do this with my patients, I assure them that there is a wide range of effective relapse strategies; our job is simply to find the right ones. Following are the basic relapse prevention strategies that I teach my patients.

### Return to the Food Plan
The first line of attack when a relapse threatens recovery is always a return to the Food Plan. If your child has binged, purged, or begun to restrict once again, you should encourage her to immediately return to the structure of the Food Plan. If your child feels she is on the brink of losing control, try to help her plan meals in detail and in advance, so that she knows exactly what she will be eating next, and when.

**Write Out a Detailed Food Plan**

Writing out the specifics of the Food Plan with your child, as we have said, is often a helpful strategy. It is important that the written plan be derived from a conversation with your child and what she thinks will help. Painstakingly devising a plan for each day that includes scheduled meals, snacks, and activities can help your child avoid long periods of unstructured time on the one hand, or "overbooking," on the other, both of which can increase the risk of relapse.

Joseph, who needed to gain weight, and his parents found a written school lunch plan helpful. Joseph's plan was posted on the refrigerator making it easy for his parents to pack his lunch. Just seeing his Food Plan every day helped Joseph remember that eating according to it was important. Some children, however, need to keep their Food Plan more private, especially from other siblings, who may use it as ammunition in the silly spats siblings often get into. I find this rarely happens in families where parents take their child's eating disorder seriously.

Joseph's written plans were instrumental in helping him and his family figure out what to do when, after having reached his goal weight, he began to lose again. The first question was whether Joseph was successful day in and day out in eating according to his plan. Yes, Joseph assured his parents, he was following the Food Plan. When this is the case it simply means the plan is no longer meeting the child's caloric needs. This happens when the child's metabolic rate takes a sudden jump upward, and is common during recovery from anorexia (see chapter 11, p. 198, for more on the hypermetabolism of anorexia). Children who are eating better start to feel better and may inadvertently become more active as well. This increased activity will increase their caloric needs and lead to weight loss if the Food Plan is not adjusted accordingly.

Because he had been following a Food Plan, it was a relatively simple process for Joseph and his parents to sit down and decide what he needed to add to turn his weight around.

**Find the Weak Points in Your Child's Food Plan**

It might be helpful for you and your child to identify what part of the Food Plan she could be executing better. Often it helps to try to recall what it was about the Food Plan that helped your child most in launching her recovery. Has your child done some backsliding in that area? You should also think about what it was that helped your child feel better about her shape and weight concerns. Some common lapses in the Food Plan are:

• **Missing breakfast.** Because of the effects of "famine metabolism" and ketone production (chapter 10, p. 166), children who skip breakfast often find that it is very easy to skip lunch as well. The problem, however, is that this seeming lack of hunger is only temporary, and sets the child up for bingeing later in the day.

• **Skipping fun foods.** Just as skipping meals, especially breakfast, often triggers a relapse, so does the temptation to skip the fun foods in the plan. Though many patients resist adding fun food into their Food Plans, when they do add them, the eating-disordered behaviors often quickly resolve.

• **Skimping on protein.** Because foods containing protein often contain fat as well, they tend to be both filling and satisfying. These qualities make protein the ideal "anti-binge" food. When a child begins to backslide from her specified Food Plan and skimp on protein, she is likely to feel overly hungry and more likely to relapse into eating-disordered behavior. Relapses usually resolve as the child returns to her Food Plan or the Food Plan is altered to better meet her needs. Most relapses are caused by undereating, either by avoiding some foods or skipping parts or all of meals or snacks.

### A Note about Self-Monitoring

In some cases, your child may have worked with a professional nutritionist or therapist who, at some point during your child's recovery, asked him to keep detailed food diaries, including records of binges and purges. If your child has found this practice (known as "self-monitoring") useful in the past, you may want to suggest resuming the diary-keeping while his eating patterns stabilize once again.

I generally do not recommend that families who are not working with a professional try this on their own, as most parents and children find it hard to be dispassionate and objective enough to look at food diaries and help their child by critiquing his approach to food. But for the child who has found food diaries helpful in the past, sometimes merely returning to the habit of monitoring his own food intake helps him turn a relapse around. (For more on how professionals use self-monitoring, see chapter 14, pp. 260 and 262.)

### A Reminder about Self-Weighing

I remind you here once again about the dangers of obsessive self-weighing, which tends to increase obsessions with body weight and can make small, natural, and insignificant variations in body weight seem important. While occasional weight checks are recommended for recovering anorexics, these are best done by professionals until the anorexic is well recovered. (For more on the advisability of weight monitoring, see chapter 11, p. 195.)

## When Should You Seek Professional Help?

There may come a point where you realize that your child's "relapses" are too severe or too frequent for you to handle alone. Here we will talk about how to know if your situation calls for professional help. Remember that relapses can also occur after a stint of professional care has ended. (For a more extensive discussion on professional care, see chapter 14.)

You should consider seeking professional help when:

• **Your child's relapse has lasted for longer than a month.** Sometimes, just the *thought* of seeking professional help is enough to get your child out of the relapse. Several times I've seen a family sit down with their child and tell her how worried they are, and how it seems that the measures they have taken as a family do not seem to be working. It might be time to consult an expert, these parents suggest. Lo and behold, the child turns the eating disorder around without any professional help.

• **Your child suffers a series of relapses.** This is an even stronger indication that your child's particular eating disorder may be more than the family can manage on its own.

• **You and your child continue to struggle and work very hard to just maintain a low level of recovery.**

• **Your child has stopped receiving professional help and then suffers a relapse that she is unable to turn around with your help alone.** Usually a medical professional will give you clear criteria for when a return to treatment is recommended. It might be when an anorexic child loses more than 5 pounds, or if parents notice an increased obsession with food or weight. Depending on the nature of your child's relapse you should consider resuming either psychological or nutritional therapy. You can gently tell your child that returning to therapy or other supportive treatment after a relapse is not a sign of failure, but of wisdom.

If you do decide to seek professional support, it is important to continue to express the conviction that recovery is possible, and that you are not giving up on your child. Telling your child that eating disorders are highly treatable and that most people recover with professional help is encouraging.

You might say, "We've done our best to help you with your eating problems. Now we want to make sure you have the best professional help possible." Or, "We're providing you with professional help because we care so much about you and want the best for you." It can also be reassuring to say,

"Because we know it's not unusual to need professional help to overcome an eating disorder and because we can see that you're struggling, consulting with professionals just makes sense."

## In Summary

The question that sooner or later faces nearly all people struggling to overcome an eating disorder is not *if* they are going to relapse, but *when* they are going to relapse. You will do any child battling an eating disorder a great favor by explaining this distinction to her. When the question changes from *if* to *when*, then suddenly (especially to a perfectionistic anorexic) the fear and pressure that she feels surrounding recovery dissipates. She realizes that relapse is just another bump on the road to recovery.

Building in this expectation makes handling relapses much easier, both for you and for your child. We have outlined all kinds of dangerous foods, moods, places, and other factors that can trigger a relapse, and we have discussed ways to get back in the saddle when this does happen. The most important message of this chapter, however, is that relapses usually occur and therefore you and your child should be prepared to deal with them.

# 14

# When You've Done All You Can:
# Professional Resources and How to Use Them

Sometimes, despite the best efforts of you, your eating-disordered child, and other members of the family, improvement and gradual resolution of the disorder may remain elusive. While the message of this book is that your efforts as parents at home can be highly effective in preventing and treating early stage eating disorders, you should know that for more entrenched eating problems professional help is usually necessary.

If, after one month—or sooner if your child has lost a dangerous amount of weight or continues to purge—you find that you and your child's efforts at adopting the Food and Exercise Plans have not worked, you should consider going outside the family and seeking the help of an experienced professional. One option open to you is to find or put together a team of professionals, which might include a physician, nutritionist, psychotherapist, and sometimes a psychiatrist and/or a family therapist. In this chapter, we will discuss how to know when you need professional help, how to decide if you need a single professional or a team of professionals, and what characteristics to look for in the various professionals you decide you need. We will also review some of the medications now being used for eating disorders that you may want to ask your child's doctor about, as well as discuss the various forms of psychotherapy that experts have found to be most effective for eating-disordered patients.

If your child's disorder is of the most serious, recalcitrant nature and outpatient therapy has not resolved it, you may need to consider inpatient or residential treatment. (See pp. 289–96 for a list of hospital and residential programs.) Included in this chapter is a checklist that will help you determine if your child really needs the round-the-clock services of an inpatient treatment facility, and some tips on how to go about finding one that will meet your child's needs.

## How to Know When You Have Done All That You Can

Meg, a high school soccer player who aspired to make the varsity team, admired Isabel, a varsity player who had lost a considerable amount of weight over the summer. Perhaps subconsciously imitating Isabel, Meg began reducing her food intake in an effort to lose weight. Her parents noticed this change, and worried it might signal the start of an eating problem. Yet despite their efforts, they could not seem to light enough of a fire under Meg to motivate her to eat adequately and stop her weight loss.

A trip to the doctor confirmed that Meg had lost enough weight to be in physical danger. Her doctor recommended that Meg see a psychologist who had a reputation of being good with young teens and was well known for her successful treatment of eating disorders, and me. This three-pronged attack on her eating disorder, by her doctor, psychologist, and me, her nutritionist, worked effectively for Meg by leaving no room in her life for the disorder to thrive.

Hearing her doctor's straightforward description of how her continued weight loss could jeopardize her bones and heart helped motivate Meg to work hard to get well. The psychologist's kind, empathetic probing into the causes of her depression led to the discovery that the suicide of one of Meg's classmates over the summer may have helped trigger the clinical depression she was suffering from. By exploring the underlying causes of her depression, and explaining to her how the depression fueled her eating problems, the psychologist helped Meg understand what was happening to her.

I was confident that I could design just the right Food Plan for Meg that would bring about steady weight gain. The explanations I provided about the importance of various nutrients, and my assurance that the Food Plan would restore her to her "healthiest thinnest" weight helped Meg follow the plan and slowly restore her lost weight.

The following are tips on how to know when you have reached that point in your battle with your child's disorder where you need to move quickly to get professional support, for your child and possibly for yourselves and the rest of your family as well. You should consider turning to professionals when:

• Your child is not making steady progress under your direction at home, or when your child's disordered behaviors are getting worse, not better. This means when your child is continuing to lose weight when she needs to be gaining, or if the frequency of your child's bingeing and/or purging is increasing, not decreasing. Parental treatment for bulimia and binge eating is particularly difficult because of the alternating feelings of shame and rebellion that affect children and adolescents suffering from these disorders.

• Your child has not made progress after one month. This is advisable even for children with less serious eating disorders, meaning they have lost less than a medically dangerous amount of weight, or only binge or purge occasionally. I recommend that parents in such situations proceed with putting a team of professionals together because eating disorders tend to either be in the state of getting better or getting worse.

• Your child's or your family's life seems to be falling apart because the eating disorder is having a profound effect on your child's ability to function academically and socially.

• Your independent-minded adolescent's natural inclination to do things her own way makes solving the disorder within the family impossible, or if not impossible, too stressful to bear. The older and more independent a child is, the less likely it is that your efforts alone will be effective. In such cases, she may make better progress working with professionals.

• You and your child have a good relationship and can work out other issues, but you find that food-related issues are impossible to see eye-to-eye on.

• You have a rocky relationship with your child. Regardless of the age of their child, some parents have a more volatile relationship with their child than others. This makes it difficult, sometimes even impossible, to work on the child's eating problems together.

• You need advice. A consultation with a qualified, experienced professional can be worth its weight in gold. He or she can help you evaluate how your child is progressing and impart wisdom gleaned from years of working with similar patients.

• Your efforts to help your child have not been well received; that is, you are having unproductive arguments, she is telling you to mind your own business, or your child is denying she has a problem. If this describes your situation, you will need the guidance of professionals to work more productively with your child.

• You and your spouse are not on the same page about how to approach your child's eating problems. In such cases, professionals can act as impartial advisors to the two of you as to how best to handle your involvement.

If you find yourselves in one of these or a similar situation, what is important is to realize that if your help has not been enough to turn around your child's eating disorder, you must find someone who can. Remember, the longer your child has an unresolved eating problem, the more difficult it will be to treat.

When it is clear that professional help is necessary, you should avail your-selves to the best treatment that your finances will allow, and that your local community has to offer.

## When Physical or Sexual Abuse Is Involved

In addition to the situations we describe in the previous section, psycho-therapy is also especially advisable for patients whose eating disorders may have been triggered by physical or sexual abuse. It is clear that such abuse is often associated with later emotional problems, including eating disor-ders. Researchers theorize that among victims of abuse, weight loss may be an attempt to arrest sexual development and to feel in control, that purg-ing may be a symbolic way of cleansing oneself, and that bingeing may dis-tract the eater from problems and numb fears, both rational and irrational, that the abuse has fostered.

It is not unusual for children who have suffered from physical or sexual abuse to be very particular about their eating and wary of rules associated with eating. They need extra support to find foods they like that allow them to maintain their health and grow normally.

My advice to families who are seeking help for an eating-disordered child who has been sexually abused is to choose a psychotherapist with experience with both abuse and eating disorders. It is particularly impor-tant for children who have experienced abuse to choose an empathetic, supportive psychotherapist.

## There Is No Stigma in Seeking Help

Having been encouraged to believe that you as parents can be effective in turning around your child's eating problem, it would not be surprising to feel guilty if you come to a point where you feel you and your child need professional help.

You should not, however, assume that you have failed, or were not strong enough to beat your child's eating disorder, or that there is something wrong with your family or your child because you have consulted outside resources. When not caught early, full-blown eating disorders are bona fide psychological disorders that can require professional treatment to turn around. Some children have such a virulent eating disorder that even if it is caught early, your child and you will benefit from the guidance of a pro-fessional.

Our point here is that there is no stigma attached to seeking professional help. Your child is ill, and you need to do whatever it takes to make her well. I have had several younger patients tell me: "I can do it myself," "Willpower should be enough," "I already know a lot about nutrition," "My eating disorder isn't bad enough to need treatment," or, "Mom and Dad don't 'believe' in therapy." Other families I have seen assert that professional help, especially psychotherapy, is only for the "real crazies," or for rich suburbanites who don't have anything better to do with their time or money. The type of analysis that the neurotic characters in Woody Allen films undergo epitomizes what some people imagine therapy being all about.

In fact, the very real benefits of getting professional help, whether it is psychotherapy or nutrition counseling are well documented. Consider:

- Children and adolescents benefit from the experience of establishing a unique relationship with and confiding in an adult other than a parent.
- Patients benefit from a confidential and therapeutic atmosphere that challenges them to change their thinking and behaviors.
- Most patients in care of a professional make the important discovery that they do have the ability to change things about themselves, and make important self-discoveries in the process. What they learn about themselves can also be put to positive use in other life situations.
- Parents benefit from having an experienced professional on their team who can advise and support them in difficult times.

Some of you may be worried that if you consult a professional, the expert will be critical of you and your child-rearing practices. You may be inclined to wait until your child seems ready or asks for treatment before providing it. While it is true that treatment will be less effective if you or your child is not keen on the idea, we advise you not to wait too long to act.

## How Will Getting Professional Help Affect Your Role as Parents?

Getting professional help does not mean that you as parents are no longer involved in your child's recovery. On the contrary, a professional or team of professionals can help you help your child in a more effective way.

If you select outpatient treatment for your child, you by necessity will fill the role of at-home nutritionist and counselor. If your child requires hospital or residential treatment, your child will eventually return home, and you will need to be there to support her recovery. Getting professional help, in other words, will not take you off the front lines of the battle against your child's eating disorder. It will be up to you to help her implement the plans that professionals have devised, encourage her to adhere to those plans, and to provide all the necessities she needs to do so.

**Using the Food and Exercise Plans in Tandem with Professional Care**

Professional treatment can help your child understand why you as parents must be involved in helping him follow a Food Plan, why you need to spend time with him after meals, and why he will benefit from sharing his fears about eating with you.

We are not suggesting that once professionals are employed that you as parents bow out of your child's treatment. Instead, we encourage an approach that allows you to be involved in an educated and wholehearted way, supporting him at home while working with professionals who will monitor your child's progress, and advise you if your child needs more intensive care.

## What Type of Professional Does Your Child Need?

When you first decide to seek professional treatment for your child, the first decision you will have to make is what type of professional you need. We will briefly outline what services each type of professional that can be seen for an eating disorder provides, and why each is beneficial. It is important to choose professionals who are experienced in treating eating disorders. In the end, doing so can make the difference between whether or not your child recovers in a timely manner.

The **medical doctor,** usually a pediatrician, a family doctor, or an internist, is an essential member of the team. You should have a doctor on your team whether you involve other professionals or not. He or she will assess and monitor your child's health with physical exams, blood tests, and, if necessary, bone density tests. If your child is underweight, the doctor will set weight goals and possibly set weights at which participation in sports is allowed. If your child's health becomes grave, the doctor will advise hospitalization for medical stabilization.

Making sure your child has regular checkups will give you the assurance that your child's health is being monitored and indeed improving, regardless of whether or not you are working with other professionals. You will want to give your doctor as much information as possible about your child's behaviors and symptoms, and make sure the doctor understands your concerns. Seeing a medical doctor (or a psychiatrist) also provides you access to promising new medications that are now being used to treat eating disorders. If your doctor is part of a team of professionals you are seeing, he or she should be in close communication with other members of the treatment team. This enables the other members of the team to help explain to your child the doctor's concerns and recommendations. The better your child understands those concerns and suggestions, the better equipped she will be to respond to them.

Seeing a **nutritionist** will keep you productively involved in your child's "food business" and reduce conflict between you and your child. The nutritionist will help your child work on behavioral goals and explain the biological underpinnings and the health consequences of a serious eating disorder. The nutritionist, who is likely to share monitoring your child's weight with the physician, can explain *why* weight goals and exercise limitations are necessary. Nutrition counseling will also help you manage your child's eating-disordered behaviors and help you and your child resolve any difficulties she is having with her Food Plan. Seeing a nutritionist can also help your child understand the benefit of your practical support at home around food and eating issues.

Seeing a **psychotherapist** can provide your child with an unbiased, insightful sounding board. A psychotherapist can help your child recognize her eating-disordered thoughts, beliefs, values, and even more important, how to actually "restructure" them.

Like a psychotherapist, a **psychiatrist** can provide psychotherapy. The psychiatrist can also prescribe medications, which a psychotherapist's license does not allow. If your child has a doctor who will prescribe psychiatric medications (medical doctors are increasingly doing this) and a psychotherapist, then a psychiatrist may not be necessary unless your child has complex psychological problems in addition to the eating disorder. In such a case, a psychiatrist might be called in for diagnosis and prescription of medications to deal with the other diagnoses.

## The Benefits of Team vs. Individual Treatment Professionals

In the United States and in countries with developed medical resources, the prevailing model for the professional treatment of serious eating disorders is the team treatment model.

This is the preferred model of treatment because studies have confirmed what I have found in my own practice, that combining counseling, medication, and nutrition therapy is the most effective approach to treating serious eating disorders. An Italian study showed that anorexics quickly and substantially improved their weight with team treatment. The study also found that after only four months of treatment, depression, anxiety, and eating-disordered attitudes were much improved. This is a considerably better and faster rate of improvement than is seen with single-focused interventions. Other research has indicated that partial treatments are less likely to lead to long-term resolution of eating problems. If your child has a serious eating disorder, it is more likely that she will need several components of the classic treatment team, if not all of them.

## Is Team Treatment Always the Way to Go? Choosing a Point of First Contact

It is clear that providing your child with the type of team treatment that I describe can pay off with a relatively quick recovery. Yet the prospect of having to assemble (and pay for) so many professionals can be daunting. You should know that not every family will need the full team that we describe. In cases that are less severe, often a child can completely resolve his eating problems with just one of the following forms of treatment alone: medical monitoring, nutrition treatment, psychotherapy, or medication. Medication is the least likely to be effective as a sole treatment.

You may, like some parents, feel most comfortable first broaching the subject of your child's disorder with your pediatrician or family doctor. The doctor can assess the seriousness of your child's eating problem and refer you, if necessary, to other respected professionals in your community.

Your child may feel most comfortable first addressing her eating disorder with a psychotherapist, although many children are especially resistant to this as the point of first contact. (The idea of having to share their deepest secrets with a stranger can be off-putting.) In cases of severe disorders, of course, counseling should not take the place of being seen by a physician, but should occur in conjunction with treatment by a medical doctor.

Many adolescents feel most comfortable talking with a nutritionist when first acknowledging their eating disorder because the nutritionist is likely to be viewed as nonthreatening, and maybe even interesting, to the food-obsessed child. My new patients often tell me, "If I could just get on a good diet, my problems will be solved." Although the problem is likely much more complex than that, if a good nutritionist is there to listen and help at the outset, your child may be willing to consider additional forms of treatment, such as counseling.

It is important to note that the type of group practice we describe in this chapter, complete with physician, psychotherapist (psychologist or psychiatrist), nutritionist, and possibly a family therapist, rarely exists outside of big cities. Nevertheless, an experienced professional in private practice, even in suburban or rural areas, will have working relationships with other qualified professionals and can help you put together your team.

In the end, it matters less which type of professional you contact first—a nutritionist, psychotherapist, or medical professional—and more whether the one you choose is experienced in treating eating disorders, can help your child gain a realistic perspective on her problems, and is someone with whom your child can form a trusting, nurturing relationship. (Again, the exception to this rule would be the severely ill child, who should be seen by a medical doctor as soon as possible.) If you do decide on team treatment, whichever professional you contact first must be a good team player, someone who works with other professionals whether or not they are involved in a group practice, and someone who can help you assess whether your child needs team treatment.

This one-professional-at-a-time approach to assembling a team is similar to what is known as the "stepped-care" approach. In this model, treatment is "stepped-up" until your child begins to make progress, beginning first with the lowest-intensity intervention and progressing as needed to gradually more intensive interventions.

A low-intensity first step, for example, would be sitting down with your child to describe your observations and expressing your concerns. If your child's eating problems continue, you would then begin working with the Food and Exercise Plans we describe in chapters 10, 11, and 12. If progress is still not forthcoming, you would arrange a visit with your child's medical doctor, who may help your child understand the potential dangerousness of her behaviors. Sometimes at this juncture medications are prescribed by the physician experienced in the care of eating-disordered patients. If this elicits no response, your child would next see a nutritionist, then a psychotherapist, or vice versa. If after all of these interventions there is still no progress, you will want to consider arranging hospital or residential care. Upon release from inpatient care the sequence of care is reversed, and is "stepped-down" as your child continues to recover.

The stepped-care approach is often effective in situations involving eating disorders of mild to moderate severity. It is the wrong approach when it is clear your child has a serious eating disorder. In such a case, there is no good reason to wait before assembling the whole team from the get-go.

## What to Look For in a Professional

When looking for a professional to help treat your eating-disordered child, it is important to find someone who is not only experienced and competent but kind, empathetic, confident, no-nonsense, and firm. The professional or professionals you select should also expect progress, express confidence that their treatment will be effective, and be hopeful for a full recovery. On the other hand, the professional should take your child's eating disorder seriously. You want to be sure that the professional recognizes that an eating disorder is a grave, potentially life-threatening disorder that must be treated with determination and effort. Professionals who cause you or your child to feel blamed for the eating disorder will be less effective. Instead, you want a professional who can express uncritical acceptance of your child and your previous efforts to help your child. In other words, you want professionals who have a strategy for treating the eating disorder that does not scapegoat you, your child, or your family.

Other attitudes and practices that are the hallmarks of a good professional are when she or he keeps you as parents informed, and is respectful of your efforts to help your child. The professional should involve you by making it clear what you can do to help and should take the time to listen to your observations, insights, and concerns. You should be informed about the techniques your child is learning, and be given an explanation of the goals of therapy.

Psychotherapist and author Steven Levenkron writes that the most effective style for professionals is to be both nurturing and authoritative, which allows them to provide a stable source of support. It is important that the professional be able to relate effectively to your child and talk in a way that is appropriate to your child's development. The professional should also be able to establish what is called a "therapeutic alliance," a trusting, independent relationship that fosters collaboration with your child.

Often children or adolescents do not begin to resolve their eating disorders until they find a professional they can talk to without feeling "judged" or "wrong." The professional should be nonjudgmental, and yet at the same time challenge the child to do better than she has been doing.

If your child is a preteen or younger expect that sessions will be a mix of individual and family meetings. Professionals should make it abundantly clear to you and your child that she or he will not keep important information from you the parents. On the other hand, your child needs to feel that her confidentiality is protected as much as possible. Although the professional is not required to protect the confidences of underage patients, respecting the young patient's privacy will help foster a collaborative relationship.

Although it may be difficult for you, it is important to remember that the primary relationship of each of the professionals your child sees, with the one exception of the family therapist, is with your child.

### Male or Female Professional, Which Is Best for Your Child?

Parents often ask me whether they should make an effort to find female professionals for their daughters or male professionals if their eating-disordered child is a boy. There is no scientific evidence that either gender is better. If your child expresses a preference, you should try to accommodate her or his wishes if possible. More important than gender is whether the professional is experienced and can make a therapeutic connection with your child.

**Credentials to Look For**

When seeking professional help, you will want to choose professionals with appropriate credentials and good reputations. Your medical professional will either be a medical doctor (M.D.) or a nurse practitioner (N.P.) or physician assistant (P.A.).

Your child's nutritionist should be a registered dietitian (R.D.). Some but not all states license nutritionists (L.R.D.). Increasingly registered dietitians also have master's (M.S.) or higher degrees in nutrition (Ph.D. or Ed.D.), though an experienced dietitian without a higher degree but with ample experience working with eating-disordered patients would also be a good choice.

The educational credentials of psychotherapists can vary from M.S.W., Ph.D., Psy.D., Ed.D., L.C.P.C. (licensed clinical professional counselors) to M.D. (for psychiatrists). States do license psychotherapists, so if you have any doubt about a psychotherapist's credentials, you can check with your state's licensing board. The bottom line is this: Is the professional experienced and do you and your child feel confident that this professional can be of help?

## How Professional Help for You Can Help Your Child's Recovery

It is important that as parents you present a united front to your child during her treatment. Stanford University psychiatrist James Lock and colleagues go so far as to assert that even the "slightest disagreement" between parents about food issues will decrease the parents' effectiveness. "You have to act as if you are one person in order to succeed," they advise parents who are attempting to refeed their anorexic children. "Acting as if you are one person," however, can be extremely challenging if you and your partner are contending with divorce, or even discord and disagreement. In such cases, professionals can be invaluable in helping both of you find common ground in your effort to support your struggling child. By providing specific direction and hints, they can help you resolve your differences more quickly than you might be able to on your own.

## Paying for Treatment: Can You Afford It?

It is the fortunate family indeed who finds that their health insurance policy covers visits to every member of an eating-disorder treatment team. Most policies, of course, cover visits to physicians, and many are willing to cover at least some visits with a qualified psychotherapist.

Policies tend to vary most in their coverage of nutrition counseling. Some policies cover nutrition as they would any other necessary medical expense. Check to see if your policy requires a written referral from your child's doctor for nutrition counseling; many do. Other medical policies are restrictive in their coverage of nutrition counseling. They may only cover such services for diabetes, or only allow three visits (which is never adequate to treat a serious eating disorder), or only allow your child to see one of their "preferred providers" (who may or may not be the best choice for your child).

You should take it upon yourselves to contact either your company's employee benefits office or the insurance company directly so that you understand your coverage. You may, like the mother of a patient of mine, decide not to take "no" for an answer. Talia's mother kept calling her insurance company, moving up the chain of command until she found the sympathetic ear of the assistant to the company's medical director. The assistant was able to arrange for a special exception for nutrition treatment for eating disorders, which remained in place for other deserving patients until the assistant retired. Another mother, whose family received state assistance, spent a day talking on the phone to everyone she could at her state's health and human services office. When she hit a dead end there, she placed a call to the governor's office, pled her case, and was soon talking to an official who was able to grant the funding she needed. Other families are not so lucky. Jeanne's limited insurance coverage did not cover nutrition counseling. Undeterred, Jeanne saved up her tips from her hairdressing job to pay for her daughter's visits. Another family had to dip into their daughter's college fund to pay for treatment. Some might view this as jeopardizing their child's future, but this family realized their daughter would not have a meaningful future unless her eating disorder was resolved.

## Playing the Role of "Case Manager"

I often advise parents to be tenacious and to take on the role of "case manager" for their child, much as Jeanne or Talia's mother did. In addition to pursuing insurance coverage, this means taking on such tasks as making sure appointments get made and following up with professionals who have not responded in a timely manner. Unfortunately, it is not unusual for even competent professionals to have less than adequate office support, or to be so busy that returning phone calls is less of a priority than it should be. You should not take it personally or assume that the professional is incompetent if you have to work hard to get appointments made or calls returned. I have had several parents recently tell me how frustrated they were waiting for a phone call back from either the doctor or the psychotherapist about an appointment. In one case the parents anxiously waited three weeks to hear back from the physician's office, which had recently experienced a big turnover in office staff. In the meantime, the parents had lost valuable time and had begun to think that they should see another physician, even though this physician was reputed to be the best in the area. I advised these parents to be proactive and to keep calling the physician's office until they had an appointment for their daughter.

It is a plus if one of the members of your child's treatment team is willing to take on some of the tasks of case manager or to advise you how best to do these things. This is particularly important if you have been referred to a team of professionals who each have independent offices, as is often the case in smaller cities and in more rural areas. I have seen parents struggling to deal with three or four different offices to get all their child's appointments booked, not to mention haggling with their insurance company, the long commutes sometimes involved in getting to the various professionals' offices, and the missed days of school and work that result. Good coordination can minimize these inconveniences, but not make them disappear. Remember that a serious eating disorder demands serious treatment and a serious commitment on the part of your family.

## Psychotherapy: What Types Are Available, and How They Can Help

Rahel, a patient of mine whose parents hail from Bombay and run a popular restaurant, is a good student. She is quick to understand the nutritional consequences of her eating disorder, but does not make real progress until she is able to connect her eating problems with her family history, her childhood, and some key events in her life. Gradually, she successfully resolves these issues with the help of a knowledgeable counselor, and is able to shed her eating disorder.

As Rahel's story illustrates, psychotherapy can sometimes be the key to unlocking the mix of motivations, defense mechanisms, and unconscious fears and desires that fuel an eating disorder, thereby paving the way for a nutrition counselor to put in place healthier eating patterns. Rahel's story is typical of some anorexics who seem compliant and able to understand the seriousness of their situation, yet are unable to change their food behaviors until they start working with a psychotherapist. The psychotherapist is able to help them uncover underlying causes of their resistance to getting well or to understand the larger meaning of their anorexia. I often tell resistant patients that a psychotherapist is like having a "paid best friend" except that you don't have to spend time on their "stuff." Like a best friend, psychotherapists give support, guidance, feedback, but with a more specific agenda.

Psychotherapy focuses on the patient's motivation, emotional needs, feelings, and beliefs. The psychotherapist, who helps the patient focus on the future as well as understanding the past, may alternately play the role of teacher, guide, or coach. A good psychotherapist should help your child understand there are good reasons for her eating-disordered behaviors and feelings but that there are more productive ways of handling food and emotions. A good psychotherapist will also help your child feel accepted, understood, and responded to and will help your child identify her needs and what kind of person she is.

The psychotherapist's goal is to help the patient develop alternate coping strategies to deal with underlying emotional issues just as the nutritionist will teach her more effective food strategies. The psychotherapist helps the patient understand how low self-esteem and societal pressures contribute to her eating problems while helping her develop a new definition of self that does not focus primarily on weight, size, and shape.

Within the research community, there is still debate over which form of psychological treatment is most effective. Here we will include a brief overview of the various types of treatments that are used for treating eating disorders. We should stress, however, that most psychotherapists do not proclaim to practice a specific form of therapy. Practitioners who are most conversant with the newest ideas in psychotherapy often incorporate aspects of the latest therapies into their unique approach, mixing and matching them to suit each individual patient.

The purpose of the following descriptions is to give you a rudimentary understanding of the theoretical underpinnings of these approaches and to enable you to have an informed discussion with prospective candidates.

### Interpersonal Psychotherapy

Interpersonal psychotherapy (IPT) is a form of short-term psychotherapy that shifts the focus from the eating disorder itself to the interpersonal problems that accompany the disorder. The IPT practitioner helps patients identify and modify any interpersonal problems they are currently grappling with, such as relationships with family and peers, as well as significant life events or conflicts that are creating stress and helping to maintain an eating disorder, or precipitate bulimic episodes.

### Psychodynamic Therapy

Psychodynamic therapy is the most prevalent counseling approach in the United States. The psychotherapist strives to understand the patient's struggles, stresses, emotional status, coping skills, interpersonal conflicts, and self-esteem issues while teaching him the value of self-acceptance and helping him develop a more realistic approach to eating disorder–related and other problems, and life in general. Psychodynamic therapy gives your child a chance to share her experiences, feelings, and fears without fear of recrimination.

### Family Treatment

There is some debate within the professional community about whether standard family therapy, which is focused on improving family dynamics, is of any help in the treatment of eating disorders.

Some professionals believe that if family therapy is not focused first and foremost on resolving the child's disorder, it can distract or, even worse, overwhelm your child by stirring up extraneous issues and emotions.

We tend to agree. Although family therapy can be effective for helping families improve communication, problem solving, as well as any difficulties your family may have dealing with problems such as divorce, separation, death, or changes in economic status, we must stress that we do *not* believe these other issues should be the focus of therapy when one member is suffering from an eating disorder. Once the eating disorder is resolved, you as parents may want to revisit the idea of whether your family would benefit from family therapy.

### The Maudsley Method

One form of family-based therapy that takes a child-focused approach, and which has been shown to be effective for anorexic patients up to age nineteen is the Maudsley method. (See chapter 4, p. 64, for a description of the Maudsley method.) Therapists in the Maudsley tradition have proven that if treatment is focused primarily on helping the patient recover from her eating disorder it can be very successful.

The advent of this effective treatment for adolescent anorexics is a significant development, since compared to bulimia and binge eating, the advances in the use of psychotherapy to treat anorexia have been more modest.

While classic Maudsley programs have not been available outside of a few U.S. research institutions or Britain, this will likely change with the 2001 publication of the first Maudsley treatment manual. Whether or not you have access to a professional familiar with the Maudsley method, however, you should look for professionals who share some of the Maudsley group's highly effective methods, such as avoidance of parent blaming, a determined approach to treatment, and encouraging parents to work as a team to take control of their child's eating and weight gain.

## Group Treatment

In many communities, group therapy is not available for the simple reason that it is difficult to get a group of busy adolescents together at the same time and place. If a professional-led group is available and your child is interested, it may be helpful. For years, I have co-led such a group for Dartmouth College students and have seen students, particularly those who suffer from bulimia or binge eating, clearly benefit from the support and input they receive. I do not, however, recommend support groups led by nonprofessionals, because poor information as well as good information can be passed on. Group treatment alone is usually not sufficient to turn around an eating disorder. If it is combined with other forms of treatment, however, it can help improve motivation for recovery.

In some communities support groups are available for parents, which may or may not be helpful, depending on the focus of the group. Support groups that have become gripe sessions about different professionals or forums for vocal members to voice their despair about the chances of their child recovering, for example, are more negative than positive. Unhelpful groups such as these can leave you feeling more discouraged and overwhelmed. If on the other hand the group helps you feel hopeful and provides you with strategies for dealing with your child's problems, then it can be a breath of fresh air.

Self-help groups such as 12-step programs may be helpful to some patients but vary in quality, and I do not recommend them as your sole form of treatment. Some 12-step groups espouse restrictive food plans such as one that, for example, excludes any food products containing flour or sugar. I do not recommend such approaches to my patients in part because following them may backfire, creating more food obsessions and increasing the tendency to binge.

## Cognitive Behavioral Therapy (CBT)

Among the various forms of counseling used to treat eating disorders, cognitive behavioral therapy (CBT) for bulimia and binge eating has been the most studied. Because many CBT techniques have become part of the standard repertoire of both psychotherapists and nutritionists treating eating disorders, we will devote some space to it here.

CBT is based on the idea that we can change negative behaviors by changing our way of thinking. In the 1950s, cognitive-behavioral approaches were developed to treat depression and other psychological problems. The theory was that negative behaviors grow out of and are influenced by negative thought processes. By examining those thought processes and correcting them, or changing the cognitive errors that give rise to those thoughts, one can alter or eradicate negative behaviors.

In the 1980s Christopher Fairburn of Oxford and colleagues developed a CBT treatment for bulimia. A bulimic patient, for example, is taught to recognize problematic thoughts such as "I am fat," or "I feel fat," and then learn how to change her thoughts to more reasonable ones such as "I can't be fat since others see me as thin," or "as being normal weight," or whatever the truth may be.

CBT has proved to be successful in treating motivated bulimic and binge-eating patients. Patients who are ambivalent usually end up being frustrated by how much work CBT requires: self-monitoring (meaning keeping detailed written records) of everything the patient eats, binge-ing and purging behaviors and associated thoughts and feelings as well as attempts at problem solving. This makes CBT more effective for a moti-vated teen, and not appropriate for children younger than twelve or thir-teen because they may not have the cognitive development necessary to make good use of CBT techniques. CBT is most effective for those who have retained some control over their bingeing. Classic CBT has proven too demanding for the usually ambivalent anorexic patient, although researchers are at work modifying CBT to make it more palatable and more effective for the anorexic patient.

As we discuss in "Nutrition Counseling," p. 262, the most up-to-date forms of nutrition counseling for eating disorders are closely modeled on CBT. Like nutrition counseling, CBT includes education components; for example, teaching patients how dieting leads to bingeing, what a normal weight range is, the medical consequences of binge eating and purging, the prescription of a Food Plan, weight monitoring, and written self-observation. These written self-observations of food intake and problematic thoughts, often called food records or food diaries, are kept daily. It is not unusual for eclectically oriented psychotherapists to employ some CBT techniques, including the suggestion to their patients to keep food diaries.

## Experience and Competence Trumps Techniques and Methods

Ideally the professionals on your team will be familiar with the various forms of psychotherapy we have described. Just because they are not, how-ever, is not good enough reason to reject them. Remember, a variety of psychological approaches have proven to be effective in treating eating dis-orders. More important than techniques or methods is that your child develops a rapport and a working relationship with an experienced, com-petent psychotherapist. This is particularly important if your child is ambivalent about therapy, since without some rapport, it will be difficult for your child to overcome that ambivalence and make progress. One study found that "feeling understood" and "feeling ready for treatment" were key precursors for recovery. In the end, what matters most is that you and your child feel confident the professional can be of help.

There is a common perception among patients that they should feel "comfortable" with any psychotherapist, that they should "click" with him or her. Feeling comfortable is not the best test of whether you have chosen the right professional. You or your child may need on occasion to be challenged, or even confronted. Although this is not always true, of course, you may do your child a disservice if you choose a professional based only on your comfort level with that person. You want to choose professionals who can help you take on the powerful force that is disrupting your child's life, the eating disorder.

## Nutrition Counseling

Nutrition counseling, or the treatment that your child receives from most registered dietitians or nutritionists, as we have noted, does exactly what we have outlined in this book: it treats eating disorders by focusing on normalizing food habits, expanding food choices, abolishing the practice of "forbidden" foods, and changing attitudes and beliefs and correcting misinformation about eating, food, and body size and shape. You want to avoid choosing a nutritionist whose approach relies only on standard nutrition educational tools such as the Food Pyramid and its emphasis on low-fat food choices.

I teach my patients that their sensations of appetite, hunger, and fullness are disturbed by their eating disorder, and that in the short run they will need to rely on the Food Plan to determine when they should start or stop eating. I explain to them how metabolism and weight management work. I help my patients develop a Food Plan that includes the most effective number of meals and snacks for their body, help them learn to keep in check out-of-control eating, and I help patients overcome their fears about certain foods and nutrients, such as fat. Sometimes I might instruct patients to keep records of food intake and eating-disordered behaviors in diaries that are reviewed in nutrition sessions. I may monitor body weight, which is essential to treatment for anorexia. By showing the bulimic or binge eater that her weight is stable, weight monitoring can help her feel confident enough to improve food intake.

Depending on your child's issues, the nutritionist may weigh patients "blindly"(standing on the scale backward) so the patient is informed of trends in weight but not the specifics. I find that this helps patients learn not to obsess about exact numbers. Weights may be taken in hospital gowns or in regular clothes. Usually if the patient is severly underweight weights are taken in gowns so that small weight changes can be detected.

Nutrition counseling usually involves the collaborative development of "homework" assignments that are reviewed and revised in sessions. Most of the homework assignments I give are focused on helping the patient improve her food intake. A common early assignment, for example, is to tell the patient to make sure she has a serving of protein at lunch and dinner. Our later nutrition sessions focus on reviewing previous homework and developing new assignments that allow the patient to deal with problems and practice new techniques during the next interval between sessions. I also explore the patient's thoughts and feelings about food and body-image issues. My goal as a nutrition counselor is to help my patients reduce dieting, which in turn directly reduces binge eating and purging. Underweight patients need encouragement, support, and practical suggestions to be able to eat enough to gain weight.

A typical course of nutrition counseling covers 8 to 15 sessions. As the patient makes progress, increasing intervals between sessions gives her a chance to practice what she is learning. Some children will need substantially more treatment than this. Parents should be ready to return to nutrition treatment any time there are signs of relapse in food behaviors.

The most up-to-date form of nutrition counseling, in short, draws on many of the principles of CBT. If your child is working with a skilled CBT therapist, she may not need a nutritionist. Conversely if your child is working with a nutritionist she may benefit more from working with a more psychodynamic-focused therapist than a heavily CBT-influenced therapist.

A good nutritionist will likely spend at least a few minutes of each individual session with you, the parents, unless your child is an independent teen or you have all agreed that this is not necessary. This time usually includes your child as well, and provides an opportunity for the nutrition counselor to summarize the treatment plan, to address your concerns, and to outline how you should be involved. You should also be able to reach the nutrition counselor for advice between sessions. Nutritionists working with teens will want to meet occasionally with parents, but most sessions will be devoted to working alone with the adolescent.

## Medications: A New Era in Eating-Disorder Treatment

For about ten years now, treating eating disorders with medications, most often the class of antidepressants known as SSRIs (serotonin selective reuptake inhibitors; examples include Prozac, Effexor, Celexa, Paxil, Lovox, and Zoloft) has been one of the most promising developments in the field.

Although scientists still debate why the SSRIs are effective in treating eating disorders, they suspect that anorexia and bulimia are caused in part by some disturbances of neurotransmitter function. Experts think in fact that the under- or overeating, obsessive perfectionism, and depression that are often part of the eating-disorder picture might have to do with unstable brain concentrations of important neurotransmitters.

The fact that there are now a variety of SSRIs for doctors to choose from (even more variations are likely to become available in the future) gives your doctor the ability to select a medicine that is most closely suited to your child, or to try a different one if your child does not respond to a particular SSRI, or has bothersome side effects. One reason SSRIs are used so widely is that for most people, side effects are nonexistent at best and at worst mild, transient, and infrequent and are usually only an issue during the first week or so of use.

We feel that it is relevant to discuss these medications here because though it is important to remember that medications alone are rarely enough treatment to turn around an eating disorder, clinical studies have shown them to be quite effective in reducing the bingeing, anxiety, and obsessing that is so characteristic of eating disorders. Still, some clinicians are hesitant to prescribe medications for younger patients, or for anorexic patients who have not gained weight. These clinicians assert that more studies need to be published before efficacy is conclusively proven. My clinical experience and that of my colleagues, however, indicates that younger patients and underweight anorexics who have been prescribed medication seem to make better progress than those who have not.

Many patients struggle with depression, anxiety, and compulsive behaviors, particularly around food and exercise. Antidepressants often are helpful in dealing with these issues, allowing the patient to direct her energy toward overcoming her eating disorder.

The patient who is most likely to be helped by medication is a normal-weight bulimic like Tenley, who took Prozac for a year and found that it reduced her urges to vomit and binge eat. When Tenley's parents first brought her to treatment she was in great distress about her frequent bingeing and purging episodes, which seemed beyond her best attempts at control. After trying several SSRIs on the recommendation of her pediatrician, she found that on Zoloft she felt more emotionally stable and hopeful and better able to control her bingeing and purging. As a result, she was able to make more progress with her psychotherapist and nutritionist.

Besides antidepressants, your eating-disordered child may be prescribed anxiety or sleeping medication if she is having trouble in those areas.

### How Can You Tell If Your Child's Medication Is Working?

Doctors must take a trial-and-error approach to prescribing and selecting the best dose of SSRI. Usually one of the SSRIs are selected and prescribed at a relatively low dose to check for any negative reactions. SSRIs are usually most effective at relatively high doses compared to doses used to treat depression. If your child seems to have no relief from intrusive thoughts or negative feelings about herself within a month's time, her doctor should be consulted. It may be time to up the dose or try another medication.

Daisy tells me that she hates the idea that she is taking medication; she wants to conquer her eating disorder without it. "I thought I would be 'prouder' of getting over my eating disorder if I did it without medication," she tells me. "I haven't even told my cousin or my best friend that I'm taking Prozac because kids my age only think that really weird people take antidepressants."

Daisy and other teens have found my "insulin" analogy helpful. I ask if they think less of diabetics for taking insulin because their bodies do not produce enough insulin. "Of course not!" Daisy exclaimed. "Well, antidepressants are similar," I explain. "Antidepressants are helpful to people who do not produce enough neurotransmitters. They help your brain keep from reabsorbing neurotransmitters too fast."

Relapse is common when patients stop taking SSRIs, which is why medical researchers recommend that patients continue taking their medication for some time (4 to 24 months) after their eating-disordered symptoms have abated.

## When Inpatient or Residential Care Should Be Considered

If your child is no longer cooperating with a treatment team, you should consider either changing treatment teams or finding a more protective environment such as a residential or hospital program. (If you find yourself switching teams more than several times you may want to reassess your own standards; are they too unrealistic?) Hospitalization can help stabilize your child medically if she is severely underweight or if her purging has become uncontrollable. Your child's low weight, especially if it is coupled with purging, is predictive of an eating disorder that may require more intensive treatment.

Short-term hospitalization can also give your family a break from the intense stress of living with and trying to help a severely eating-disordered child, and help jump-start more appropriate eating. Keep in mind that once your child is released from the hospital, continued outpatient care is crucial to support the improvements made in the hospital.

Following is a checklist to help you determine whether or not your child needs more intensive treatment than she is now getting. If you check any of the problems listed and your child is unwilling to try to solve them outside a hospital or treatment facility setting, you should recruit your doctor or the professionals on your team to help you find either a short-term hospital stay to stabilize your child's condition or a longer-term residential program.

## Behaviors and Attitudes That Indicate More Intensive Treatment

❑ If your child is not progressing with outpatient treatment.

❑ If there is continued weight loss, especially if accompanied by fainting and/or a significant decrease in energy. Since relentless weight loss is so dangerous, especially in younger patients, hospitalization should be considered if outpatient care has not been able to arrest it.

❑ If your child is extremely low weight. This can be dangerous and is associated with sudden death in eating-disordered patients. Your doctor can help you know when your child's low weight indicates the need for more intensive treatment.

❑ If your anorexic child needs to have her activity curtailed in order to gain necessary weight, and all other methods of doing so have failed.

❑ If your bulimic child needs to control her bingeing and purging, and all other methods of doing so have failed.

❑ If laboratory tests reveal dangerous medical findings. Your doctor will advise you if your child's malnutrition, vital signs, or electrolytes are reasons for hospitalization.

❑ If frequent hospitalizations are necessary to stabilize your child's weight or labs. For example, when the weight your child gains in the hospital or other behavioral improvements she achieves are quickly lost upon release.

❑ If your child has attempted suicide or exhibited an increase in self-harm, such as cutting. These behaviors are more likely in bulimic patients. Children who are engaging in these types of self-destructive behaviors should be in treatment with a psychotherapist, who can advise parents when a safer environment like a hospital or residential setting is necessary.

All of these behaviors should be taken very seriously, although parents should keep in mind that if the child is willing to cooperate, they can be handled by outpatient treatment.

### The Pros and Cons of Residential Treatment
Residential treatment usually provides experienced staff and a peer (other patients) group that is understanding. Your child may also feel that it is safer and less stressful to be in a residential treatment facility than in a hospital or at home.

The drawbacks to hospitalization and residential treatments are that they are costly and they disrupt family life and school. Some experts wonder if institutional treatment increases the patient's sense of ineffectiveness, and sends the patient and the family the message that an eating disorder is something that requires "professionals to do something to the patient" rather than professionals supporting the patient and her family in their efforts to change.

Since it is normal to feel fear and hesitation when confronted with the choice of putting a child in a hospital or residential program, it helps to talk to other parents who have chosen such treatment for their children, or to professionals who have had patients enrolled in similar programs. Most programs and local professionals can put you in touch with other parents who are willing to talk to you about their experiences. I advise parents to approach every stage of treatment for their child's eating disorder with the philosophy that the eating disorder can be treated and overcome. The trick is to provide enough treatment so that your child can master her eating problems. When it becomes clear hospital or residential treatment is necessary for her to be successful, I suggest you approach this decision the same way you have made every decision necessary to ensure her recovery each step of the way: by providing whatever is necessary to beat the disorder.

If your child has an effective outpatient team, then a short visit to a more structured program may serve as a "shot in the arm" that moves treatment forward. It can help the resistant patient see that parents and treatment team are serious about stepping up treatment if necessary. I have seen patients do very well in outpatient treatment after a few days in a hospital program because they know if they do not make progress they will be spending an extended time in an inpatient program.

In other cases, though, short stints of inpatient treatment have not brought about observable progress. Instead, the child seems to take two steps backward for every step forward. In this situation, making plans for a longer residential stay is usually more effective. Once he is enrolled in such a program, you need to rely on the expertise of the residential treatment providers to advise you what the optimal length of stay for him is.

### What to Look For in an Inpatient or Residential Care Facility

Whatever facility you choose for your child, it should be a facility where you feel respected, are kept informed, and are not blamed for her eating disorder. Staff and administrators at the facility should give you hope about the future and your child's recovery, and give you advice on how you can be helpful to her.

To find the best facility for your child, ask local respected practitioners which facilities they recommend and whether they can put you in touch with families who have used these facilities. You should talk to these families about their experiences, and pay attention to any warnings they may have to offer about the facility. I also suggest you visit potential institutions if you can manage it. Since you will want to be as involved as possible with her treatment, you will want to choose the closest and best facility. Most residential programs encourage family participation by providing group and counseling sessions for family members. In some parts of the country it may not be possible to find a quality local facility. Then placing your child in the best facility you can find is what you should do.

## In Summary

We have described in this chapter how sometimes, despite your best efforts to turn around your child's eating disorder, the disorder is simply too powerful and entrenched, she is too resistant to your attempts to help, or you have such difficulties communicating with her that you must look to professionals for help. For some of you, all of these may be true.

We have outlined the services that the various professionals available to you can provide, and described how a single professional or a team of professionals not only can be highly effective in difficult situations but can also enhance your own ability to help your child.

Whether your child's situation requires a short stint seeing a nutritionist or a psychotherapist, or a longer course of outpatient or inpatient treatment, remind yourself that turning around the disorder quickly is your number-one priority. Your job, simply put, is to provide whatever it takes to do that.

# 15

# In Closing

Nothing is as heartbreaking as being the parent of a child who is suffering, whether it is from a raging flu, a broken heart, or an eating disorder. Children, we believe, are meant to absorb the richness of life and radiate good health, not to suffer fainting spells, self-starvation, compulsions to binge or purge, or insecurities about their own bodies and self-worth.

To watch in frustration as your child picks at her dinner or rejects it outright, to wake up in the middle of the night seized by terror, wondering whether your child's heart will give out while she is sleeping, or whether the sounds you hear in the bathroom are those of your child forcing herself to purge—these are not feelings or experiences you ever anticipated when you became parents.

We hope that reading this book has first of all helped you to feel that you are not alone in your struggle. Next, we hope that it has helped you move beyond the stage of self-blame and recriminations ("What did we do wrong?") and to feel confident that you as parents can play a vital role in helping your child regain her former health and radiance.

During the fifteen years I have spent as a nutritionist helping children suffering from eating disorders and their parents, I have been privileged to work with hundreds of families, to witness the cycle of shock, frustration, despair, hope, and, ultimately, recovery, occur again and again. I have witnessed profound illness and the immense strain it places on the family, but also countless remarkable recoveries. Often, as we have noted, children and families emerge from their battle with an eating disorder stronger, a more cohesive unit, and with a better sense of who they are and what they want from life.

I have also repeatedly seen eating-disordered children, often the classic high-achieving, people-pleasing, perfectionistic students, attack their disorder just as they have attacked every other challenge in their life: with determination and a burning desire to emerge triumphant. The very qualities that have made them vulnerable to their disorder are those that enable them to recover.

I will never forget Lucy, a second-generation American whose doctor parents emigrated from Southeast Asia. On the fast track from preschool on, Lucy appeared to all observers to be an all-American success story. Though not as athletically gifted as she wished (one heartbreak was not making the cut for her high school soccer team), she resigned herself to serving as team manager and took up jogging.

Where Lucy excelled was in the classroom. No matter what the subject was, she almost always pulled down the top score. For Lucy's junior and senior years of high school, her parents enrolled her as a day student at the well-respected private boarding school in the next town. Lucy was not thrilled with this plan. She loved her life, her friends, her school. Yet she had to admit her parents' plan made sense; she dreamed of entering medical school some day, and a more competitive high school could increase her chances of getting into a good college and help make those plans a reality.

The decision was made one summer evening as the family sat on their front porch and discussed the pros and cons of this big step. The transition that fall, however, was harder than either Lucy or her parents had imagined. Lucy found it difficult to break into her new school's social network. It didn't help that she was a day student (Lucy had been adamant that she did not want to board at her new school) and the soccer team's manager position was already filled.

The first couple of months were also tough academically, as the courses at her new school were more rigorous. Before long, though, Lucy had caught up with her classmates and was once again consistently placing at the top of her class.

No longer feeling an integral part of her old group of friends, yet with no new friends to take their place, Lucy found herself somewhat at loose ends during the afternoons and on weekends.

In retrospect, it was hard for Lucy to point to any one factor that triggered her eating disorder. Was it having time on her hands or feeling lonely for the first time in her life? Was her effort to improve her appearance a response to her lack of social standing?

Although she still does not know the answers to these questions, she does know that her occasional jogs gradually became a major part of each day.

Before long, she was religiously counting fat grams and calories. With a sense of gratification, she charted her longer and longer runs and her decreasing weight. By spring, Lucy's overly busy parents became aware of her downward spiral when warm-weather tank tops and shorts revealed the nearly 15 pounds Lucy had lost.

Tempted to replay the decision to change schools, and to blame themselves for their lack of insight, her parents instead focused their energies on rising to the occasion and grappling with the disorder head-on.

It was an unusually warm spring day that found the family again gathered on their front porch. This time, Lucy's parents mapped out the strategies they would employ to get Lucy's eating and exercise problems under control. First on the list was an appointment with Lucy's doctor. There were the expected ups and downs, and Lucy did take a leave of absence from school that spring semester. She chose later to re-enroll in her old high school for her senior year. The next spring, in her valedictory speech for the graduating class, Lucy talked openly about her ordeal with anorexia, and its effect on her family. By the end of her speech, the audience was in tears. I heard later that away at college (a top private California university), Lucy wrote her senior thesis on the challenges of growing up female in modern-day America. I also heard she gave another valedictory speech, in which she again told her story. This one earned a standing ovation.

I recently heard that Lucy was graduating from medical school, once again at the head of her class. Whenever I hear about another of Lucy's accomplishments, I feel proud of her and what she has accomplished. No matter how many glittering achievements Lucy amasses, I have no doubt that her victory over anorexia will be among those that she cherishes most.

We leave you now with this final case history to remind you of two things: the incredible strength that lies within every child, no matter how sick she or he is, and of the power that lies within every parent, no matter how worried and helpless you feel.

We hope that you are now better educated about your role in your child's recovery, armed with practical strategies that can help your entire family achieve a more balanced attitude toward food, eating, exercise, and your bodies, and a sense of perspective about the ordeal that you are going through, or have gone through.

There are a few points that we hope will stay with you, whether your child grows into adulthood eating-disorder free or whether eating and food issues remain a challenge that requires an occasional return to the Food and Exercise Plans. The first is that the best gift you can give a child struggling with eating issues is the ability to eat in an organized, carefree fashion, to give up diets, and to be educated enough to make sound, confident food choices.

Remember, recovery from an eating disorder, whether it is anorexia, bulimia, or binge-eating disorder, is predicated on accepting and practicing normal eating and exercise. The Food and Exercise Plans provide your child with a blueprint for regular eating and exercise. Ideally, once your child has internalized the structure and organization of these plans, she will be ready to discard these "training wheels," and embark upon a life where normal eating and exercise are second nature to her.

We also remind you that the sooner you address and turn around an eating problem, the easier it is. Most of the physical symptoms and consequences of a serious eating disorder are reversible upon weight gain, but there are two significant exceptions to this rule: bone mass changes and brain abnormalities. Anorexia-related bone loss can occur in as little as six months, and brain changes have been detected within an even shorter span of time. While you can expect some recovery in these areas, it now appears that full recovery is unlikely.

Yet another of the central themes in our book is the influential roles that you as parents and our culture at large play in the development of your child's self-esteem and body image. We have talked about the pervasive, negative influence of a culture that promotes an unrealistic ideal of thinness, what some have called "the Western toxin effect." We hope that you will take to heart the strategies we offer that will help you combat those effects.

We have offered suggestions on how to transform any negative messages you may be sending your child about food, body shape, and size into positive messages. If you are comfortable and accepting of your own bodies and adopt food and exercise behaviors that are relaxed and healthy, you will have gone a long way in protecting your child from an eating disorder.

We hope this book has left you with a vivid sense of the complexity of the modern-day eating disorder, the impossibility of boiling it down to a simple cause-and-effect equation. Accusations and self-recriminations crumble under the weight of the overwhelming evidence that tells us that eating disorders are multifactorial: no one thing, circumstance, action, or parenting behavior alone can be held responsible for your child's predicament. Equally clear should be that there is no "magic bullet" cure, no one medicine, therapy, infusion, or potion that is going to solve your child's disorder. Recovery requires the effort of the entire family, hard work, patience, and perseverance. We hope that this book has played a role in giving you the tools, as well as the hope and the faith, necessary to accomplish your goal.

# Diagnosing Eating Disorders

Professionals diagnose eating disorders using the guidelines published in the American Psychiatric Association's (APA) *Diagnostic and Statistical Manual of Mental Disorders,* 4th Edition (Washington, D.C.: American Psychiatric Association, 1994). This manual is known as the *DSM-IV.* Its clear descriptions of the various eating disorders, which we have included below, are helpful to any reader who wants to grasp the full range of eating-disordered behaviors and attitudes.

Before a diagnosis of anorexia or bulimia can be made all the criteria outlined must be present. When a person has serious eating problems but does not exhibit all the criteria of either anorexia or bulimia, then eating disorder not otherwise specified (EDNOS) is the standard diagnosis. The APA's diagnostic criteria for binge-eating disorder are still provisional, which means that binge-eating disorder is included in the latest *DSM,* published in 1994, as a *proposed* classification that will require further study before it is considered a full-fledged eating disorder. Despite its provisional status, the diagnosis of binge-eating disorder is used by most professionals.

**Diagnostic Criteria for Anorexia Nervosa**

A. Refusal to maintain body weight at or above a minimally normal weight for age and height (e.g., weight loss leading to maintenance of body weight less than 85% of that expected; or failure to make expected weight gain during a period of growth, leading to body weight less than 85% of that expected). [See Appendix B for growth charts that will help you determine "normal" weights for your child's age. If your child has lost weight, the growth charts will help you determine what percentage of body weight has been lost.]

B. Intense fear of gaining weight or becoming fat, even though underweight.

C. Disturbance in the way in which one's body weight or shape is experienced, undue influence of body weight or shape on self-evaluation, or denial of the seriousness of the current low body weight.

D. In postmenarcheal females, amenorrhea, i.e., absence of at least three consecutive menstrual cycles. (A woman [or a girl] is considered to have amenorrhea if her periods occur only following hormone, e.g., estrogen administration.)

## Diagnostic Criteria for Bulimia Nervosa

A. Recurrent episodes of binge eating. An episode of binge eating is characterized by both of the following:

 (1) eating, in a discrete period of time (e.g., within any 2-hour period), an amount of food that is definitely larger than most people would eat during a similar period of time and under similar circumstances

 (2) a sense of lack of control over eating during the episode (e.g., a feeling that one cannot stop eating or control what or how much one is eating)

B. Recurrent inappropriate compensatory behavior in order to prevent weight gain, such as self-induced vomiting; misuse of laxatives, diuretics, enemas, or other medications; fasting; or excessive exercise.

C. The binge eating and inappropriate compensatory behaviors both occur, on average, at least twice a week for 3 months.

D. Self-evaluation is unduly influenced by body shape and weight.

E. The disturbance does not occur exclusively during episodes of Anorexia Nervosa.

## Diagnostic Criteria for Binge-Eating Disorder

A. Recurrent episodes of binge eating. An episode of binge eating is characterized by both of the following:

 (1) eating, in a discrete period of time (e.g., within any 2-hour period), an amount of food that is definitely larger than most people would eat in a similar period of time under similar circumstances

 (2) a sense of lack of control over eating during the episode (e.g., a feeling that one cannot stop eating or control what or how much one is eating)

B. The binge-eating episodes are associated with three (or more) of the following:
   (1) eating much more rapidly than normal
   (2) eating until feeling uncomfortably full
   (3) eating large amounts of food when not feeling physically hungry
   (4) eating alone because of being embarrassed by how much one is eating
   (5) feeling disgusted with oneself, depressed, or very guilty after overeating
C. Marked distress regarding binge eating is present.
D. The binge eating occurs, on average, at least 2 days a week for 6 months.
E. The binge eating is not associated with the regular use of inappropriate compensatory behaviors (e.g., purging, fasting, excessive exercise) and does not occur exclusively during the course of Anorexia Nervosa or Bulimia Nervosa.

**Eating Disorder Not Otherwise Specified (EDNOS)**
The Eating Disorder Not Otherwise Specified category is for disorders of eating that do not meet the criteria for any specific Eating Disorder. Examples include
   1. For females, all of the criteria for Anorexia Nervosa are met except that the individual has regular menses.
   2. All of the criteria for Anorexia Nervosa are met except that, despite significant weight loss, the individual's current weight is in the normal range.
   3. All of the criteria for Bulimia Nervosa are met except that the binge eating and inappropriate compensatory mechanisms occur at a frequency of less than twice a week or for a duration of less than 3 months.
   4. The regular use of inappropriate compensatory behavior by an individual of normal body weight after eating small amounts of food (e.g., self-induced vomiting after the consumption of two cookies).
   5. Repeatedly chewing and spitting out, but not swallowing, large amounts of food.
   6. Binge-eating disorder: recurrent episodes of binge eating in the absence of the regular use of inappropriate compensatory behaviors characteristic of Bulimia Nervosa.

## Body Weight Assessments

**Body Mass Index**

Body Mass Index (BMI) is the best tool available to professionals for assessing degrees of underweight and overweight. Yet because it does not take into account the individual's natural rate of growth, body build, or genetic predisposition, it is a less than perfect method of assessment.

It is best to have your doctor or nutritionist weigh, measure, and calculate a BMI for your child because he or she is more likely to be able to take the measurements accurately and will know what factors to take into account to determine if your child's weight is healthy. Whoever measures your child should do it sensitively. Many professionals believe it is best if the child is kept from knowing her weight, particularly if she is at risk for, or has an eating disorder.

If you choose to weigh your child, have her dress in lightweight clothes (e.g., light pajamas) and use a reliable, relatively new scale. Have your child stand on the scale backward so she cannot see her weight. If you want to compare weight measurements, make sure weights are taken on the same scale and at approximately the same time of day, since body weight naturally fluctuates over the course of a day.

To measure height, have your child take off her shoes and stand against a wall. Heels, buttocks, shoulders, and back of head should touch the wall. The child should be told to put her heels together, to "stand tall," and to look straight ahead. Place a ruler or book on top of the child's head, then use a yardstick or nonstretchable measuring tape to measure up from the floor to the ruler.

With accurate height and weight measurements, you can mathematically calculate BMI as we describe below or estimate BMI using the charts on pp. 279 and 280. If you prefer, you can use the BMI calculator found on the Centers for Disease Control (CDC) Web site (http://www.cdc.gov/nccdphp/dnpa/bmi/calc-bmi.htm).

To calculate BMI, use this formula: BMI = weight/height$^2$ × 703. We have used the conversion factor (703) recommended by the CDC in the BMI calculation. Some professionals use a slightly different conversion factor; the resulting differences are not clinically significant. An easy way to do this calculation is as follows: BMI = weight (in pounds) divided by height (in inches), divided by height (in inches) × 705. The decimal point should be fully carried out. Height is entered into the BMI formula in inches:

$$3 \text{ feet} = 36 \text{ inches}$$
$$4 \text{ feet} = 48 \text{ inches}$$
$$5 \text{ feet} = 60 \text{ inches}$$
$$6 \text{ feet} = 72 \text{ inches}$$

Fractions of inches and pounds are entered into the BMI formula as decimal values:

⅛ inch or ⅛ pound = .125          ⅝ inch or ⅝ pound = .625
¼ inch or ¼ pound = .25           ¾ inch or ¾ pound = .75
⅜ inch or ⅜ pound = .375          ⅞ inch or ⅞ pound = .875
½ inch or ½ pound = .5

For example: a person who weighs 99.5 pounds and is 5'2¼" tall has a BMI of 18.05, or rounded to the nearest whole number, 18.

The calculation looks like this:

Pounds/Height = x
99.5/62.25 = 1.5983935743

x/Height = y
1.5983935743/62.25 = .02567700521

y × 703 = BMI
.02567700521 × 703 = 18.05 ÷ BMI = 18

Your doctor is likely to do the BMI calculation in metrics. The metric calculation looks like this: BMI = weight (in kilograms)/height (in meters) squared.

**BMI for weights (in pounds) and heights 3' through 4' 9"**

| BMI | 13 | 14 | 15 | 16 | 17 | 18 | 19 | 20 | 21 | 22 | 23 | 24 | 25 | 30 |
|---|---|---|---|---|---|---|---|---|---|---|---|---|---|---|
| 3' | 24 | 26 | 28 | 29 | 31 | 33 | 35 | 37 | 39 | 40 | 42 | 44 | 46 | 55 |
| 3'1" | 25 | 27 | 29 | 31 | 33 | 35 | 37 | 39 | 41 | 43 | 45 | 47 | 49 | 58 |
| 3'2" | 27 | 29 | 31 | 33 | 35 | 37 | 39 | 41 | 43 | 45 | 47 | 49 | 51 | 61 |
| 3'3" | 28 | 30 | 32 | 35 | 37 | 39 | 41 | 43 | 45 | 47 | 50 | 52 | 54 | 65 |
| 3'4" | 30 | 32 | 34 | 36 | 39 | 41 | 43 | 45 | 48 | 50 | 52 | 55 | 57 | 68 |
| 3'5" | 31 | 33 | 36 | 38 | 41 | 43 | 45 | 48 | 50 | 52 | 55 | 57 | 60 | 72 |
| 3'6" | 33 | 35 | 38 | 40 | 43 | 45 | 48 | 50 | 53 | 55 | 58 | 60 | 63 | 75 |
| 3'7" | 34 | 37 | 39 | 42 | 45 | 47 | 50 | 52 | 55 | 58 | 60 | 63 | 66 | 79 |
| 3'8" | 36 | 38 | 41 | 44 | 47 | 49 | 52 | 55 | 58 | 60 | 63 | 66 | 69 | 82 |
| 3'9" | 37 | 40 | 43 | 46 | 49 | 52 | 55 | 57 | 60 | 63 | 66 | 69 | 72 | 86 |
| 3'10" | 39 | 42 | 45 | 48 | 51 | 54 | 57 | 60 | 63 | 66 | 69 | 72 | 75 | 90 |
| 3'11" | 41 | 44 | 47 | 50 | 53 | 56 | 60 | 63 | 66 | 69 | 72 | 75 | 78 | 94 |
| 4'0" | 43 | 46 | 49 | 52 | 56 | 59 | 62 | 65 | 69 | 72 | 75 | 78 | 82 | 98 |
| 4'1" | 44 | 48 | 51 | 55 | 58 | 61 | 65 | 68 | 72 | 75 | 78 | 82 | 85 | 102 |
| 4'2" | 46 | 50 | 53 | 57 | 60 | 64 | 67 | 71 | 75 | 78 | 82 | 85 | 89 | 106 |
| 4'3" | 48 | 52 | 55 | 59 | 63 | 66 | 70 | 74 | 78 | 81 | 85 | 89 | 92 | 111 |
| 4'4" | 50 | 54 | 58 | 61 | 65 | 69 | 73 | 77 | 81 | 84 | 88 | 92 | 96 | 115 |
| 4'5" | 52 | 56 | 60 | 64 | 68 | 72 | 76 | 80 | 84 | 88 | 92 | 96 | 100 | 120 |
| 4'6" | 54 | 58 | 62 | 66 | 70 | 75 | 79 | 83 | 87 | 91 | 95 | 99 | 103 | 124 |
| 4'7" | 56 | 60 | 64 | 69 | 73 | 77 | 82 | 86 | 90 | 94 | 99 | 103 | 107 | 129 |
| 4'8" | 58 | 62 | 67 | 71 | 76 | 80 | 85 | 89 | 93 | 98 | 102 | 107 | 111 | 134 |
| 4'9" | 60 | 65 | 69 | 74 | 78 | 83 | 88 | 92 | 97 | 101 | 106 | 111 | 115 | 138 |

**BMI for weights (in pounds) and heights 4'10" through 6'4"**

| BMI | 13 | 14 | 15 | 16 | 17 | 18 | 19 | 20 | 21 | 22 | 23 | 24 | 25 | 30 |
|-----|----|----|----|----|----|----|----|----|----|----|----|----|----|----|
| 4'10" | 62 | 67 | 72 | 76 | 81 | 86 | 91 | 96 | 100 | 105 | 110 | 115 | 119 | 143 |
| 4'11" | 64 | 69 | 74 | 79 | 84 | 89 | 94 | 99 | 104 | 109 | 114 | 119 | 124 | 148 |
| 5'0" | 66 | 72 | 77 | 82 | 87 | 92 | 97 | 102 | 107 | 112 | 118 | 123 | 128 | 153 |
| 5'1" | 69 | 74 | 79 | 85 | 90 | 95 | 100 | 106 | 111 | 116 | 122 | 127 | 132 | 158 |
| 5'2" | 71 | 76 | 82 | 87 | 93 | 98 | 104 | 109 | 115 | 120 | 126 | 131 | 136 | 164 |
| 5'3" | 73 | 79 | 85 | 90 | 96 | 101 | 107 | 113 | 118 | 124 | 130 | 135 | 141 | 169 |
| 5'4" | 76 | 81 | 87 | 93 | 99 | 105 | 110 | 118 | 122 | 128 | 134 | 140 | 145 | 174 |
| 5'5" | 78 | 84 | 90 | 96 | 102 | 108 | 114 | 120 | 126 | 132 | 138 | 144 | 150 | 180 |
| 5'6" | 80 | 87 | 93 | 99 | 105 | 111 | 118 | 124 | 130 | 136 | 142 | 148 | 155 | 186 |
| 5'7" | 83 | 89 | 96 | 102 | 108 | 115 | 121 | 128 | 134 | 140 | 146 | 153 | 159 | 191 |
| 5'8" | 85 | 92 | 98 | 105 | 112 | 118 | 125 | 131 | 138 | 144 | 151 | 158 | 164 | 197 |
| 5'9" | 88 | 95 | 101 | 108 | 115 | 122 | 128 | 135 | 142 | 149 | 156 | 162 | 169 | 203 |
| 5'10" | 90 | 97 | 104 | 111 | 118 | 125 | 132 | 139 | 146 | 153 | 160 | 167 | 174 | 209 |
| 5'11" | 93 | 100 | 107 | 114 | 122 | 129 | 136 | 143 | 150 | 158 | 165 | 172 | 179 | 215 |
| 6'0" | 96 | 103 | 110 | 118 | 125 | 132 | 140 | 147 | 154 | 162 | 169 | 177 | 184 | 221 |
| 6'1" | 98 | 106 | 114 | 121 | 129 | 136 | 144 | 151 | 159 | 166 | 174 | 182 | 189 | 227 |
| 6'2" | 101 | 109 | 117 | 124 | 132 | 140 | 148 | 156 | 163 | 171 | 179 | 186 | 194 | 234 |
| 6'3" | 104 | 112 | 120 | 128 | 136 | 144 | 152 | 160 | 168 | 176 | 184 | 192 | 200 | 240 |
| 6'4" | 107 | 115 | 123 | 131 | 140 | 148 | 156 | 164 | 172 | 180 | 189 | 197 | 205 | 246 |

# Recommended BMI Cutoff Values for Adolescents

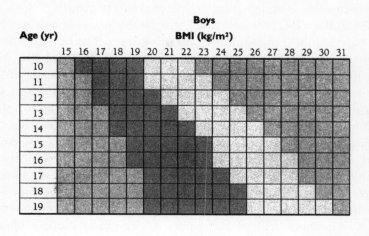

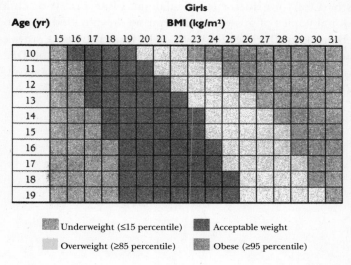

Underweight (≤15 percentile)    Acceptable weight

Overweight (≥85 percentile)    Obese (≥95 percentile)

Note: Values for BMI are rounded to the nearest integer for simplicity; any loss of accuracy is unlikely to be clinically significant.

Source: Adapted from A. Must, G. E. Dallal, and W. H. Dietz, Reference data for obesity: 85th and 95th percentiles of body mass index (wt/ht²) and triceps skinfold thickness, *American Journal of Clinical Nutrition* 53 (1991): 839–46. Reprinted with permission from F. Sizer and E. Whitney, *Nutrition: Concepts and Controversies* (Belmont, Calif.: Wadsworth, 2000, 8th ed., p. Z).

**Growth Charts**

You may have seen the growth charts that doctors use to monitor the growth patterns of children ages 2 to 20. These include gender-specific growth curves because boys and girls have different rates of growth.

In 2000, the CDC recommended that health professionals use growth charts based on BMI to monitor children's growth. The new growth charts for boys and girls ages 2 to 20 are reprinted on pp. 283 and 284. Because height is hard to measure accurately in children under the age of 2, BMI curves are not used for younger children. Normal growth curves show a decrease during the preschool years, when most children have a spurt of growth in height, and then gradually increase beginning about ages 4 to 6 into adulthood as both height and weight increase. For most children, healthy BMI values fall somewhere between the 15th and the 85th percentile-for-age. The chart on p. 281 gives the BMI cutoff values for various ages for these CDC percentile categories. A BMI value that is at or below the 5th percentile-for-age is equivalent to the DSM weight loss criterion for anorexia of "85% of that expected." We cannot emphasize enough that it is best for your doctor to calculate and interpret your child's BMI.

Additional copies of growth charts can be downloaded by going to the CDC Web site. Growth charts for boys can be found at: http://www.cdc.gov/nchs/about/major/nhanes/growthcharts/set2/chart%2015.PDF. Growth charts for girls can be found at: http://www.cdc.gov/nchs/about/major/nhanes/growthcharts/set2/chart%2016.PDF.

## CDC Growth Charts: United States

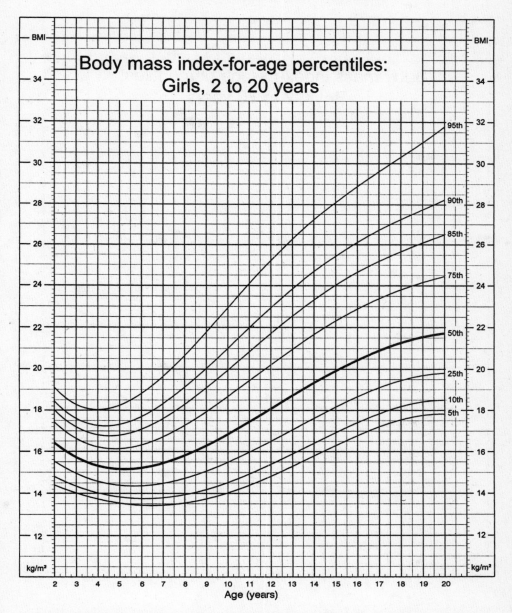

Body mass index-for-age percentiles:
Girls, 2 to 20 years

Source: Developed by the National Center for Health Statistics in collaboration with the National
Center for Chronic Disease Prevention and Health Promotion (2000).

## CDC Growth Charts: United States

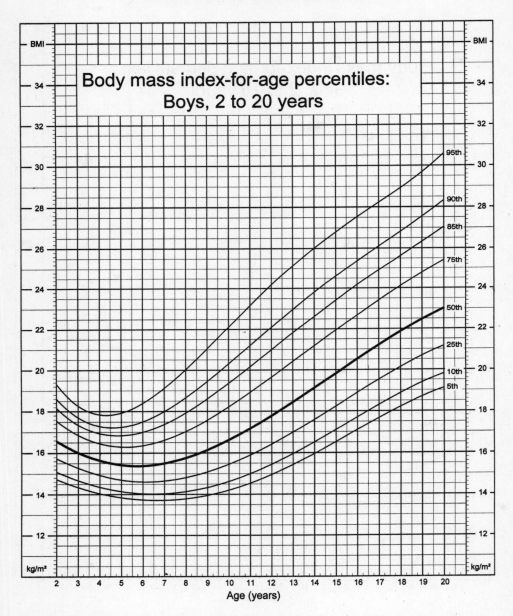

Body mass index-for-age percentiles:
Boys, 2 to 20 years

Source: Developed by the National Center for Health Statistics in collaboration with the National Center for Chronic Disease Prevention and Health Promotion (2000).

# Further Reading

Andersen, A. E., Cohn, L., and Holbrook, T. (2000). *Making Weight: Men's Conflicts with Food, Weight, Shape and Appearance*. Carlsbad, Calif.: Gürze Books.

Brumberg, J. J. (1988). *Fasting Girls*. Cambridge, Mass.: Harvard University Press.

Fairburn, C. G. (1995). *Overcoming Binge Eating*. New York: Guilford Press.

Kilbourne, J. (1999). *Can't Buy My Love: How Advertising Changes the Way We Think and Feel*. New York: Touchstone.

Pipher, M. (1994). *Reviving Ophelia: Saving the Selves of Adolescent Girls*. New York: G. P. Putnam's Sons.

Pope, H. G., Jr., Phillips, K. A., and Olivardia, R. (2000). *The Adonis Complex: The Secret Crisis of Male Body Obsession*. New York: The Free Press.

Sizer, F., and Whitney, E. (2000). *Nutrition: Concepts and Controversies*, (8th ed.). Belmont, Calif.: Wadsworth.

Stone, D., Patton, B., and Heen, S. (1999). *Difficult Conversations: How to Discuss What Matters Most*. New York: Penguin Books.

Vandereycken, W., and Noordenbos, G., eds. (1998). *The Prevention of Eating Disorders*. New York: New York University Press.

## Resources for Professionals

American Psychiatric Association. (1994). *Diagnostic and Statistical Manual of Mental Disorders* (4th ed.). Washington, D.C.

American Psychiatric Association. (2000). *Practice Guidelines for the Treatment of Patients with Eating Disorders* (2nd ed.). Washington, D.C.

Fairburn, C. G., Marcus, M. D., and Wilson, G. T. (1993). "Cognitive-Behavioral Therapy for Binge Eating and Bulimia Nervosa: A Comprehensive Treatment Manual," in C. G. Fairburn and G. T. Wilson, eds., *Binge Eating: Nature, Assessment and Treatment*. New York: Guilford Press.

Garner, D. M., and Garfinkel, P. E., eds. (1997). *Handbook of Treatment for Eating Disorders* (2nd ed.). New York: Guilford Press.

Herrin, M. M. (in press). *Nutrition Counseling in the Treatment of Eating Disorders.* New York: Brunner-Routledge.

Johnson, N. G., Roberts, M. C., and Worell, J., eds. (1999). *Beyond Appearance: A New Look at Adolescent Girls.* Washington, D.C.: American Psychological Association.

Lask, B., and Bryant-Waugh, R., eds. (2000). *Anorexia Nervosa and Related Eating Disorders in Childhood and Adolescence* (2nd ed.). East Sussex, U.K.: Psychology Press.

Levy-Warren, M. H. (1996). *The Adolescent Journey: Development, Identity Formation, and Psychotherapy.* Northvale, N.J.: Jason Aronson.

Lock, J., LeGrange, D., Agras, W. S., and Dare, C. (2001). *Treatment Manual for Anorexia Nervosa: A Family-Based Approach.* New York: Guilford Press.

Mehler, P. S., and Andersen, A. E., eds. (1999). *Eating Disorders: A Guide to Medical Care and Complications.* Baltimore: Johns Hopkins Press.

Piran, N., Levine, M. P., and Steiner-Adair, C. (1999). *Preventing Eating Disorders: A Handbook of Interventions and Special Challenges.* Philadelphia: Brunner/Mazel.

Yates, A. (1991). *Compulsive Exercise and the Eating Disorders: Toward an Integrated Theory of Activity.* New York: Brunner/Mazel.

# Informational, Support, and Advocacy Organizations and Web Sites

**UNITED STATES**

*Anorexia Nervosa and Related Eating Disorders (ANRED)*
P.O. Box 5102
Eugene, OR 97405
541-344-1144
www.anred.com

*Eating Disorder Awareness and Prevention (EDAP)*
603 Stewart Street, Suite 803
Seattle, WA 98101
800-931-2237 (Hotline)
www.edap.org

*Gürze Books*
P.O. Box 2238
Carlsbad, CA 92018
800-756-7533
www.bulimia.com

*Harvard Eating Disorders Center*
356 Bolyston Street
Boston, MA 02116
617-236-7766
www.hedc.org

*Healing Connections, Inc.*
212-585-3450
www.healingconnections.org

*International Association of Eating Disorder Professionals (IAEDP)*
800-800-8126
www.iaedp.com

*Massachusetts Eating Disorders Association, Inc. (MEDA)*
92 Pearl Street
Newton, MA 02158
888-525-MEDA
www.medainc.org

*National Association of Anorexia Nervosa and Associated Disorders (ANAD)*
P.O. Box 7
Highland Park, IL 60035
847-831-3438
e-mail: Anad20@aol.com

*National Eating Disorders Organization (NEDO)*
6655 S. Yale Avenue
Tulsa, OK 74136
918-481-4044

National Eating Disorders Screening
Program (NEDSP)
One Washington Street, Suite 304
Wellesley Hills, MA 02481
781-239-0071
www.mentalhealthscreening.org

## CANADA

*ANAD (Association for Awareness and
Networking Around Disordered Eating)*
2040 W. 12th Avenue, Suite 109
Vancouver, BC V6J 2G2
604-739-2070
877-288-0877 (toll-free)
www.anad.bc.ca
e-mail: anad@direct.ca

*BCEDA (British Columbia Eating
Disorder Association)*
526 Michigan Street
Victoria, BC V8V 1S2
250-383-2755
e-mail: bceda@direct.ca

*Eating Disorder Resource Centre of BC*
1081 Burrard Street
Room 2C-213
Vancouver, BC V6Z 1Y6
604-806-9000
800-655-1822 (toll-free in BC)

*The National Eating Disorder
Information Center*
CW 1-211
200 Elizabeth Street
Toronto, ON M5G 2C4
416-340-4156
www.nedic.on.ca
e-mail: nedic@uhn.on.ca

## ONLINE RESOURCES

http://www.eatingdisorders.
mentalhelp.net
http://www.somethingfishy.org
http://www.caringonline.com

### CANADIAN AND INTERNATIONAL LINKS

http://www.eating-disorder.org

# Residential and Hospital Programs

In most cases, local outpatient treatment (physician, psychotherapist, and nutritionist) that allows your child to live at home is not only sufficient to treat an eating disorder but is the preferable first approach to treatment. If outpatient treatment proves ineffective, however, a residential or hospital-based program should be considered. Finding a suitable program can seem like a daunting task when one has to not only consider the program's reputation, but also determine whether the cost of the program will be covered by insurance. Local outpatient professionals and hospital staff are your best resource for names of good regional programs. Your insurance company may be able to provide a list of programs for which they will cover at least some of the costs.

We have searched our files and the Internet in an effort to compile a list of treatment programs or centers in both the United States and Canada. In the few areas where we could not find contact information for inpatient programs, we have listed outpatient treatment centers. We do not endorse any specific programs, nor can we vouch for the quality of any of the programs we have listed. Additional listings can be found by clicking on "Treatment Centers" at: http://www.somethingfishy.org/treatmentfinder.php or http://www.caringonline.com. For additional Canadian treatment centers, click on "Treatment" at http://www.eating-disorder.org.

## UNITED STATES

**ARKANSAS**
*Levi Hospital Eating Disorders Clinic*
300 Prospect Avenue
Hot Springs, AR 71901
501-624-1281
www.levihospital.com

**ARIZONA**
*The Meadows*
1655 North Tegner Street
Wickenberg, AZ 85390
520-684-3926
800-MEADOWS

*Mirasol*
5931 North Oracle Road
Tucson, AZ 85704
888-520-1700
www.mirasol.net
e-mail: support@mirasol.net

*Remuda Ranch*
One East Apache Street
Wickenburg, AZ 85390
800-445-1900
www.remuda-ranch.com

*Rosewood*
36075 South Rincon Road
Wickenburg, AZ 85390
520-684-9594
800-845-2111
800-280-1212
e-mail: rosewranch@aol.com

*Sierra Tucson*
39580 South Lago del Oro Parkway
Tucson, AZ 85739
800-842-4487
www.sierratucson.com

**CALIFORNIA**
*Center for Discovery and Adolescent Change*
4136 Ann Arbor Road
Lakewood, CA 90712
562-425-7418
www.centerfordiscovery.com
e-mail:
eatingdisorders@centerfordiscovery.com

*Healthy Within* (outpatient services only)
4510 Executive Drive, #102
San Diego, CA 92121
858-622-0221
877-500-5151
www.healthywithin.com

*Monte Nido*
27162 Sea Vista Drive
Malibu, CA 90265
310-457-9958
www.montenido.com
e-mail: mntc@montenido.com

*Montecatini*
2524 LaCosta Avenue
Rancho La Costa, CA 92009
760-436-8930
www.montecatinieatingdisorder.com
e-mail: monte@tns.net

*The Neuropsychiatric Institute and Hospital*
University of California, Los Angeles
760 Westwood Plaza, Suite B8-213
Los Angeles, CA 90024
310-794-1022
800-825-9989
www.mentalhealth.ucla.edu

*Rader Programs*
Pacific Shores Hospital
2130 Ventura Road
Oxnard, CA 93030
800-841-1515
www.raderprograms.com

**COLORADO**
*Bethesada Psychiatric Health Center*
4400 East Cliff Avenue
Denver, CO 80222
303-759-6159

**CONNECTICUT**
*Institute of Living*
400 Washington Street
Hartford, CT 06106
800-673-2411

*The Renfrew Center of Connecticut*
436 Danbury Road
Wilton, CT 06897

800-RENFREW
www.renfrew.org
e-mail: info@renfrewcenter.com

*Wellspring*
21 Arch Bridge Road
Bethlehem, CT 06751
203-266-8000
203-266-8030
www.wellspring.org

**DELAWARE**
*The Brandywine Center, LLC*
2500 Grubb Road, Suite 240
Wilmington, DE 19810
302-475-1880
www.brandywinecenter.com
e-mail: info@brandywinecenter.com

**FLORIDA**
*Canopy Cove*
2300 Killearn Center Boulevard
Tallahassee, FL 32308
800-236-7524
www.canopycove.com
e-mail: info@canopycove.com

*The Renfrew Center of Miami*
151 Majorca Avenue, Suite B
Coral Gables, FL 33134
800-RENFREW
www.renfrew.org
e-mail: info@renfrewcenter.com

*The Renfrew Center of Southern Florida*
7700 Renfrew Lane
Coconut Creek, FL 33073
800-RENFREW
www.renfrew.org
e-mail: info@renfrewcenter.com

*The Willough at Naples*
9001 Tamianmi Trail East
Naples, FL 33962
800-722-0100

**GEORGIA**
*Ridgeview Institute*
3995 South Cobb Drive

Smyrna, GA 30080
770-434-4567
800-329-9775
www.ridgeviewinstitute.com

**HAWAII**
*Aloha Hawaii Healing Retreats*
400 Hualani, #325
Hilo, HI 96720
888-967-8622
808-969-9622
e-mail: keala@nethawaii.net

**ILLINOIS**
*Linden Oaks Hospital*
852 West Street
Naperville, IL 60540
630-305-5500

**INDIANA**
*Eating Disorders Center of Indiana*
3945 Eagle Creek Parkway, Suite C
Indianapolis, IN 46254
317-329-7071
877-794-1491
www.edci.net
e-mail: mr@edci.net

**IOWA**
*University of Iowa Hospitals and Clinics*
200 Hawkins Drive
Iowa City, IA 52242-1009
319-356-2406

**KANSAS**
*Menninger Clinic*
P.O. Box 829
Topeka, KS 66601-0829
800-351-9058
785-350-5553
www.menninger.edu

*University of Kansas School of Medicine, Wichita*
8901 East Orme
Wichita, KA 67207
800-322-8901

**LOUISANA**
*DePaul-Tulane Behavioral Health Center*
1040 Calhoun Street
New Orleans, LA 70118
800-548-4183
www.depaultulane.com

**MAINE**
*Westbrook Community Hospital*
40 Park Road
Westbrook, ME 04092
207-854-8464, ext. 3136
800-779-8444, ext. 3136
e-mail:
ppuchalski@westbrookhospital.org

**MARYLAND**
*Center for Eating Disorders*
7601 Osler Drive
Towson, MD 21204
410-427-2100
www.eating-disorder.com

*Eating Disorders Program*
The Johns Hopkins Hospital
600 Wolfe Street
Baltimore, MD 21287
410-955-3863

**MASSACHUSETTS**
*Deaconess Waltham Hospital*
Hope Avenue
Waltham, MA 02453
781-647-6000 (ask operator for "PAES")
781-647-6507

*Laurel Hill Inn*
131 Woburn Street
Medford, MA 02155
781-396-1116
www.laurelhillinn.com
e-mail: lhi@laurelhillinn.com

*Massachusetts General Hospital*
12 Parkman Street
Boston, MA 02114
617-726-2724

*McLean Hospital*
115 Mill Street
Belmont, MA 02178
617-855-2000

**MICHIGAN**
*Sparrows' Haven, Inc.*
1611 West Centre
Portage, MI 49024
616-329-1223
www.sparrowshaven.com
e-mail: sparrows@net-link.net

**MINNESOTA**
*Eating Disorders Institute at Methodist Hospital*
6490 Excelsior Boulevard, Suite E315
St. Louis Park, MN 55426
952-993-6200
www.methodisthospital.com/
eating_disorders

*University of Minnesota Eating Disorder Program*
Department of Psychiatry
2701 University Avenue S.E., Suite 206
Minneapolis, MN 55414
612-627-4498
e-mail: welle005@maroon.tc.umn.edu

**MISSISSIPPI**
*The Best of Both Worlds Therapy Center*
(outpatient services only)
8378 Ham Road
Meridian, MS 39305
601-679-1527
e-mail: carlacurry4@aol.com

**MISSOURI**
*Castlewood*
800 Holland Road
St. Louis, MO 63021
636-386-6611
888-822-8938
www.castlewoodtc.com

*La Montagne*
P.O. Box 300
Crystal City, MO 63019
636-931-3883
www.lamontagne.org
e-mail: lamontedtx@aol.com

**MONTANA**
*Rimrock Foundation*
1231 North 29th Street
Billings, MT 59101
800-227-3953
406-248-3175
www.rimrock.org
e-mail: comm@rimrock.org

**NEBRASKA**
*Richard Young Center*
515 South 26th Street
Omaha, NE 68105
402-354-6690

**NEVADA**
*Lake Mead Hospital Medical Center*
1409 East Lake Mead Boulevard
North Las Vegas, NV 89030
702-649-7711
www.lakemeadhospital.com
e-mail:
annette.kinsman@tenethealth.com

**NEW HAMPSHIRE**
*Cheshire Medical Center Adolescent Program*
Dartmouth-Hitchcock Keene
580 and 590 Court Street
Keene, NH 03431
603-352-4111

*Hampstead Hospital*
218 East Road
Hampstead, NH 03841
603-329-5311
800-600-5311
www.hampsteadhospital.com
e-mail: cgove@hampsteadhospital.com

**NEW JERSEY**
*The Renfrew Center of Northern New Jersey*
70 West Allendale Avenue, Suite D
Allendale, NJ 07401
800-RENFREW
www.renfrew.org
e-mail: info@renfrewcenter.com

*Somerset Medical Center*
110 Rehill Avenue
Somerville, NJ 08876
908-685-2200
www.somersetmedicalcenter.com

**NEW MEXICO**
*The Life Healing Center of Santa Fe*
P.O. Box 6758
Santa Fe, NM 87502
800-989-7406
505-989-7436
www.life-healing.com
e-mail: lhc@life-healing.com

**NEW YORK**
*The Eating Disorders Clinic*
*New York State Psychiatric Institute*
*Columbia Presbyterian Medical Center*
Unit 98
1051 Riverside Drive
New York, NY 10032
212-543-5316
www.columbia.edu/~ea12
e-mail: edru@pi.cpmc.columbia.edu

*Four Winds Saratoga*
30 Cresent Avenue
Saratoga Springs, NY 12866
800-959-1287
www.fourwindshospital.com
e-mail: markets@fourwindshospital.com

*Four Winds Syracuse*
650 South Salina Street
Syracuse, NY 13202
315-476-2161
800-647-6479
www.fourwindshospital.com

*Four Winds Westchester*
800 Cross River Road
Katonah, NY 10536
914-763-8151
800-546-1770
www.fourwindshospital.com
e-mail: marketk@fourwindshospital.com

*The Renfrew Center of New York City*
11 East 36th Street
New York, NY 10016
800-RENFREW
www.renfrew.org
e-mail: info@renfrewcenter.com

**NORTH CAROLINA**
*Structure House*
3017 Pickett Road
Durham, NC 27705
800-553-0052
919-493-4205
www.structurehouse.com
e-mail: info@structurehouse.com

**NORTH DAKOTA**
*University of North Dakota*
*Neuropsychiatric Research Institute*
P.O. Box 1415
Fargo, ND 58107
877-299-3511
701-293-1335
www.nrifargo.com
e-mail: mburgard@nrifargo.com

*Eating Disorders Institute*
120 South 8th Street, Suite 1
Fargo, ND 58103
800-437-4010, ext. 4111
701-234-4111

**OHIO**
*River Centre Clinic*
5465 Main Street
Sylvania, OH 43560
419-885-8800
www.river-centre.org

*University Hospitals Health System (UHHS)*
*Laurelwood Hospital and Counseling Centers*
35900 Euclid Avenue
Willoughby, OH 44094
440-953-3000
216-595-0500, ext. 45, Dr. Lucene
Wisniewski
www.laurelwoodhospital.com
e-mail: access@laurelwoodhospital.com

**OKLAHOMA**
*Laureate Psychiatric Clinic and Hospital*
6655 South Yale Avenue
Tulsa, OK 74136
918-491-3702
800-322-5173
www.laureate.com

*Rader Programs*
Brookhaven Hospital
201 South Garnett Road
Tulsa, OK 74128-1800
800-841-1515

**OREGON**
*Providence St. Vincent Medical Center*
9205 S.W. Barnes Road
Portland, OR 97225
503-216-1234

**PENNSYLVANIA**
*Center for Overcoming Problem*
*Eating (COPE)*
Western Psychiatric Institute and Clinic
University of Pittsburgh Medical Center
3811 O'Hara Street
Pittsburgh, PA 15213
412-624-0012

*Hershey Medical Center*
500 University Drive
Hershey, PA 17033
717-531-3841
www.hmc.psu.edu
e-mail: lraimo@psu.edu

*The Renfrew Center of Philadelphia*
475 Spring Lane
Philadelphia, PA 19128
215-482-5353
800-RENFREW
www.renfrew.org
e-mail: info@renfrewcenter.com

*The Renfrew Center of Bryn Mawr*
735 Old Lancaster Road
Bryn Mawr, PA 19010
800-RENFREW
www.renfrew.org
e-mail: info@renfrewcenter.com

**SOUTH CAROLINA**
*Institute of Psychiatry*
Medical University of South Carolina
67 President Street
P.O. Box 250861
Charleston, SC 29425
843-792-0092
www.musc.edu
e-mail: brewertt@musc.edu

**TENNESSEE**
*Mercy Ministries of America*
P.O. Box 111060
Nashville, TN 37222-1060
615-831-6987
www.mercyministries.com
e-mail: mercymin@voy.net

**TEXAS**
*Presbyterian Hospital of Dallas*
8200 Walnut Hill Lane
Dallas, TX 75231
800-477-3729
214-345-6789
www.phscare.org/presbydallas

*Shades of Hope*
402-A Mulberry Street
Buffalo Gap, TX 79508
800-588-HOPE (4673)
915-572-3843
www.shadesofhope.com
e-mail: info@shadesofhope.com

**UTAH**
*Center for Change*
1790 North State Street
Orem, UT 84057
801-224-8255
www.centerforchange.com

**VERMONT**
*Brattleboro Retreat*
Anna Marsh Lane
P.O. Box 803
Brattleboro, VT 05302
800-738-7328
802-257-7785
www.bratretreat.org

**VIRGINIA**
*Medical Associates of Reston*
(outpatient services only)
1800 Town Center Drive, Suite 212
Reston, VA 20190
703-435-2227
www.mar.nova.org

*Walnut Avenue Associates* (outpatient services only)
16 Walnut Avenue W.
Roanoke, VA 24016
540-345-6468
e-mail: zentago@aol.com

**WASHINGTON**
*Swedish Medical Center, Ballard*
Eating Disorder Program
5300 Tallman Avenue N.W.
Seattle, WA 98107-1507
206-781-6345
www.swedish.org

**WASHINGTON, D.C.**
*Eating Disorders Recovery Center of WATS*
4455 Connecticut Avenue N.W.,
Suite A400
Washington, DC 20008
202-537-1780, ext. 99

**WISCONSIN**
*Rogers Memorial Hospital*
34700 Valley Road
Oconomowoc, WI 53066
800-767-4411
www.rogershospital.org

**WYOMING**
*Mercer House* (outpatient services only)
435 CY Avenue
Casper, WY 82601
307-265-7366

## CANADA

### ALBERTA

*University of Alberta Hospital Eating Disorders Program*
Subunit 4F4, 8440-112 Street
Edmonton, AB T6G 2B7
780-407-6114
780-407-6239
www.cha.ab.ca/healthsite/pk3940sh.asp
e-mail: lshobe@cha.ab.ca

### BRITISH COLUMBIA

*St. Paul's Hospital*
Eating Disorder Program
1081 Burrard Street
Vancouver, BC V62 1Y6
604-682-2344
www.eatingdisorders-sph.org

*Eating Disorders Program in the Capital Region/Mental Health*
(outpatient services only)
Ministry of Children and Family
Development
302-2955 Jutland Road
Victoria, BC V8T 5J9
250-387-0000

### MANITOBA

*Westwind Eating Disorder Recovery Centre*
458-14th Street
Brandon, MB R7A 4T3
204-728-2499
888-353-3372
www.westwind.mb.ca
e-mail: gusdalb@mb.sympatico.ca

### NOVA SCOTIA

*Eating Disorders Action Group*
(outpatient group only)
150 Bedford Highway, #2614
Halifax, NS B3M 3J5
902-443-9944
www.e-d-a-g.com
e-mail:
iamworthmyweight@hotmail.com

### ONTARIO

*Homewood Health Centre*
150 Delhi Street
Guelph, ON N1E 6K9
519- 824-1010
www.homewoodhealth.com

*The Hospital for Sick Children*
555 University Avenue
Toronto, ON M5G 1X8
416-813-7195
www.sickkids.on.ca
e-mail: heather.graham@sickkids.ca
(for information only, not advice)

*Sheena's Place*
87 Spadina Road
Toronto, ON M5R 2T1
416-927-8900
www.sheenasplace.org

### QUEBEC

*Carpe Diem*
Centre therapeutique des troubles
alimentaires
380 Chemin du Domaine
Saint-Ludger, PQ G0M 1W0
819-548-5841
www.centrecarpediem.qc.ca
e-mail: info@centrecarpediem.qc.ca

*Douglas Hospital*
Adolescent Psychiatric Department
6875 Lasalle Boulevard
Montreal, PQ H4H 1R3
514-761-6131, ext. 2117

*Eating Disorder Clinic*
*Adolescent Medicine Service*
Ste-Justine Hospital
3175 Côte Ste-Catherine
Montreal, PQ H3T 1C5
514-345-4721
e-mail: jean_wilkins@ssss.gouv.qc.ca

### SASKATCHEWAN

*BridgePoint Center for Eating Disorders*
P.O. Box 190
Milden, SK S0L 2L0
306-935-2240
e-mail: www.bridgepointcenter.ca

# References

*Preface: My Own Story*

Heatherton, T. F., Nichols, P., Mahamedi, F., and Keel, P. (1995). Body weight, dieting, and eating disorder symptoms among college students, 1982 to 1992. *American Journal of Psychiatry* 152, 1623–29.

Rosen, J. C., Compas, B. E., and Tacy, B. (1993). The relation among stress, psychological symptoms, and eating disorder symptoms: A prospective analysis. *International Journal of Eating Disorders* 14, 153–62.

Neumark-Sztainer, D., and Hannan, P. J. (2000). Weight-related behaviors among adolescent girls and boys. *Archives of Pediatric and Adolescent Medicine* 154, 569–77.

Childress, A. C., Brewerton, T. D., Hodges, E. L., and Jarrell, M. P. (1993). The kids' eating disorder survey (KEDS): A study of middle school students. *Journal of American Academy of Child and Adolescent Psychiatry* 32, 843–50.

Califano, J. A. (January 2001). *Food for thought: Substance abuse and eating disorders.* CASA Conference presented by the National Center on Addiction and Substance Abuse at Columbia University.


*1. At Risk: Recognizing an Eating Disorder and Spotting Early Warning Signs*

Brumberg, J. J. (1988). *Fasting girls.* Cambridge, Mass.: Harvard University Press.

Striegel-Moore, R. H., and Steiner-Adair, C. (1998). Primary prevention of eating disorders: Further considerations from a feminist perspective. In W. Vandereycken and G. Noordenbos, eds., *The prevention of eating disorders* (pp. 1–22). New York: New York University Press.

Lask, B., and Bryant-Waugh, R., eds. (2000). *Anorexia nervosa and related eating disorders in childhood and adolescence* (2nd ed.). East Sussex, U.K.: Psychology Press.

Lucas, A. R., Beard, C. M., O'Fallon, W. M., and Kurland, L. T. (1991). Fifty-year trends in the incidence of anorexia nervosa in Rochester, Minn.: A population-based study. *American Journal of Psychiatry* 148, 917–22.

American Psychiatric Association. (2000). *Practice guideline for the treatment of patients with eating disorders* (2nd ed.). Washington, D.C.

Carlat, D. J., Camargo, C. A., Jr., and Herzog, D. B. (1997). Eating disorders in males: A report on 135 patients. *American Journal of Psychiatry* 154, 1127–32.

Russell, G. F. M. (1997). The history of bulimia nervosa. In D. M. Garner and P. E. Garfinkel, eds., *Handbook of treatment for eating disorders* (2nd ed., pp. 11–24). New York: Guilford Press.

Herzog, D. B., Keller, M. B., Lavori, P. W., and Bradburn, I. S. (1991). Bulimia nervosa in adolescence. *Journal of Developmental Behavior in Pediatrics* 12, 191–95.

Bulik, C. M. (1987). Drug and alcohol abuse by bulimic women and their families. *American Journal of Psychiatry* 144, 1604–6.

American Psychiatric Association. (1994). *Diagnostic and statistical manual of mental disorders* (4th ed.). Washington, D.C.

Society for Adolescent Medicine (1995). Eating disorders in adolescents. *Journal of Adolescent Health* 16, 476–80.

Braun, D. L., Sunday, S. R., Huang, A., and Halmi, K. A. (1999). More males seek treatment for eating disorders. *International Journal of Eating Disorders* 25, 415–24.

Stunkard, A. J. (1993). A history of binge eating. In C. G. Fairburn and G. T. Wilson, eds., *Binge eating: Nature, assessment, and treatment* (pp. 15–34). New York: Guilford Press.

Hetherington, M. M., Stoner, S. A., Andersen, A. E., and Rolls, B. J. (2000). Effects of acute food deprivation on eating behavior in eating disorders. *International Journal of Eating Disorders* 28, 272–83.

Garner, D. M. (1997). Psychoeducational principles in treatment. In D. M. Garner and P. E. Garfinkel, eds., *Handbook of treatment for eating disorders* (2nd ed., pp. 145–77). New York: Guilford Press.

Spitzer, R. L., Yanovski, S., Wadden, T., Wing, R. Marcus, M. D., Stunkard, A., Devlin, M., Mitchell, J., Hasin, D., and Horne, R. L. (1993). Binge-eating disorders: Its further validation in a multisite study. *International Journal of Eating Disorders* 13, 137–53.

## 2. Bad Habit or Dangerous Behavior?: When to Worry about Disordered Eating

Herzog, D. B., Hopkins, J. D., and Burns, C. D. (1993). A follow-up study of 33 subdiagnostic eating disordered women. *International Journal of Eating Disorders* 14, 261–67.

Striegel-Moore, R. H., and Cachelin, F. M. (1999). Body-image concerns and disordered eating in adolescent girls: Risk and protective factors. In N. G. Johnson, M. C. Roberts, and J. Worell, eds., *Beyond appearance: A new look at adolescent girls* (pp. 85–108). Washington, D.C.: American Psychological Association.

Rodin, J., Silberstein, L., and Striegel-Moore, R. (1985). Women and weight: A normative discontent. In T. B. Sonderegger, ed., *Nebraska symposium on motivation: Psychology and gender,* 24, vol. 32 (pp. 267–308). Lincoln: University of Nebraska Press.

Schur, E. A., Sanders, M., and Steiner, H. (2000). Body dissatisfaction and dieting in young children. *International Journal of Eating Disorders* 27, 74–82.

Maloney, M. J., McGuire, J., Daniels, S. R., and Specker, B. (1989). Dieting behavior and eating attitudes in children. *Pediatrics* 84, 482–89.

Huon, G., and Lim, J. (2000). The emergence of dieting among female adolescents: Age, body mass index, and seasonal effects. *International Journal of Eating Disorders* 28, 221–25.

Hsu, L. K. G. (1997). Can dieting cause an eating disorder? *Psychological Medicine* 27, 509–13.

Brewerton, T. D., Dansky, B. S., Kilpatrick, D. G., and O'Neal, P. M. (2000). Which comes first in the pathogenesis of bulimia nervosa: Dieting or bingeing? *International Journal of Eating Disorders* 28, 259–64.

Eccles, J., Barber, B., Jozefowicz, D., Malenchuk, O., Vida, M. (1999). Self-evaluations of competence, task values, and self-esteem. In N. G. Johnson, M. C. Roberts, and J. Worell, eds., *Beyond appearance: A new look at adolescent girls* (pp. 53–83). Washington, D.C.: American Psychological Association.

Graber, J. A., Archibald, A. B., and Brooks-Gunn, J. (1999). The role of parents in the emergence, maintenance, and prevention of eating problems and disorders. In N. Piran, M. P. Levine, and C. Steiner-Adair, eds., *Preventing eating disorders: A handbook of interventions and special challenges* (pp. 44–62). Philadelphia: Brunner/Mazel.

Shisslak, C. M., Crago, M., Gray, N., Estes, L. S., McKnight, K., Parnaby, O. G., Sharpe, T., Bryson, S., Killen, J., and Taylor, C. B. (1998). The McKnight Foundation prospective study of risk factors for the development of eating disorders. In W. Vandereycken and G. Noordenbos, eds., *The prevention of eating disorders* (pp. 57–74). New York: New York University Press.

Bryant-Waugh, R. (2000). Overview of the eating disorders. In B. Lask and R. Bryant-Waugh, eds. *Anorexia nervosa and related eating disorders in childhood and adolescence* (2nd ed., pp. 27–40). East Sussex, U.K.: Psychology Press.

Huon, G. F., and Walton, C. J. (2000). Initiation of dieting among adolescent females. *International Journal of Eating Disorders* 28, 226–30.

Smolak, L., Levine, M. P., and Schermer, F. (1999). Parental input and weight concerns among elementary schoolchildren. *International Journal of Eating Disorders* 25, 263–71.

## 3. Prevention: The Power of the Preemptive Strike

Striegel-Moore, R. H., and Cachelin, F. M. (1999). Body-image concerns and disordered eating in adolescent girls: Risk and protective factors. In N. G. Johnson, M. C. Roberts, and J. Worell, eds., *Beyond appearance: A new look at adolescent girls* (pp. 85–108). Washington, D.C.: American Psychological Association.

Eccles, J., Barber, B., Jozefowicz, D., Malenchuk, O., and Vida, M. (1999). Self-evaluations of competence, task values, and self-esteem. In N. G. Johnson, M. C. Roberts, and J. Worell, eds., *Beyond appearance: A new look at adolescent girls* (pp. 53–83). Washington, D.C.: American Psychological Association.

Swarr, A. E., and Richards, M. H. (1996). Longitudinal effects of adolescent girls' pubertal development, perceptions of pubertal timing, and parental relations on eating problems. *Developmental Psychology* 32, 636–46.

Huon, G. F., and Walton, C. J. (2000). Initiation of dieting among adolescent females. *International Journal of Eating Disorders* 28, 226–30.

Gowers, S. G., North, C. D., Byram, V., and Weaver, A. B. (1996). Life event precipitants of adolescent anorexia nervosa. *Journal of Child Psychology and Psychiatry and Allied Disciplines* 37, 469–77.

Murray, C., Waller, G., and Legg, C. (2000). Family dysfunction and bulimic psychopathology: The mediating role of shame. *International Journal of Eating Disorders* 28, 84–89.

Striegel-Moore, R. H., and Steiner-Adair, C. (1998). Primary prevention of eating disorders: Further considerations from a feminist perspective. In W. Vandereycken and G. Noordenbos, eds., *The prevention of eating disorders* (pp. 1–22). New York: New York University Press.

Silverstein, B., and Perlick, D. (1995). *The cost of competence: Why inequality causes depression, eating disorders, and illness in women.* New York: Oxford University Press.

Nasser, M., and Katzman, M. (1999). Eating disorders: Transcultural perspectives inform prevention. In N. Piran, M. P. Levine, and C. Steiner-Adair, eds., *Preventing eating disorders: A handbook of interventions and special challenges* (pp. 26–43). Philadelphia: Brunner/Mazel.

Chiu, A. (May 20, 1999). Study finds rise in signs of eating disorders after TV comes to Fiji. *OnlineAthens: News,* online, http://www.onlineathens.com/stories/052099/new_0520990021.shtml.

Kilbourne, J. Personal communication, April 19, 2000.

Birch, L. L. (1998). Psychological influences on the childhood diet. *Journal of Nutrition* 128, 407S–10S.

Birch, L. L., and Fisher, J. O. (2000). Mothers' child-feeding practices influence daughters' eating and weight. *American Journal of Clinical Nutrition* 71, 1054–61.

Fisher, J. O., and Birch, L. L. (1999). Restricting access to foods and children's eating. *Appetite* 32, 405–19.

Rozin, P., Ashmore, M., and Markwith, M. (1996). Lay American conceptions of nutrition: Dose insensitivity, categorical thinking, contagion, and the monotonic mind. *Health Psychology* 15, 438–47.

## 4. The Family on the Front Lines

Bostic, J. Q., Muriel, A. C., Hack, S., Weinstein, S., and Herzog, D. (1997). Anorexia nervosa in a 7-year-old girl. *Journal of Developmental and Behavioral Pediatrics* 18, 331–33.

Liebman, R., Minuchin, S., and Baker, L. (1974). The role of the family in the treatment of anorexia nervosa. *Journal of the American Academy of Child Psychiatry* 13, 264–74.

Coons, H. (2001). Fat girl: thin girl. Unpublished manuscript.

Sharpe, T. M., Killen, J. D., Bryson, S. W., Shisslak, C. M., Estes, L. S., Gray, N., Crago, M., and Taylor, C. B. (1998). Attachment style and weight concerns in preadolescent and adolescent girls. *International Journal of Eating Disorders* 23, 39–44.

Lock, J., LeGrange, D., Agras, W. S., and Dare, C. (2001). *Treatment manual for anorexia nervosa: A family-based approach.* New York: Guilford Press.

Steiner, H., and Lock, J. (1998). Anorexia nervosa and bulimia nervosa in children and adolescents: A review of the past 10 years. *Journal of the American Academy of Child and Adolescent Psychiatry* 37, 352–59.

## 5. Boys at Risk

Field, A. E., Colditz, G. A., and Peterson, K. E. (1997). Racial/ethnic and gender differences in concern with weight and in bulimic behaviors among adolescents. *Obesity Research* 5, 447–54.

Braun, D. L., Sunday, S. R., Huang, A., and Halmi, K. A. (1999). More males seek treatment for eating disorders. *International Journal of Eating Disorders* 25, 415–24.

Carlat, D. J., and Camargo, C. A., Jr. (1991). Review of bulimia nervosa in males. *American Journal of Psychiatry* 148, 831–43.

Pope, H. G., Jr., Olivardia, R., Gruber, A., and Borowiecki, J. (1999). Evolving ideals of male body image as seen through action toys. *International Journal of Eating Disorders* 26, 65–72.

Siever, M. D. (1994). Sexual orientation and gender as factors in socioculturally acquired vulnerability to body dissatisfaction and eating disorders. *Journal of Consulting and Clinical Psychology* 62, 252–60.

Carlat, D. J., Camargo, C. A., Jr., and Herzog, D. B. (1997). Eating disorders in males: A report on 135 patients. *American Journal of Psychiatry* 154, 1127–32.

Keel, P. K., Klump, K. L., Leon, G. R., and Fulkerson, J. A. (1998). Disordered eating in adolescent males from a school-based sample. *International Journal of Eating Disorders* 23, 125–32.

Sharp, C. W., Clark, S. A., Dunan, J. R., Blackwood, D. H. R., and Shapiro, C. M. (1994). Clinical presentation of anorexia nervosa in males: 24 new cases. *International Journal of Eating Disorders* 15, 125–34.

Spitzer, R. L., Yanovski, S., Wadden, T., Wing, R., Marcus, M. D., Stunkard, A., Devlin, M., Mitchell, J., Hasin, D., and Horne, R. L. (1993). Binge-eating disorders: Its further validation in a multisite study. *International Journal of Eating Disorders* 13, 137–53.

Pope, H. G., Jr., Phillips, K. A., and Olivardia, R. (2000). *The Adonis complex: The secret crisis of male body obsession.* New York: The Free Press.

Farrow, J. A. (1992). The adolescent male with an eating disorder. *Pediatric Annals* 21, 769–74.

Andersen, A. E., Watson, T., and Schlechte, J. (June 3, 2000). Osteoporosis and osteopenia in men with eating disorders. *The Lancet* 355, 1967–68.

French, S. A., Story, M., Neumark-Sztainer, D., Downes, B., Resnick, M., and Blum, R. (1997). Ethnic differences in psychosocial and health behavior correlates of dieting, purging, and binge eating in a population-based sample of adolescent females. *International Journal of Eating Disorders* 22, 315–22.

Davis, C., and Katzman, M. A. (1999). Perfection as acculturation: Psychological correlates of eating problems in Chinese male and female students living in the United States. *International Journal of Eating Disorders* 25, 65–70.

## 6. *Understanding the Medical Consequences of an Eating Disorder*

Stashwick, C. (1996). When you suspect an eating disorder. *Contemporary Pediatrics* 13, 124–53.

Nussbaum, M., Baird, D., Sonnenblick, M., Cowan, K., and Shenker, I. R. (1985). Short stature in anorexia nervosa patients. *Journal of Adolescent Health Care* 6, 453–55.

Warren, M. P., Holderness, C. C., Lesobre, V., Tzen, R., Vossoughian, F., and Brooks-Gunn, J. (1994). Hypothalamic amenorrhea and hidden nutritional insults. *Journal of the Society for Gynecologic Investigation* 1, 84–88.

Atkins, D. M., and Silber, T. J. (1993). Clinical spectrum of anorexia nervosa in children. *Journal of Developmental and Behavioral Pediatrics* 14, 211–16.

Hall, A., Delahunt, J. W., and Ellis, P. M. (1985). Anorexia nervosa in the male: Clinical features and follow-up of nine patients. *Journal of Psychiatric Research* 19, 315–21.

Waldholtz, B. D. (1999). Gastrointestinal complaints and function in patients with eating disorders. In P. S. Mehler and A. E. Andersen, eds., *Eating disorders: A guide to medical care and complications* (pp. 86–99). Baltimore: Johns Hopkins University Press.

Andersen, A. E. (1999). The diagnosis and treatment of eating disorders in primary care medicine. In P. S. Mehler and A. E. Andersen, eds., *Eating disorders: A guide to medical care and complications* (pp. 1–26). Baltimore: Johns Hopkins University Press.

Schocken, D. D., Holloway, J. D., and Powers, P. S. (1989). Weight loss and the heart: Effects of anorexia nervosa and starvation. *Archives of Internal Medicine* 149, 877–81.

Katzman, D. K., and Zipursky, R. B. (1997). Adolescents with anorexia nervosa: The impact of the disorder on bones and brains. *Annals of the New York Academy of Sciences* 817, 127–37.

Grinspoon, S., Herzog, D., and Klibanski, A. (1997). Mechanisms and treatment options for bone loss in anorexia nervosa. *Psychopharmacology Bulletin* 33, 399–404.

Andersen, A. E. (1999). Using medical information psychotherapeutically. In P. S. Mehler and A. E. Andersen, eds., *Eating disorders: A guide to medical care and complications* (pp. 192–201). Baltimore: Johns Hopkins University Press.

Carmichael, K. A., and Carmichael, D. H. (1995). Bone metabolism and osteopenia in eating disorders. *Medicine* 74, 254–67.

Morgan, J. F. (1999). Eating disorders and reproduction. *Australian and New Zealand Journal of Obstetrics and Gynaecology* 39, 167–73.

Franko, D. L., and Walton, B. E. (1993). Pregnancy and eating disorders: A review and clinical implications. *International Journal of Eating Disorders* 13, 41–47.

Conti, J., Abraham, S., and Taylor, A. (1998). Eating behavior and pregnancy outcome. *Journal of Psychosomatic Research* 44, 465–77.

Schlechte, J. A. (1999). General endocrinology. In P. S. Mehler and A. E. Andersen, eds., *Eating disorders: A guide to medical care and complications* (pp. 132–43). Baltimore: Johns Hopkins University Press.

Fairburn, C. G. (1995). Physiology of anorexia nervosa. In K. D. Brownell and C. G. Fairburn, eds., *Eating disorders and obesity: A comprehensive handbook* (pp. 251–60). New York: Guilford Press.

Touyz, S. W., and Beumont, P. J. V. (1994). Neuropsychological assessment of patients with anorexia and bulimia nervosa. In S. Touyz, D. Byrne, and A. Gilandas, eds., *Neuropsychology in clinical practice* (pp. 305–26). San Diego, Calif.: Academic Press.

Bachrach, L. K., Guido, D., Katzman, D., Litt, I. F., and Marcus, R. (1990). Decreased bone density in adolescent girls with anorexia nervosa. *Pediatrics* 86, 440–47.

Mehler, P. S. (1999). Nutritional rehabilitation: Practical guidelines for refeeding the anorectic patient. In P. S. Mehler and A. E. Andersen, eds., *Eating disorders: A guide to medical care and complications* (pp. 63–75). Baltimore: Johns Hopkins University Press.

McComb, R. J. (1993). Dental aspects of anorexia nervosa and bulimia nervosa. In A. S. Kaplan and P. E. Garfinkel, eds., *Medical issues and the eating disorders: The interface* (pp. 101–22). New York: Brunner/Mazel.

Fairburn, C. G. (1995). *Overcoming binge eating.* New York: Guilford Press.

Russell, G. (1979). Bulimia nervosa: An ominous variant of anorexia nervosa. *Psychological Medicine* 9, 429–48.

Kaye, W. H., Weltzin, T. E., Hsu, L. K. G., McConaha, C. W., and Bolton, B. (1993). Amount of calories retained after binge eating and vomiting. *American Journal of Psychiatry* 150, 969–71.

Bo-Linn, G. W., Santa Ana, C. A., Morawski, S. G., and Fordtran, J. S. (1983). Purging and calorie absorption in bulimic patients and normal women. *Annals of Internal Medicine* 99, 14–17.

Garner, D. M. (1997). Psychoeducational principles in treatment. In D. M. Garner and P. E. Garfinkel, eds., *Handbook of treatment for eating disorders* (2nd ed., pp. 145–77). New York: Guilford Press.

Woodside, D. B. (1995). Review of anorexia nervosa and bulimia nervosa. *Current Problems in Pediatrics* 25, 67–89.

Mitchell, J. E., Specker, S., and Edmonson, K. (1997). Management of substance abuse and dependence. In D. M. Garner and P. E. Garfinkel, eds., *Handbook of treatment for eating disorders* (2nd ed., pp. 415–23). New York: Guilford Press.

Crow, S. J., Keel, P. K., and Kendall, D. (1998). Eating disorders and insulin-dependent diabetes mellitus. *Psychosomatics* 39, 233–43.

Rydall, A. C., Rodin, G. M., Olmsted, M. P., Devenyi, R. G., and Daneman, D. (1997). Disordered eating behavior and microvascular complications in young women with insulin-dependent diabetes mellitus. *New England Journal of Medicine* 336, 1849–54.

Yanovski, S. Z., Nelson, J. E., Dubbert, B. K., and Spitzer, R. L. (1993). Association of binge eating disorder and psychiatric comorbidity in obese subjects. *American Journal of Psychiatry* 150, 1472–79.

Mitchell, J. E. (1995). Medical complications of bulimia nervosa. In K. D. Brownell and C. G. Fairburn, eds., *Eating disorders and obesity: A comprehensive handbook* (pp. 271–75). New York: Guilford Press.

## 8. Avoiding Parent Traps: How Improving Your Relationship to Food and Your Body Can Help Your Child

Woodside, D. B., Field, L. L., Garfinkel, P. E., and Heinmaa, M. (1998). Specificity of eating disorders diagnoses in families of probands with anorexia nervosa and bulimia nervosa. *Comprehensive Psychiatry* 39, 261–64.

Strober, M., Freeman, R., Lampert C., Diamond, J., and Kaye, W. (2000). Controlled family study of anorexia nervosa and bulimia nervosa: Evidence of shared liability and transmission of partial syndromes. *American Journal of Psychiatry* 157, 393–401.

Lilenfeld, L. R., Kaye, W. H., Strober, M. (1997). Genetics and family studies of anorexia nervosa and bulimia nervosa. *Baillière's Clinical Psychiatry* 3, 177–97.

Lilenfeld, L. R., Kaye, W. H., Greeno, C. G., Merikangas, K. R., Plotnicov, K., Pollice, C., Rao, R., Strober, M., Bulik, C. M., and Nagy, L. (1998). A controlled family study of anorexia nervosa and bulimia nervosa. *Archives of General Psychiatry* 55, 603–10.

Stice, E., Agras, W. S., and Hammer, L. D. (1999). Risk factors for the emergence of childhood eating disturbances: A five-year prospective study. *International Journal of Eating Disorders* 25, 375–87.

Levenkron, S. Personal communication, February 20, 2001.

Levenkron, S. (1978). *The best little girl in the world.* New York: Warner Books.

Levenkron, S. (2000). *Anatomy of anorexia.* New York: W. W. Norton.

Smolak, L., Levine, M. P., and Schermer, F. (1999). Parental input and weight concerns among elementary school children. *International Journal of Eating Disorders* 25, 263–71.

Pike, K. M., and Rodin, J. (1991). Mothers, daughters, and disordered eating. *Journal of Abnormal Psychology* 100, 198–204.

Edmunds, H., and Hill, A. J. (1999). Dieting and the family context of eating in young adolescent children. *International Journal of Eating Disorders* 25, 435–40.

Graber, J. A., Archibald, A. B., Brooks-Gunn, J. (1999). The role of parents in the emergence, maintenance, and prevention of eating problems and disorders. In N. Piran, M. P. Levine, and C. Steiner-Adair, eds., *Preventing eating disorders: A handbook of interventions and special challenges* (pp. 44–62). Philadelphia: Brunner/Mazel.

Koff, E., and Rierdan, J. (1991). Perceptions of weight and attitudes toward eating in early adolescent girls. *Journal of Adolescent Health* 12, 307–12.

Schur, E. A., Sanders, M., and Steiner, H. (2000). Body dissatisfaction and dieting in young children. *International Journal of Eating Disorders* 27, 74–82.

Levy-Warren, M. H. (1996). *The Adolescent journey: Development, identity formation, and psychotherapy.* Northvale, N.J.: Jason Aronson.

Striegel-Moore, R. H., and Cachelin, F. M. (1999). Body-image concerns and disordered eating in adolescent girls: Risk and protective factors. In N. G. Johnson, M. C. Roberts, and J. Worell, eds., *Beyond appearance: A new look at adolescent girls* (pp. 85–108). Washington, D.C.: American Psychological Association.

Attie, I., and Brooks-Gunn, J. (1989). Development of eating problems in adolescent girls: A longitudinal study. *Developmental Psychology* 25, 70–79.

Byely, L., Archibald, A. B., Graber, J., and Brooks-Gunn, J. (2000). A prospective study of familial and social influences on girls' body image and dieting. *International Journal of Eating Disorders* 28, 155–64.

## 9. Beyond the Family Circle: Friends, School, and Summer Camp

Paxton, S. J. (1999). Peer relations, body image, and disordered eating in adolescent girls: Implications for prevention. In N. Piran, M. P. Levine, and C. Steiner-Adair, eds., *Preventing eating disorders: A handbook of interventions and special challenges* (pp. 134–47). Philadelphia: Brunner/Mazel.

Striegel-Moore, R. H., and Cachelin, F. M. (1999). Body-image concerns and disordered eating in adolescent girls: Risk and protective factors. In N. G. Johnson, M. C. Roberts, and J. Worell, eds., *Beyond appearance: A new look at adolescent girls* (pp. 85–108). Washington, D.C.: American Psychological Association.

Lask, B., and Bryant-Waugh, R., eds. (2000). *Anorexia and related eating disorders in childhood and adolescence* (2nd ed.) East Sussex, U.K.: Psychology Press.

Wertheim, E. H., Paxton, S. J., Schutz, H. K., and Muir, S. L. (1997). Why do adolescent girls watch their weight? An interview study examining sociocultural pressures to be thin. *Journal of Psychosomatic Research* 42, 345–55.

Vohs, K. D., Heatherton, T. F., and Herrin, M. (2001). Disordered eating and the transition to college: A prospective study. *International Journal of Eating Disorders* 29, 280–88.

## 10. Normalizing Eating with a Food Plan

Rolls, B. J., Hetherington, M., and Burley, V. J. (1988). The specificity of satiety: The influence of foods of different macronutrient content on the development of satiety. *Physiology and Behavior* 43, 145–53.

Garrow, J. S. (1985). The contribution of protein synthesis to thermogenesis in man. *International Journal of Obesity* 9 (Suppl. 2), 97–101.

Kreipe, R. E. (1995). Eating disorders among children and adolescents. *Pediatrics in Review* 16, 370–79.

Gendall, K. A., Joyce, P. R., and Abbott, R. M. (1999). The effects of meal composition on subsequent craving and binge eating. *Addictive Behaviors* 24, 305–15.

Winocur, J. (1990). Nutrition therapy. In N. Piran and A. S. Kaplan, eds., *A day hospital group treatment program for anorexia nervosa and bulimia nervosa* (pp. 61–78). New York: Brunner/Mazel.

## 11. Getting the Most out of the Food Plan

Touyz, S. W., and Beumont, P. J. V. (1985). A comprehensive, multidisciplinary approach for the management of patients with anorexia nervosa. In S. W. Touyz and P. J. V. Beumont, eds., *Eating disorders: Prevalence and treatment* (pp. 11–22). Belgowlah, Australia: Williams and Wilkins.

Obarzanek, E., Lesem, M. D., and Jimerson, D. C. (1994). Resting metabolic rate of anorexia nervosa patients during weight gain. *American Journal of Clinical Nutrition* 60, 666–75.

Dempsey, D. T., Crosby, L. O., Pertschuk, M. J., Feurer, I. D., Buzby, G. P., and Mullen, J. L. (1984). Weight gain and nutritional efficacy in anorexia nervosa. *American Journal of Clinical Nutrition* 39, 236–42.

Salisbury, J. J., Levine, A. S., Crow, S. J., and Mitchell, J. E. (1995). Refeeding, metabolic rate, and weight gain in anorexia nervosa: A review. *International Journal of Eating Disorders* 17, 337–45.

Fairburn, C. G., Marcus, M. D., and Wilson, G. T. (1993). Cognitive-behavioral therapy for binge eating and bulimia nervosa: A comprehensive treatment manual. In C. G. Fairburn and G. T. Wilson, eds., *Binge eating: Nature, assessment and treatment* (pp. 361–404). New York: Guilford Press.

Bo-Linn, G. W., Santa Ana, C. A., Morawski, S. G., and Fordtran, J. S. (1983). Purging and calorie absorption in bulimic patients and normal women. *Annals of Internal Medicine* 99, 14–17.

Kaye, W. H., Weltzin, T. E., Hsu, L. K. G., McConaha, C. W., and Bolton, B. (1993). Amount of calories retained after binge eating and vomiting. *American Journal of Psychiatry* 150, 969–71.

Garner, D. M. (1997). Psychoeducational principles in treatment. In D. M. Garner and P. E. Garfinkel, eds., *Handbook of treatment for eating disorders* (2nd ed., pp. 145–77). New York: Guilford Press.

Fairburn, C. G., Jones, R., Peveler, R. C., Hope, R. A., and O'Connor, M. (1993). Psychotherapy and bulimia nervosa: The longer-term effects of interpersonal psychotherapy, behavior therapy, and cognitive behavior. *Archives of General Psychiatry* 50, 419–28.

Agras, W. S., and Apple, R. F. (1997). *Overcoming eating disorder: Therapist guide.* San Antonio: The Psychological Corporation.

## 12. Normalizing Exercise

Davis, C., Kennedy, S. H., Ravelski, E., and Dionne, M. (1994). The role of physical activity in the development and maintenance of eating disorders. *Psychological Medicine* 24, 957–67.

American College of Sports Medicine. (1998). Position stand: The recommended quantity and quality of exercise for developing and maintaining cardiorespiratory and muscular fitness, and flexibility in healthy adults. *Medicine and Science in Sports and Exercise* 30, 975–91.

Yates, A. (1991). *Compulsive exercise and the eating disorders: Toward an integrated theory of activity.* New York: Brunner/Mazel.

Klibanski, A., Biller, B. M. K., Schoenfeld, D. A., Herzog, D. B., and Saxe, V. C. (1995). The effects of estrogen administration on trabecular bone loss in young women with anorexia nerovsa. *Journal of Clinical Endocrinology and Metabolism* 80, 898–904.

Joyce, J. M., Warren, D. L., Humphries, L. L., Smith, A. J., and Coon J. S. (1990). Osteoporosis in women with eating disorders: Comparison of physical parameters, exercise, and menstrual status with SPA and DPA evaluation. *Journal of Nuclear Medicine* 31, 325–31.

## 14. When You've Done All You Can: Professional Resources and How to Use Them

Brambilla, F., Draisci, A., Peirone, A., Brunetta, M. (1995). Combined cognitive-behavioral, psychopharmacological and nutritional therapy in eating disorders. *Biological Psychiatry* 32, 59–63.

Fairburn, C. G., Norman, P. A., Welch, S. L., O'Connor, M. E., Doll, H. A., and Peveler, R. C. (1995). A prospective study of outcome in bulimia nervosa and the long-term effects of three psychological treatments. *Archives of General Psychiatry* 52, 304–12.

Garner, D. M., Vitousek, K. M., and Pike, K. M. (1997). Cognitive-behavioral therapy for anorexia nervosa. In D. M. Garner and P. E. Garfinkel, eds., *Handbook of treatment for eating disorders* (2nd ed., pp. 94–144). New York: Guilford Press.

Levenkron, S. (1982; reissued 1997). *Treating and overcoming anorexia nervosa.* New York: Warner Books.

Waller, G., and Katzman, M. A. (1998). Female or male therapists for women with eating disorders? A pilot study of experts' opinions. *International Journal of Eating Disorders* 23, 117–23.

Lock, J., LeGrange, D., Agras, W. S., and Dare, C. (2001). *Treatment manual for anorexia nervosa: A family-based approach.* New York: Guilford Press.

Wilson, G. T. (1999). Cognitive behavior therapy for eating disorders: Progress and problems. *Behavior Research and Therapy* 37, S79–S95.

Bulik, C. M., Sullivan, P. F., Carter, F. A., McIntosh, V. V., and Joyce, P. R. (1999). Predictors of rapid and sustained response to cognitive-behavioral therapy for bulimia nervosa. *International Journal of Eating Disorders* 26, 137–44.

Kaplan, C. A., Thompson, A. E., and Searson, S. M. (1995). Cognitive behaviour therapy in children and adolescents. *Archives of Disease in Childhood* 73, 472–75.

Hsu, L. K. G., Crisp, A. H., and Callender, J. S. (1992). Psychiatric diagnoses in recovered and unrecovered anorectics 22 years after onset of illness: A pilot study. *Comprehensive Psychiatry* 33, 123–27.

Herrin, M. M. (in press). *Nutrition counseling in the treatment of eating disorders.* New York: Brunner/Routledge.

Kaye, W., Gendall, K., and Strober, M. (1998). Serotonin neuronal function and selective serotonin reuptake inhibitor treatment in anorexia and bulimia nervosa. *Biological Psychiatry* 44, 825–38.

Gowers, S. G., Weetman, J., Shore, A., Hossain, F., and Elvins, R. (2000). Impact of hospitalisation on the outcome of adolescent anorexia nervosa. *British Journal of Psychiatry* 176, 138–41.

Wooley, S. C. (1994). Sexual abuse and eating disorders: The concealed debate. In P. Fallon, M. A. Katzman, and S. C. Wooley, eds., *Feminist perspectives on eating disorders* (pp. 171–211). New York: Guilford Press.

# Index

# About the Authors

MARCIA HERRIN, Ed.D., M.P.H., R.D., is the founder and codirector of the Dartmouth College Eating Disorders Prevention, Education, and Treatment Program, one of the most respected programs of its kind in the nation. She also has a private practice specializing in eating disorders. Having conquered the problem herself as a teenager, she speaks with authority and compassion. Dr. Herrin received her doctorate in nutrition from Columbia University. She has been featured in *People* magazine and has appeared on *Today* and *48 Hours*.

NANCY MATSUMOTO is a freelance writer based in Toronto. She is a former correspondent for *People* magazine who has written frequently on eating disorders, and whose work has appeared in *Time, Newsweek, The New York Times,* and the *Los Angeles Times,* among other publications.